DEPARTMENT OF PHYSICAL EDUCATION
UNIVERSITY OF CALIFORNIA
DAVIS, CALIFORNIA

SO-ALF-350

THIS B

DEPARTMENT OF PHYSICAL EDUCATION
DEPARTMENT OF PHYSICAL EDUCATION
UNIVERSITY OF CALIFORNIA
DAVIS, CALIFORNIA

EXERCISE AND
HEART DISEASE

A Progress in Cardiovascular Diseases Reprint

EXERCISE AND HEART DISEASE

Edited by

Edmund H. Sonnenblick, M.D.

Professor of Medicine, and
Chief, Division of Cardiology
Albert Einstein College of Medicine
Bronx, New York

Michael Lesch, M.D.

Magerstadt Professor of Medicine
Northwestern University School of Medicine
Director, Section of Cardiology
Northwestern Memorial Hospital
Chicago, Illinois

GRUNE & STRATTON

A Subsidiary of Harcourt Brace Jovanovich, Publishers

New York   San Francisco   London

The chapters of this book appeared originally in the July/August 1972 (Vol. XV, No. 1), January/February 1975 (Vol. XVII, No. 4), January/February, May/June, July/August and September/October 1976 issues (Vol. XVIII, No. 4 and No. 6 and Vol. XIX, No. 1 and No. 2), May/June 1977 (Vol. XIX, No. 6) of *Progress in Cardiovascular Diseases,* a bimonthly journal published by Grune and Stratton, Inc., and edited by Edmund H. Sonnenblick, M.D., and Michael Lesch, M.D.

Grune & Stratton, Inc.
111 Fifth Avenue
New York, New York 10003

Distributed in the United Kingdom by
Academic Press, Inc. (London) Ltd.
24/28 Oval Road, London NW 1

Library of Congress Catalog Number 77-75709
International Standard Book Number 0-8089-1016-7

Printed in the United States of America

CONTENTS

Integrated Mechanisms of Cardiovascular Response and Control During Exercise in the Normal Human

Elvin E. Smith, Arthur C. Guyton, R. Davis Manning, and Ronald J. White

PHYSICAL exercise is one of the most stressful conditions imposed on the cardiovascular system of man. Full participation and adaptability of the various neural, humoral, and hydraulic components of the circulation are of paramount importance in enabling man to meet the demands for oxygen and substrate delivery, in addition to carbon dioxide and metabolite removal. In heavy physical exercise, the cardiac output may reach six to eight times the resting value, and in the accomplished marathon runner, may be maintained above 85% of these values in excess of 2 hr.

With the background of the current interest in exercise as a preventive regimen for coronary heart disease, in the use of the exercise stress test for the early diagnosis of acquired coronary heart disease, and in the possibility of exercise as a therapeutic adjunct in the treatment of coronary heart disease, an adequate understanding of normal circulatory function during exercise is essential.

Several excellent reviews have recently appeared addressed to problems of cardiovascular adjustment to exercise.[1-3] It is not the purpose of this paper to duplicate these reviews. Rather, we hope to develop a coherent and workable concept of the over-all dynamics and regulation of the circulation during exercise. Discrete functions of individual segments of the circulation in exercise will be discussed in other articles of this series.

While the responses of the cardiovascular system during exercise involve virtually every circulatory component, these responses fall basically into three categories. The first of these is the large reduction in resistance in the working musculature produced by local vasodilatation.[4] This local vasodilatation is the one absolutely essential response common to the performance of exercise. However, were this the only response, one result of the vasodilatation would be a drastic fall in arterial pressure, and collapse would ensue. Fortunately, a second group of responses mediated by the sympathetic nervous system is directed toward maintaining an arterial perfusion pressure sufficient to insure adequate blood flow to the working musculature.[5] The third major response pattern is maintenance of an acceptable body temperature, which becomes an important consideration in the regulation of the circulation if exercise continues until body temperature begins to rise significantly.[3] These three responses are to some extent interrelated. Moreover, each has effector or activating components as well as feedback, monitoring, and regulatory components. Before proceeding with an analysis of the circulatory changes involved in exercise, let us first define and discuss these various effector and feedback components, an understanding of which is essential to the development of a coherent concept of the responses of the cardiovascular system during exercise.

EFFECTOR AND FEEDBACK COMPONENTS

Figure 1 displays the various effector and feedback components of the circulatory system during exercise. To simplify this analysis and Fig. 1, the following definitions have been employed: local regulation is defined as the process by which each individual tissue or organ regulates its blood flow in response to its metabolic need. The term "sympathetic stimulation" as used here means the combination of sympathetic stimulation and parasym-

From the Department of Physiology, Texas A&M University, College of Medicine, College Station, Tex. and the Department of Physiology and Biophysics, University of Mississippi School of Medicine, Jackson, Miss.

Supported in part by NIH Grant HL11678.

Reprint requests should be addressed to Dr. Elvin E. Smith, Department of Physiology, College of Medicine, Texas A&M University, College Station, Tex. 77843.

© 1976 by Grune & Stratton, Inc.

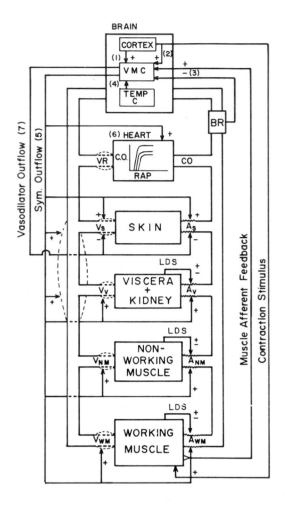

Fig. 1. Schematic representation of the interrelationship of the various effector and control mechanisms operative during exercise and discussed throughout the text.

Symbols: TEMP C, temperature regulating center; BR, baroreceptor; VR, venous return; +, increased resistance or tone; /\/\/ , resistance; VMC, vasomotor center; CO, cardiac output; LDS, local vasodilation stimulus; −, decreased resistance or tone; $<\mathrm{\_\_\_}>$, capacitance. A_s, A_v, A_{nm}, A_{wm}: arterial inflow to the skin$_{(s)}$, viscera$_{(v)}$, nonworking muscle$_{(nm)}$, and working muscle$_{(wm)}$, respectively; V_s, V_v, V_{nm}, V_{wm}: venous outflow from the skin$_{(s)}$, viscera$_{(v)}$, nonworking muscle$_{(nm)}$, and working muscle$_{(wm)}$, respectively. (1) Anticipatory signal for exercise from cortex to vasomotor center. This signal is not universally present in exercise. (2) Cortical radiation or spillover to vasomotor center and linked to the contraction signal to muscle. (3) Output from baroreceptor considered in this schema to oppose the rise in arterial pressure occurring in exercise. The baroreceptor signal may be modified or biased in the vasomotor center. (4) Output from temperature regulating center to vasomotor center in response to a rising body temperature. Result is increased sympathetic outflow to nonskin areas and decreased sympathetic outflow and increased dilator outflow to skin. (5) Sympathetic outflow equals the algebraic sum of sympathetic constrictor effects minus sympathetic dilator effects (?) and minus parasympathetic effects. (6) Heart rate effects and stroke volume effects lumped into family of curves responsive to sympathetic outflow. (7) Vasodilator outflow equals the algebraic sum of sympathetic vasodilator effects minus sympathetic constrictor effects and minus parasympathetic effects.

pathetic withdrawal. The effects of an accumulating heat load are those cardiovascular adjustments which redistribute blood to the skin areas in order to maintain body temperature at an acceptable level.

Effector Components

Local Vasodilatation

The unique event occurring in muscular exercise is the large decrease in resistance of the vasculature of the working muscle. While stimulation of certain areas within the brain may produce cardiovascular alterations similar in many aspects to the response of the circulation to exercise,[6] no facet of sympathetic stimulation can possibly duplicate this large decrease in resistance occurring at the local level. Blood flow to an active muscle may be increased more than 15-fold during exercise,[7] and this cannot be explained purely on the basis of sympathetic stimulation. It is a well known fact that when all of the nerves to a muscle area have been

blocked and the muscle has then been activated, blood flow to that muscle begins to increase almost immediately.[1,8] This increase in blood flow is due entirely to a decrease in the intrinsic vascular resistance of the muscle vasculature. This decrease in vascular resistance is the primary mechanism by which increased oxygen and metabolic foodstuffs are delivered to the working muscle. Furthermore, the effects of this vasodilatation are not limited only to the working muscle, for the vasodilatation causes secondary effects in the entire circulation. That is, as the resistance to flow in the muscle decreases, the resistance to venous return also decreases, and this results in increased venous return to the heart.[4] Thus a large increase in venous return and in cardiac output can occur during exercise, even when the only primary effect is decreased resistance to blood flow in the working musculature. This has been demonstrated in studies in which, during exercise, total sympathetic blockade has been initiated and yet in which the cardiac output still increases, though much less than normally.[9-11]

While the decline in resistance can be mathematically related to the intensity of work (oxygen consumption),[12,13] the precise cause of the metabolic vasodilatation in active muscle is yet unknown. Many different suggestions have been offered. The more notable of these are K^+, H^+, lactate, various nucleotide breakdown products, and oxygen lack.[14-16] It is beyond the scope of this article to attempt to settle the question of which factor regulates blood flow in the working muscle. However, it is very clear that muscle blood flow begins to increase almost simultaneously with the onset of muscular activity through a local vasodilator mechanism, even when all of the nerves to the active muscles have been blocked.[8] And, while a separation of the roles of the various metabolic vasodilators in producing and regulating muscle blood flow may not be possible, one fact is clear. Local muscle blood flow, and indeed, even cardiac output are directly related to work loads and to O_2 consumption[12] (Fig. 2). Using this principle, it is permissible to use oxygen demand or even muscle oxygen tension as the regulated variable in an analysis of flow changes during exercise. From a systems analysis standpoint, it matters little to the over-all function of the circulation whether the relationship between muscle partial pressure of oxygen and blood flow be a direct one, or one mediated through another metabolite released during exercise proportional to tissue oxygen tension or oxygen demand.

One aspect of importance of local vasodilatation in distributing blood flow during exercise may be seen when one compares blood flow through working muscles with blood flow through nonworking muscles. While sympathetic stimulation during exercise tends to increase the resistance to blood flow in both areas, the resistance to blood flow in the working muscles is greatly reduced, while resistance in the nonworking muscles is increased.[1,8] This effect can be seen in human beings when one compares leg blood flow to arm blood flow during exercise on a bicycle ergometer.[1,8] The increase in blood flow to the working leg muscles is the result of a decrease in leg vascular resistance mediated by the local vasodilatation mechanism. However, an increase in arterial pressure, as a result of sympathetic stimulation, maintains and even enhances the muscle perfusion pressure head, thus markedly increasing the flow through the greatly decreased

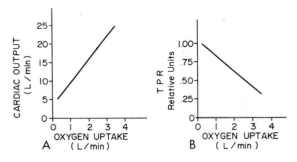

Fig. 2. Relationship between cardiac output (A) and total peripheral resistance (B) to oxygen consumption in normal humans.

vascular resistance network of the leg. Since the muscles of the arm are not working, there is no vasodilatory stimulus to dilate the arm vasculature or to counterbalance the effect of sympathetic stimulation to increase the arm resistance. Therefore, the arm blood flow decreases. But were it not for the increase in resistance in nonworking muscle areas, blood flow in these areas would actually increase because of the elevated pressure, and thus subtract from the blood flow available for the working muscle.

While the importance of sympathetic stimulation during exercise has been heavily stressed, one cannot disregard the overriding importance of local vasodilatation in producing the exercise response. When these two effects, local vasodilatation and sympathetic stimulation, are considered simultaneously, one can see how they are integrated to produce the cardiovascular pattern seen in exercise. It would certainly be a poorly designed system that would allow over-all sympathetic stimulation to constrict the arterioles in the working muscle. Local vasodilatation provides a mechanism by which the effects of increased blood pressure produced by sympathetic stimulation may be directed to those areas of the body whose needs are greatly increased during muscle exercise. Thus, through integrated action of both mechanisms, blood flow to working areas is increased, while blood flow to nonworking muscle is maintained at control levels or even decreased.

Sympathetic Stimulation

One of the best known of all circulatory reactions is the classic fight, fright, or flight sympathetic response to stress. It is well documented that this autonomic outpouring can be triggered by psychic or emotional stimuli, as well as by various

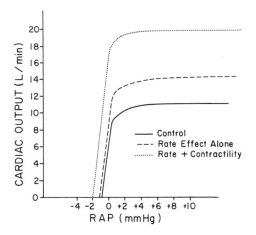

Fig. 3. Effect of rate and increased contractility on the cardiac function curve. Increased rate and contractility together are far more effective in increasing the pumping ability of the heart than increased rate alone. RAP; right atrial pressure.

neural mechanisms.[6,17-20] The effect of intense sympathetic stimulation on the exercising cardiovascular system may be divided into cardiac effects and peripheral effects.

Cardiac effects. Figure 3 displays the effects of sympathetic stimulation on the heart. This figure illustrates that sympathetic stimulation of the heart during exercise increases the effectiveness of the heart as a pump through two mechanisms: an increase in heart rate and an increase in contractile ability of the heart. Studies in isolated heart preparations indicate that an increasing heart rate per se, independent of sympathetic stimulation, increases the ability of the heart to pump blood; that is, with the given right atrial pressure held exactly constant, the output will increase as the heart rate increases up to a critical rate.[21-23] However, at very high rates, the output then declines due to insufficient ventricular filling time, to allow complete filling of the ventricles during diastole.[21-22]

A second cardiac effect of sympathetic stimulation during exercise is an increase in the myocardial contractility.[21,23,24] The studies of Sarnoff[24] show that an increase in sympathetic stimulation of the myocardium results in increased contractile force of the myocardium for a given right atrial pressure.

In essence, the heart under the influence of sympathetic stimulation during exercise becomes a stronger pump with enhanced output characteristics. Maximal sympathetic stimulation of the heart is capable of elevating the plateau level of the

cardiac output curve by more than 70% of the control value.[4] The results of these two effects, increased heart rate and increased contractility of the myocardium, are illustrated in the curves of Fig. 3. It is evident from this figure that as sympathetic stimulation excites the heart, the cardiac function curve shifts upward and to the left. The reader is reminded that the curves of Fig. 3 represent only examples from a family of curves that portray the effect of varying degrees of sympathetic stimulation on the heart. For mild levels of sympathetic stimulation, the cardiac function may well be intermediate; i.e., between the control curve and the upper curve displayed in Fig. 3.

A third effect of sympathetic stimulation upon the heart during exercise has nothing directly to do with the pumping characteristics of the heart, but does significantly alter peripheral circulatory function. That is, sympathetic stimulation decreases both the diastolic and systolic volumes of the ventricles.[6,25,26] This decrease in cardiac blood volume displaces blood from the heart into the peripheral circulation, and, in effect, amounts to an infusion of blood into the peripheral circulation, with the following effects.

Peripheral effects. Major peripheral effects of sympathetic stimulation are constriction of both the resistance and capacitance vessels.[1,8,27-33] These are very important effects in exercise, since if they do not occur, the arterial pressure falls precipitiously at the onset of exercise because of the decreased vascular resistance of the working muscle,[9,10,34,35] Mellander[36] showed that the constrictor fibers of the sympathetic nervous system can accomplish approximately an eightfold increase in arteriolar resistance. He also showed that intense sympathetic stimulation will expel approximately 40% of the blood contained in the capacitance vessels. The effects of sympathetic stimulation on the peripheral circulation have a profound effect on the mean circulatory pressure,[4] as illustrated in Fig. 4. The graphic convention of Fig. 4 is such that the intersection of the venous return curve with the abscissa is equal to the mean circulatory pressure. Mean circulatory pressure is the name given to the driving force tending to return blood from the periphery to the heart.[4] Sympathetic stimulation increases the degree of "tightness" with which the capacitance vessels press upon the blood contained within them. This results in elevation of peripheral venous pressure and

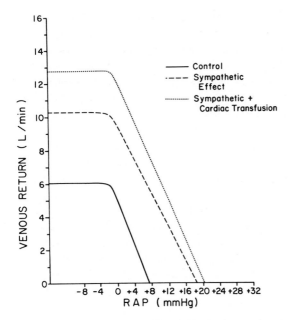

Fig. 4. Venous return plotted as a function of right atrial pressure (RAP). Sympathetic stimulation through its effect on mean circulatory pressure (MCP) (intercept of abscissa) increases venous return. The third curve shows that blood expelled from the heart into the peripheral circulation as heart size decreases under sympathetic stimulation promotes an additional increase in MCP and in venous return.

an increase in the pressure drop from the veins to the right atrium. The result of intense sympathetic stimulation, as in Fig. 4, is an increase in mean circulatory pressure from its control value of 7 mm Hg up to a value greater than 18 mm Hg. The resistance to venous return can be deduced by the slope of the venous return curve, where a decrease in the slope is indicative of an increased resistance to venous return, and an increase in the slope is indicative of a decreased resistance to venous return.[23] In Figure 4, sympathetic stimulation has resulted in constriction of the major veins and increased resistance to venous return. However, the increase in mean circulatory pressure is greater than the increase in resistance to venous return, and the result is a twofold increase in the plateau value of venous return. But as in the section on cardiac effects of sympathetic stimulation, the reader is here reminded that a family of curves exists and that the curve indicative of any particular example is dependent on the absolute degree of sympathetic stimulation. The third curve of Fig. 4 illustrates that, concomitant with the decrease in vascular capacitance elicited by the sympathetic

stimulation, the volume of blood expelled from the heart by the decrease in heart size under sympathetic influence is translocated to the peripheral circulation. When this cardiac "transfusion" is added to the peripheral circulation, an additional increase in mean circulatory pressure of several mm Hg occurs.

Combined cardiac and peripheral effects. It is axiomatic that, except possibly for beat-to-beat variations, cardiac output and venous return must be equal. This principle is used in the technique of analysis of circulatory changes, using the equilibrium point of cardiac function and venous return curves as in Fig. 5, which combines the cardiac and peripheral effects of exercise-sympathetic stimulation.[4,23]

The normal cardiac output curve and the normal venous return curve intercept each other at a single point, A, when the right atrial pressure is near 0 mm Hg and the cardiac output and venous return are equal at 5 l per min. If the effectiveness of the heart as a pump is increased without any peripheral effects, the maximal increase in cardiac output may be only 15%–20% above the control value (A'). This is so because the venous return curve flattens at a level slightly above the control value for venous return because of collapse of the veins when the central venous pressure falls below atmospheric pressure. Therefore, regardless of the effectiveness of the heart as a pump, or regardless of the increased capability of the heart to handle large outputs, cardiac output and venous return

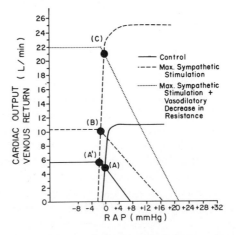

Fig. 5. Cardiac function and venous return curves displayed simultaneously to illustrate changes in cardiac output during exercise. Equilibrium points A, A', B, and C are explained in the text.

can equal each other at no point higher than the plateau level of the venous return curve.

On the other hand, maximum peripheral effects of sympathetic stimulation, with no cardiac involvement, can result in only a twofold increase in the plateau level of the venous return curve, and since venous return and cardiac output cannot rise above the venous return plateau level no matter how powerful the heart is, the cardiac output is limited to this level of venous return. Therefore, sympathetic nerve stimulation of the heart or of the peripheral circulation—or even of both at the same time—can have only moderate effects on cardiac output. Point B of Fig. 5 represents the equilibrium point between the cardiac function curve and the venous return curve under approximately maximum sympathetic stimulation. It can be seen in this figure that the cardiac output has risen approximately twofold as the result of the increase in venous return and a simultaneous shift in the cardiac function curve to the left. The increase in venous return is primarily the result of decreased capacitance of the venous vessels and the increase of mean circulatory pressure up to 18 mm Hg.

Combined Sympathetic Stimulation and Local Vasodilatation

Point C of Fig. 5 graphically displays the circulatory response to exercise. Note that the difference between B and C is mainly the result of a large decrease in resistance to venous return (which causes the slope of the venous return curve to increase); this allows the venous return to be considerably higher for any given right atrial pressure. This increased tendency for venous return is the result of the decrease in resistance to venous return caused by local vasodilatation.[4] Point B of Fig. 5 shows that maximum sympathetic stimulation by itself results in only a doubling cardiac output. However, when local vasodilatation is added to the effects of the sympathetic stimulation, as occurs during exercise, the cardiac output is now more than 4 times normal. Thus, to fully explain the cardiovascular events of maximum exercise, one must simultaneously consider the effects of local vasodilatation and of sympathetic stimulation.

Heat Load Effects

The cardiovascular effects of exercise of short duration may be explained by simultaneous consideration of the effects of local vasodilatation and of sympathetic stimulation. However, exercise of longer duration must also consider a third factor: the effect of an accumulating heat load on the cardiovascular system.[2,3] Muscular exercise, and the resultant increase in energy usage by the working muscles, produce large quantities of heat that must be eliminated from the body. This heat elimination is accomplished mainly by selective vasodilatation of the skin vasculature. When exercise is mild, the cardiovascular reserve is sufficient to allow for flow both to exercising muscles and to allow for increased flow to the skin area. However, when exercise is maximum, the cardiovascular system no longer has sufficient reserve to meet the added stress of heat on it, so that a pronounced cardiovascular drift, to be discussed later, becomes evident.[2] The basic mechanism of the thermal response is dilatation of the skin vasculature. However, as the skin vessels dilate and their blood volume increases, there is also a simultaneous decrease in blood volume elsewhere in the circulation, and the arterial pressure and resistances in the peripheral circulation are altered in a manner that affects exercise performance. Thus, in any analysis of cardiovascular function during exercise, consideration must be given to those mechanisms connected with thermal regulation that alter the cardiovascular response to exercise. A recent review by Rowell deals extensively with these thermal regulatory mechanisms.[2]

Control Mechanisms

The precision with which the cardiovascular system is regulated in response to varying work loads placed on it by exercise is convincing evidence for the existence of control mechanisms that match the cardiovascular "effort" to the needs of the working musculature. The exact nature of all the controls operative during exercise is perhaps the largest unanswered question in exercise physiology. While several different types of control mechanisms have been postulated, confirmatory evidence for some of these is not yet available, or is at best inconclusive.

Hydrodynamic Feedback Control System

A hydrodynamic feedback system that is well documented, but often unrecognized as a feedback system, is basic to all circulatory control during exercise.[4] It functions in every type of muscle activity, even when the entire sympathoadrenal system has been blocked,[9,10,35] when the spinal cord has been cut,[37] or when an animal has been rendered totally decrebrate.[38] This hydrodynamic feedback has its origin in two facts: (1) total venous return is the sum of flow through all the tissue of the body, and (2) the Frank–Starling law of the heart which, in effect, states that the heart, within physiologic limits, acts as a sump pump and will propel forward all of the blood returned to it. During exercise, the vasculature of the working muscle dilates via the local vasodilator mechanisms discussed in previous section (*Effector Components*). The increased flow through these areas increases total venous return. The heart then pumps this increased venous return as cardiac output, which is distributed to peripheral beds according to the resistance of each bed. Since the local vasodilator mechanism is graded in response to metabolic need,[39] the increase in cardiac output and the increase in flow to each active muscle will also be graded in response to exercise intensity. In mild to moderate degrees of exercise, this hydrodynamic feedback can be sufficient to meet the cardiovascular demands.[34,35] In more stressful situations, the decrease in total peripheral resistance during exercise will exceed the ability of the hydrodynamic feedback to maintain arterial pressure; in this case, sympathetic support becomes necessary.[9,10] Nevertheless, this hydrodynamic feedback is the primary basis of circulatory regulation during exercise. The other control mechanisms are necessary mainly to maintain or increase arterial pressure.

Cortical Radiation

The simplest type of sympathetic control that has been postulated states that as the somatomotor cortex sends activating impulses to the muscular system during exercise, collateral impulses are directed to the diencephalic and medullary vasomotor areas of the brain to activate and sustain an "exercise" cardiovascular response. Perhaps the strongest basis for this argument comes from the laboratory of Rushmer and associates.[6,40] Their studies demonstrate that stimulation in the H_2 fields of Forel and in the periventricular gray matter initiates cardiovascular changes that strongly resemble those seen in exercising dogs. And it has been shown in man that a cerebral stimulus for contraction, even when the muscular response has

been blocked, can initiate cardiovascular changes in the absence of muscular contraction.[41] It is enticing to some physiologists to believe that the nervous system sets up an "integrated pattern" of neural outflow to the cardiovascular center during exercise, and that this "pattern" regulates the response of the cardiovascular system.[42]

However, the major drawback to this theory lies in the apparent lack of discovery of any cardiovascular feedback to the neural area to apprise the neural hierarchy of the effectiveness with which the cardiovascular system is meeting its needs. Thus, this postulated system amounts basically to an open-ended, no-feedback system.

Humoral Feedback

A very attractive theory of feedback control is concerned with the level of oxygen, of carbon dioxide, or of various humoral factors in the blood, the changes in which are indicative of and related to the level of exercise. That is, as one exercises, the venous oxygen tension falls and venous carbon dioxide concentration rises, and one or both of these variables are postulated to be monitored to serve as a feedback stimulus for regulating cardiovascular performance.[43] However, no functional sensor for these substances has been located in the venous side of the circulation. And, indeed, when one looks at carbon dioxide and oxygen levels in arterial blood even during heavy levels of exercise, one sees that the carbon dioxide concentration does not increase perceptibly and may even be below normal. Furthermore, the oxygen level in the arterial blood does not fall to a level sufficient to produce the observed cardiovascular response. Thus, while this hypothesis may have much appeal, from a theoretical standpoint, the practical view influenced by available data, reveals that the hypothesis has almost no substantive backing.[44,45]

Baroreceptor Feedback

Warner's studies and analyses indicated that upon initiation of exercise, the events in the working muscles resulted in an almost immediate arteriolar vasodilatation and a decrease in total peripheral resistance.[46,47] Thus arterial pressure began to fall, and baroreceptor activation of the sympathetics commenced. The essence of this theory is that regulation of the circulation during exercise is controlled by changes in the total peripheral resistance acting back through the arterial pressure baroreceptors. That is, as the total peripheral resistance begins to fall, the arterial pressure begins to fall, the baroreceptor reflex is activated, and sympathetic stimulation of the heart and vasculature ensues. This results in shifts in blood volume, a change in venous capacitance, and an increase in cardiac output—all of which restore the arterial pressure to its "set point." While this theory has a definite appeal, two factors argue against it. First, a decline in arterial pressure upon initiation of exercise is by no means a constant finding.[12,13,48] Secondly, available information in man shows that the sensitivity of the baroreceptors may even be diminished in the well trained athlete.[5,49]

Acceptance of the baroreceptor feedback theory is of necessity connected with a postulation that the "set point" of the baroreceptor reflex must be reset during exercise. That is, as exercise is initiated, the "set point" of the baroreceptor is elevated to a new level; for instance, to 140 mm Hg. Then, as exercise begins and total peripheral resistance falls, the baroreceptor reflex now detecting that the arterial pressure is 120 mm Hg (20 points below the set point) activates sympathetic activity sufficiently to result in higher heart rate, increased cardiac contractility, and generalized vasoconstriction—all of which raise the arterial pressure near to the set point level. However, most of the available information, while admittedly limited to a study of the reflex control of heart rate, tends to indicate that, if anything, the baroreceptor reflex is suppressed during exercise.[49,50] No available information seems to point definitely toward a resetting of the baroreceptor reflex during exercise.[5]

Muscle Afferent Feedback

The muscle afferent feedback hypothesis basically states that when muscle contraction occurs, afferent signals are sent by reflex action from receptors in the exercising muscle to the brain.[51-56] These signals excite the sympathetic centers at various autonomic levels. The presence of such a reflex from exercising muscle has been demonstrated by Coote et al.[51] They electrically stimulated the cut peripheral ends of spinal ventral root nerves and obtained marked rises in blood pressure that were proportional to the stimulation strength or to the tension developed in the muscles. If the muscle was treated with curare to prevent contraction, there was no central cardiovascular change

when the nerve was stimulated, thus indicating that muscle contraction itself is necessary for the reflex to occur. Additional evidence for a graded nature of the response was obtained when the ventral root was stimulated and a constrictor was placed around the arterial inflow to the contracting muscle. A much larger increase in blood pressure was obtained for a given stimulus strength or a given tension development when the muscle was rendered ischemic. Additional evidence for the reflex nature of this response was shown when the reflex was abolished if the dorsal roots were cut. From a systems analysis standpoint, this reflex is ideal for the regulation of the central circulation, since it is proportional to the metabolic needs of the exercising muscle.

Evidence that this reflex exists in man has been demonstrated by several investigators.[55,56] The most commonly used example is that of sustained static contraction of forearm muscles. In these studies, using only the muscles of one arm, cardiac output climbs to double the control value within 2 min of a handgrip exercise of 50% of the maximum voluntary contraction. Additionally, the response in man has been shown to be graded, since the responses of the central circulation are proportional to the degree of tension developed during the handgrip. If the arterial inflow is interrupted by an occlusion cuff, the response in terms of heart rate, arterial blood pressure, and cardiac output is increased over an equal contraction with no occlusion present. Furthermore, if the occluding cuff remains in place after the termination of the contraction, the central cardiovascular variables will remain elevated until after removal of the cuff. That the same reflex as demonstrated by Coote et al.[51] is involved can be shown in the studies performed on subjects with peripheral afferent information abolished. In a study of patients with syringomyelia[55,56] involving only one arm, it was found that the usual cardiovascular responses were obtained from the unaffected arm, but that the responses obtained when the affected forearm contracted were greatly reduced or even abolished.

The exact anatomic correlate of this reflex remains undetermined at the present time. It is obvious from the studies in which contraction was abolished that contraction itself is necessary for this response to occur.[51] Furthermore, a decrease in oxygen tension of itself is not sufficient to evoke the reflex. The studies of Lind et al.[55] show that 20 min of occlusion of the resting arm has no pressor effect. It has been suggested by Donald et al.[56] that the intensity of the reflex is related to the metabolic status of the muscle, as indicated by the graded response in the two studies cited above. Moreover, McCloskey and Mitchell[57] give evidence that the reflex is not mediated by the muscle spindles, the tendon receptors, or proprioceptive receptors in the joints, but rather are excited through a metabolic mechanism. Studies in dinitrophenol-induced hypermetabolism lend support to this hypothesis.[58]

PHASES OF EXERCISE

Analysis of data from exercise studies indicates that the cardiovascular responses to exercise may be considered in four phases. These are: (1) The anticipatory or expectant phase in which various neural, humoral, and even mechanical factors act in concert to ready the cardiovascular system for the upcoming exertion. (2) The on-transient or initial phase in which large changes in the various cardiovascular variables occur simultaneously with the onset of exercise. Reflex adjustments are rapidly involved in this initial phase, as are rapid shifts of intravascular volume from one compartment to another. Mechanical factors are very important in the early increases in cardiac output. (3) The adjustment, or fine tuning phase in which continual readjustment of flow and volume distribution may occur to insure adequate flow to active areas. (4) The "drift" period during which the gradual diminution of metabolic foodstuffs, the accumulation of an oxygen debt, accumulation of metabolic by-products, and the increasing effects of heat load predominate. The end-point of this phase, if the work load is sufficiently high or the duration sufficiently long, is exhaustion.

Anticipatory Phase

The anticipatory phase of exercise is that phase occurring immediately prior to the actual initiation of exercise. While afferent reflexes may initiate or maintain central cardiovascular involvement during the actual exercising phase, it is difficult to conceive how afferent information could be used to trigger sympathetic outpouring before exercise has actually begun. However, it is well documented that an autonomic outpouring can be triggered by psychic or emotional stimuli, and that these might set the various cardiovascular compensations into effect before actual physical work has begun.[20,28,40] Concrete, definitive work on the anticipation response to exercise has been difficult to obtain because of the very nature of the mental involvement. However, increases in heart rate, cardiac output, and arterial pressure, as well as a decrease in venous compliance have all been shown to begin prior to the actual initiation of muscular contraction. While a recorded anticipation response is not present in every exercise condition, it is easily seen in those exercise studies in which a high degree of emotional involvement occurs. Examples are a well conditioned runner standing at the starting line in an important race, or the racing greyhound standing at the starting gate, anxiously awaiting the appearance of the "rabbit."[19,35]

While some investigators have questioned the importance of an anticipation reaction during exercise on the grounds that the same level of reactivity of the cardiovascular variables will be reached in any event immediately after the initiation of exercise,[5] it is highly likely that priming the cardiovascular system prior to the actual start of exercise may well furnish an extra margin of performance. This may well decrease the time needed to reach peak performance, thus making the difference between succeeding or failing a given task, such as running a race, escaping danger, and so on.

The anticipation response almost certainly appears to be of cerebral origin, and the effector limb of the response most certainly lies within the autonomic nervous system. Indeed, studies in which the anticipation response has been removed by surgical or chemical sympathectomy show a definite lag in starting speed.[34,35,59,60] However, it is difficult to determine how much of this decreased response is due to loss of the anticipation response, versus the loss of responses during the initiation of exercise. This latter phenomenon is discussed in the following.

When an anticipatory response to exercise is simulated on a complex circulatory model (Guyton et al.),[61] the model predicts an increase in cardiac output of 75%–80% caused by an anticipatory reflex sympathetic stimulation of the cardiovascular system. An additional prediction is an increase in arterial pressure of 50–60 mm Hg. When the anticipatory response occurs, the muscles have not yet begun to work, and there is not yet any decrease in the resistance to blood flow in the muscle or nonmuscle areas. However, both muscle and nonmuscle blood flows increase transiently because of the increase in perfusion pressure.

While there has been some evidence for the existence of sympathetic vasodilator activation prior to muscle contraction,[62] the role played by this neurogenic vasodilatation in the anticipatory response is questionable. Indeed, Uvnas has been unable to ascertain the existence of sympathetic vasodilatory fibers in nonhuman primates, or to definitely delineate their role in the normal human being during exercise.[62]

Initiation Phase

For purposes of discussion, the initiation phase will be defined as those events occurring within the first few seconds of the beginning of exercise. If one examines the various cardiovascular variables during this period, it is impressive to note the rapidity with which many of them change. Within a matter of seconds, heart rate and cardiac output can increase to 2–3 times normal, and arterial pressure can rise by 50 mm Hg.[63-67] Although the steady-state values of these variables may eventually rise to above these levels, the extreme rapidity of this early on-transient response deserves comment. The factors responsible for these fast adaptations of the cardiovascular system to exercise appear to be a combination of mechanical and neural factors.

Mechanical Compression

One of the first factors contributing to these early rapid changes in cardiovascular dynamics is mechanical compression of the vessels in the working muscles and of intra-abdominal vessels compressed by contraction of the abdominal wall.[37,55,68,69] Contraction of the exercising muscle raises the pressure in the muscle veins and capillaries in proportion to the degree of muscular compression. Pressure generated by contraction of the abdominal wall compresses the abdominal veins, and this pressure is in turn transmitted to the blood. These effects cause an increase in the mean circulatory pressure and in the pressure gradient for venous return of up to 4 times normal.[37] In studies in which the gradient for venous return was elevated fourfold and in which the pumping ability of the heart is not increased by sympathetic stimulation, the venous return and, con-

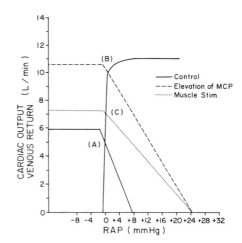

Fig. 6. Effect of muscular compression on mean circulatory pressure (intercept of venous return curves with the abscissa) and on the equilibrium point of the cardiac function and venous return curves. A is the control point. B is the cardiac output obtained when MCP is increased without muscular compression. C illustrates that an equal increase in MCP caused by electrical stimulation of the hindlimbs results in a lesser increase in cardiac output because of the increased resistance to venous return caused by muscular compression.

sequently, the cardiac output increased 120%. However, in studies in which the effect of exercise was duplicated by electrical stimulation of the leg musculature of the dog, an increase of only 40% in cardiac output was observed. This discrepancy appears to have been due to the increase in resistance to venous return occasioned by compression of the vessels, particularly the abdominal veins.[37] This effect is illustrated in Fig. 6.

Neural Participation

It is obvious to any observer of cardiovascular variables during exercise that regardless of whether an anticipation response has or has not been present prior to exercise, an intense and significant neural autonomic component is present almost immediately upon initiation of exercise. The precise cause of this autonomic outpouring has been debatable for some time, as discussed in the introductory section. However, while the exact nature of activation of the sympathetic nervous system during the initiation phase of exercise is unclear, there is proof of the importance of the autonomic component in this phase. Studies in which the total effect of sympathetic activation has been abolished by surgical or pharmacologic means show that the animal initiating exercise without the sympathetic nervous system is indeed operating under a very large handicap.[9-11,34] The autonomic activation effect may best be discussed under the various hemodynamic variables upon which it exerts its influence.

Heart rate. Without a doubt, the most widely measured cardiovascular variable during exercise is the heart rate. The increase in heart rate upon the initiation of exercise may be seen frequently within 1 sec, and often the increase amounts to twofold or more within 10-15 sec. The initial increase in heart rate is most likely due to vagal withdrawal, while the additional increase in rate seen 8-10 sec later has a large sympathetic cardio-accelerator component.[15] The neural, or reflex nature of this initial increase in heart rate is evidenced by (1) its rapidity, and (2) by a frequent overshoot effect.[64] That is, the heart rate may frequently peak rapidly and then decline by several percentage points. However, if exercise persists, the heart rate may climb upward as effort and body temperature increase. The temperature effects will be discussed later. The importance of this early neurogenic component can probably best be seen in those studies in which it has been blocked. In studies of cardiac denervation, the heart rate increases more slowly.[34,35,59,60] However, after a delay allowing circulating catecholamines to reach the myocardium, the heart rate increases substantially. Pure cardiac denervation handicaps the system mainly in the first $\frac{1}{2}$ min of effort.[34] However, if both the cardiac nerves and the remainder of the sympathoadrenal system are blocked, the heart rate may fail to increase substantially in the early phases of exercise.[35] Experimental studies indicate that animals may perform with only minor curtailments of flow and oxygen delivery up to moderate levels of effort. However, at heavy levels of effort, a considerable deficit in cardiovascular performance is observed. At mild and moderate levels of exercise, these results may be explained by the Frank-Starling mechanism, which appears to be able, by an increase in stroke volume, to offset the failure of heart rate to increase. However, at heavy levels of effort, the Starling mechanism is unable, unaided, to offset the effects of complete sympathoadrenal blockade on heart rate.[21]

Right atrial pressure. Right atrial pressure, in short-term conditions, is basically determined by the balance between venous return and right ventricular pumping ability.[23] As illustrated in Fig. 3, sympathetic stimulation shifts the cardiac function curve upward and to the left in such a manner that a larger cardiac output occurs at any given right atrial pressure. Figure 4 illustrates that sympathetic stimulation increases mean circulatory pressure and the pressure gradient for venous return in such a manner that, for a given right atrial pressure, venous return is enhanced. Stated otherwise: if myocardial pumping ability increases without a concurrent increase in venous return, right atrial pressure will fall. In addition, if venous return is enhanced without an increase in myocardial pumping ability, right atrial pressure will rise. Thus, right atrial pressure during the initiation of exercise is determined by the relative time courses of the changes in the peripheral circulation and the changes in myocardial pumping ability. In Fig. 5, sympathetic stimulation has shifted right atrial pressure from the control of 0 mm Hg to -1 mm Hg. A slight decrease of right atrial pressure in all but the most severe levels of exercise is a constant finding. At very severe levels of exercise, a slight increase in right atrial pressure is predicted in order to balance venous return and cardiac output.

Total peripheral resistance. Within $\frac{1}{2}$ sec after the initiation of exercise, a progressive decline in total peripheral resistance begins. This decline can be directly related to the level of work[70] (oxygen consumption), Fig. 2. As shown in Fig. 1, the cardiovascular system can be considered to be a network of parallel vascular flow channels. The change in total peripheral resistance during exercise is an algebraic summation of the changes in resistance in all these parallel beds.

A decrease in resistance, or vasodilatation, can be detected in working musculature within $\frac{1}{2}$ sec of the initiation of exercise.[1,59] This suggests that the dilatation occurs almost instantaneously with muscle contraction. Furthermore, the time course of vasodilatation is similar in persons with sympathectomized forearms.[8] This data suggests that the vasodilatation is of local origin, without neural involvement. The exact cause of this local vasodilatation is undecided at the present, as discussed in the introductory section. It is known, however, that the decrease in resistance in the working muscle is directly related to the metabolic needs of that muscle.[71] The vascular resistances of vessels located in nonexercising muscle areas increase with the onset of exercise.[8] Here again, the degree of increase in resistance is related to the level of exercise, the increase being small in mild levels of exercise and large in severe levels of exercise. Were it not for the increase in resistance in the nonexercising areas, blood flow to these areas would increase as the arterial pressure increased, thus subtracting from flow available for working muscle. This effect can most easily be seen in human beings when measurements of forearm vascular resistance are made during leg exercise.[1,8] In such studies, there is both an increase in resistance and a decrease in the vascular capacitance of the forearm. In addition, resistance to skin blood flow initially increases, with the result that skin blood flow tends to decrease early in exercise. As a heat load is accumulated by the body when exercise persists, skin flow then increases considerably in the later stages of exercise, as thermal demands increase.[1,8]

A major compensatory reaction to exercise occurs in the splanchnic area. Blood flow to the kidney, spleen, liver, and, notably, to the intestines decreases markedly with exercise.[2,31,72-76] In addition, sympathetic outflow results in venoconstriction and a decrease in the vascular volume in these organs. Once again, the increase in resistance and the decrease in capacitance in these organs is proportional to the level of effort or to the metabolic needs of the working muscle.[2] These organs all represent areas where function can be temporarily curtailed in order to make additional blood volume and flow available to the working muscle. In addition to the early reduction in flow to the splanchnic area, a more pronounced reduction in flow may appear if the exercise persists and if the thermal load on the body increases. This will be discussed in detail later.

Cardiac output. Many studies in human beings during exercise have shown that cardiac output increases rapidly almost immediately upon initiation of exercise. Cardiac output appears to approach a plateau usually in less than a minute. In general the time of the plateau, but not its level is independent of the work load.[70] The most rapid early increase in cardiac output is due to the effects of muscle and abdominal compression of the peripheral veins, as discussed previously.[37] A remarkable feature of this response is that the initial changes in cardiac output occur at a faster rate than does the initial change in oxygen uptake.

However, the plateau level appears to be determined by the metabolic needs of the working musculature.[70] It is useless to argue whether the increase in cardiac output during this phase is the result of an increase in heart rate or an increase in stroke volume. But rather the role of the heart should be considered as that of a force-feed pump. That is, because of the decrease in resistance to venous return and the increase in mean circulatory pressure, the venous return increases, and the heart, acting through the combined effects of the Frank-Starling mechanism, cardioacceleration, and the inotropic effect of sympathetic stimulation is capable of pumping this increased venous return to the periphery as cardiac output. The decrease in total peripheral resistance occurring during this phase is necessary to achieve the high levels of cardiac output during exercise.

Arterial pressure. Evidence on the arterial pressure changes during the initiation of exercise has been somewhat contradictory. By careful selection of references one can show that (1) the arterial pressure falls upon initiation of exercise,[47] (2) the arterial pressure remains stable during the initiation phase,[77] or (3) the arterial pressure increases by 15-20 mm Hg at the beginning of exercise.[48,78,79] If, as mentioned in the introductory section, there is no resetting of the baroreceptors, and if the vagal effects of the baroreceptor response to a rising arterial pressure are considered to be modified by central mechanisms, then arterial pressure during the initiation phase of exercise may be considered to be the passive product of resistance and cardiac output. That is, the arterial pressure may not be closely regulated, but is determined by the output of the left ventricle and the resistance into which this output is flowing. If, indeed, arterial pressure is not considered to be regulated during the increased flow state of exercise, then it becomes axiomatic that (1) if the venous return and cardiac output initially increase proportionally more than arterial resistance falls, the arterial pressure will increase; (2) if venous return (cardiac output) and resistance change equally but in opposite directions, arterial pressure may remain unchanged; (3) if resistance decreases more rapidly than output from the left heart increases, the arterial pressure may initially fall.

The initial change in arterial pressure, therefore, depends upon the relative relationships of the time constants for the increase in venous return; the time constants for the movement of the increased venous return through the cardiac chambers, the pulmonary circuit, and into the aorta; and the time constants for the decrease in arterial resistance induced by local vasodilator mechanisms.

The importance of the rapid sympathetic response to the initiation of exercise can be demonstrated when the sympathetic response has been removed or altered. If the neural cardioaccelerator response is removed by total cardiac denervation, the arterial pressure tends to fall with the initiation of exercise.[60] In these animals, the decrease in arterial resistance precedes the increase in cardiac output. However, within a few seconds, cardiac output begins to increase substantially, and the arterial pressure begins to rise above control levels. If both the neural component and the circulating catecholamine component are removed through sympathoadrenal blockade, the combined effect of the loss of the neural cardioaccelerator response and the loss of the increased resistance in nonworking muscle and nonmuscle areas can result in a decrease in arterial pressure sufficient to produce collapse.[9,10] Additionally, if mitral stenosis or other cardiac pathology is present and retards the cardiac output response to exercise, a decrease in mean arterial pressure is seen upon initiation of exercise.[80] If, on the other hand, an artificial resistance is imposed to prevent the decrease in arterial pressure, a large increase in arterial pressure is seen.[47]

In the normal human being an initial increase in arterial pressure is usually seen, indicating that the factors which increase the venous return and the pumping ability of the heart precede the factors which decrease the total peripheral resistance. The increase in arterial pressure during the initial 10–15 sec of exercise is usually mild, averaging 10–20 mm Hg. A decrease in pressure upon initiation of exercise is usually indicative of a pathologic condition.[80]

Stroke volume. The literature on exercise physiology is filled with contradictory statements concerning the role of stroke volume during exercise. Until the late 1950s, most circulatory physiologists believed that the intrinsic regulatory properties of the circulation were sufficient to explain almost entirely the increase in cardiac output during exercise. Their concept was based upon the opinion that the increase in venous return automatically increased cardiac output through the Frank–Starling mechanism, and that the increase in cardiac output was primarily the result of in-

creased stroke volume. However, in the 1950s, data from Rushmer's lab began to show that, in unanesthetized dogs, the increase in cardiac output in mild exercise occurred mainly through an increase in heart rate, with little change in stroke volume.[6,20,25] The controversy was compounded when extensive investigations were begun in human beings. This occurred as a result of data from exercising human beings in the supine position being used interchangeably with data from exercising human beings in the erect position. Further complications occurred when control data obtained in the supine position were compared with exercise data obtained in the erect position. The stroke volume reserve in the supine position appears to be minimal, because stroke volume approaches its maximum value in the supine human. There is normally a decrease in stroke volume in the human being upon transition from the supine to the erect posture.[21] Therefore, any increase in stroke volume as the result of exercise may be masked by the postural change in stroke volume.

The divergent findings in studies dealing with stroke volume changes during exercise may be explained when one considers that stroke volume is not an independently controlled variable, but rather, a variable that is dependent upon factors related to venous return, cardiac pumping ability, and heart rate. Stroke volume can be considered to be a resultant variable determined by the interrelationships and time constants of these factors. As an example, if the venous return increases more rapidly due to the sympathetic stimulation of exercise than does heart rate due to muscular compression of the legs and abdomen, then stroke volume will abruptly increase upon initiation of exercise. On the other hand, if heart rate increases more rapidly than venous return, stroke volume may fall upon initiation of exercise. If the time constants are equal, stroke volume may remain unchanged.

The controversy in this area appears to be reasonably well solved on the basis of the data which is available today. In mild to moderate exercise, the increase in heart rate may of itself be sufficient to account for the increase in cardiac output, without any change in stroke volume.[6,20] On the other hand, if heart rate is not allowed to increase or if the heart is paced at a constant rate, the stroke volume increase is sufficient to account for the increase in cardiac output in mild and moderate exercise.[60,81] Therefore, in mild to moderate exercise, either one of these mechanisms—increase in heart rate or stroke volume augmentation—can provide the increase in cardiac output. In severe exercise this is not the case. In severe exercise, the heart rate may increase up to $2\frac{1}{2}$–3 times normal. If there is no increase in stroke volume, the maximum increase in cardiac output will amount to 2.5–3-fold. The maximum increase in stroke volume appears to be 2 times the resting value.[21] Therefore, if heart rate is held constant, the maximum increase in cardiac output will be two times the normal value. Thus while either one of these mechanisms may be capable of handling the increased venous return in mild to moderate exercise, neither is individually capable of elevating the cardiac output to the values seen in severe exercise. If the change in heart rate and the increase in stroke volume are both maximal, then the cardiac output may increase 5–6 times the normal value. This agrees quite well with the data obtained in exercising normal humans.

In conclusion, in the normal human being in erect posture, stroke volume generally increases upon initiation of exercise.[21] The absolute magnitude of this increase is related to the relative intensity of the effort.[12] The initial increase may be as large as 50%. However, in severe exercise, the steady-state increase in stroke volume has been recorded as high as 100% above the control value.[21] The plateau level of stroke volume appears to be reached at 40% of maximum oxygen uptake and at a heart rate of 110.[82]

Adjustment Phase

General Energy Balance

Most cardiovascular variables reach a steady-state condition if the level of exercise is submaximal. As discussed in the last section, the initiation of exercise is attendant with very rapid changes in cardiac output, arterial pressure, mean circulatory pressure, and so on. However, in all but the most severe levels of exercise, most of these variables plateau with only minor changes in their absolute quantitative levels after the first few minutes of exercise.[70] During this steady-state phase, many of the minor variations appear to be of a fine tuning nature, as evidenced by frequent overshoot in early exercise, and then drop to plateau, as occurs with cardiac output and heart rate. It may be argued, that there is no steady-state phase, since one observes that even mild exercise cannot continue indefinitely. Mueller, for

instance, has shown that no true steady state in heart rate will appear if the level of exercise is above what he terms the "endurance level."[83] The endurance level, as defined by Mueller, is a level of exercise that can be tolerated continuously for 8 hr. For the untrained human, this amounts to no more than mild walking. Mueller has shown that if the level of exercise is above this endurance level, heart rate will continue to rise throughout the period of exercise. While Mueller's thesis may be essentially correct, there is also evidence that many of the controlled cardiovascular variables do become reasonably steady for periods ranging from several minutes to more than 2 hr, depending upon the absolute degree of exertion. It is this reasonably steady-state period that we should now like to discuss.

The appearance of a steady state in the cardiovascular system during exercise implies that a balance of forces has been achieved. That is, the the needs of the working musculature have been balanced, or matched by the adjustments of the circulation to supply these needs. If the metabolic needs of the working musculature exceed the delivery by the cardiovascular system, then appropriate reactions take place to reinstitute proper balance. There is one factor with which the various measured cardiovascular variables will quantitate in very close relationship during exercise. This common denominator appears to be the level of effort as indicated by the oxygen uptake.[12,84] Oxygen uptake per se correlates well with various cardiovascular variables in a homogenous population. However, in a heterogenous population—that is, one with individuals of varying degrees of fitness—oxygen uptake no longer is a good predictor. However, if one measures the maximum oxygen uptake of each person in that heterogenous population and also finds the oxygen uptake at a given level of exercise, then a plot of any cardiovascular variable against the *per cent of maximum oxygen uptake* will restore the relationship. To achieve comparability between individuals of a heterogenous population, the per cent increase in a cardiovascular variable must be plotted against the per cent of maximum oxygen uptake achieved at that level of exercise. For instance, Rowell has shown that the splanchnic blood flow at a given level of exercise is much greater in well trained athletes than in normal individuals or in individuals with mitral stenosis at the same level of exercise (Fig. 7A).[31] If the absolute level of effort

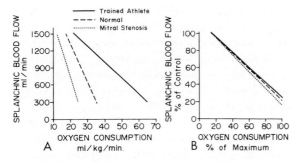

Fig. 7. Splanchnic blood flow as a function of (A) actual oxygen consumption and (B) per cent of maximum oxygen consumption of each group. Adapted from Rowell.[31]

is not considered, but rather, the per cent of maximum oxygen uptake achieved, as the common comparator, plots of splanchnic blood flow versus per cent of maximum oxygen uptake achieved in athletes, normal individuals, and patients with mitral stenosis are superimposed as shown in Fig. 7B.[2,31] As another example, the maximum heart rate during exercise in well trained individuals is not very much different from the maximal heart rate during exercise in untrained individuals. However, the oxygen uptake and the cardiac output are considerably higher in trained individuals,[85] and the heart rate in an untrained individual will be higher than the heart rate in an athlete at an equal work load.[86] Again, if one plots the per cent change in heart rate versus the per cent of maximum oxygen uptake, the two individuals can then be compared. Therefore, to discuss the steady-state phase of exercise, one needs to keep in mind both the absolute level of exertion as indicated by the oxygen uptake at that workload, and the per cent of maximum oxygen uptake for that individual.

Adjustment Mechanisms

The considerations cited above lead one to conclude that the primary regulation of central cardiovascular dynamics during the steady-state phase is based on the degree of completeness with which the circulation is meeting the metabolic requirements of the working muscles. Any discrepancy between need and supply is corrected by two mechanisms, one local and one central. The local mechanism occurs in the working musculature and relates to the local vasodilator system discussed in the introductory section. If flow is insufficient to supply the metabolic needs, a decrease in resistance to flow in that vascular bed will result. This results in an increased flow to that

muscular area, and thus increases venous return and cardiac output.

The central mechanism may well operate through the graded characteristics of muscle-afferent activation of the sympathetic system. That is, if a discrepancy exists between need and flow, the feedback signals of the muscle-afferent system are supposedly increased, and an increase in sympathetic outflow results. This increased sympathetic outflow increases myocardial contractility, heart rate, venomotor tone, mean circulatory pressure, and resistance to flow in nonworking muscle and nonmuscle areas, such as the renal and splanchnic circulation. These effects achieve not only an increase in venous return and cardiac output, but also achieve redistribution of flow directed toward the working musculature.

Evidence exists that the increased sympathetic constrictor effect may also be directed toward the working muscle, but the local vasodilator mechanism appears to have a sympatholytic effect.[8] Thus in working muscle, a balance is achieved between the local vasodilatation and the tendency for sympathetic vasoconstriction. The two contrasting stimuli are not comparable, in that a small vasodilator signal may counteract a large sympathetic constrictor stimulus. This balance between the local vasodilator system and the sympathetic constrictor system serves to direct the sympathetic constrictor outflow effects to nonworking areas, yet at the same time negates the need for a complicated sympathetic outflow distribution from the higher centers. No need for multiple pathways of sympathetic outflow exists. Rather, a generalized sympathetic outflow can occur, and this balance between local and central stimuli will automatically direct the effects of the generalized sympathetic outflow to areas of the body where an increase in resistance will not interfere with exercise performance, but will enhance the distribution of blood volume and flow toward the active muscles.

Splanchnic Volume Shifts

The splanchnic bed can serve as another reservoir from which volume and flow may be redistributed during the steady-state phase of exercise, even though the gross circulatory variables such as arterial pressure and cardiac output appear to be reasonably constant. As shown in Fig. 5, if the equilibrium point between the cardiac function curve and the venous return curve is located either on the plateau area of the venous return curve or on the plateau area of the cardiac function curve, no further increase in cardiac output is possible. An increased availability of oxygen can then be furnished to the working muscles only through a redistribution of the cardiac output—which redistribution results in a larger per cent of the available cardiac output being directed toward the working muscles. In addition to blood flow that can be directed away from the nonworking muscle, the splanchnic area offers a potential reservoir for the redistribution of blood flow. Rowell[2,31] and others[72,73] have shown in human studies that blood flow may be severely curtailed to the liver and to the other splanchnic areas during exercise. Blood flow to the visceral areas may fall to as low as 30% of control.

Numerous studies have attempted to calculate the increased amount of oxygen that may be made available to working muscle by redistributing a given quantity of blood from the splanchnic area.[2] Most of these calculations are made on the basis of the amount of oxygen contained in the blood flow that is redistributed. However, the circulatory model of Coleman et al.[87] indicates that a much larger increase in cardiac output to the peripheral area can occur than would be calculated on the basis of the blood flow that has been shifted—provided that the heart has not yet reached its pumping limit. This results from the shift of blood volume in addition to the shift in flow, and may be explained as follows. Volume is shifted from the splanchnic area by two mechanisms: one is active venoconstriction induced by the sympathetic response to exercise, and the other is a passive contraction of the visceral vessels caused by the drop in the perfusion pressure resulting from increased visceral arterial resistance. Coleman's model showed that a 2.5-fold increase in arterial resistance of the splanchnic bed is sufficient to translocate 220 ml of blood from the visceral area to the remainder of the circulation, and that this amount of translocated blood is sufficient to increase peripheral flow by 85%, which is a considerably greater increase in arterial supply to the working muscle than would be calculated on the basis of the oxygen contained in 220 ml of blood. However, in the model, this large increase in peripheral flow is the result of a very large increase in arterial pressure. Thus during exercise, when the arterial pressure does not rise to very high levels, the increase in peripheral flow as a result of

visceral vasoconstriction may well be intermediate between that predicted by the model and that calculated from the decrease in visceral blood flow.

Mechanisms by which the arterial resistance is increased and venoconstriction occurs in the visceral area appear to be purely sympathetic in origin, brought about by both increased sympathetic neural activity and increased levels of circulating catecholamines. From the studies of Rowell[2,31] relating visceral blood flow to per cent of maximum oxygen uptake required during exercise, it also becomes readily apparent that there is an inverse relationship between visceral blood flow and muscular work effort (Fig. 7). Furthermore, the absolute amount of the decrease in visceral flow is dependent upon the degree of sympathetic stimulation, which in turn is determined by the flow requirements of the working muscle.

Plasma Volume Regulation

Another regulatory phenomenon that occurs during the steady-state phase of exercise relates to the regulation of plasma volume. Studies in which the plasma volume is measured during exercise show that fluid begins to leave the capillaries almost immediately upon the initiation of exercise and continues to filter outward from the vascular bed during the first 10–15 min.[88–94] At this point, the decrease in plasma volume appears to cease. And the final decrease in plasma volume has been measured at between 10% and 15%. These findings pose two interesting questions: (1) what are the factors that result in the rapid loss of fluid from the circulation? (2) what factors terminate the loss of fluid from the circulation and prevent further loss?

The reasons for the rapid initial loss of fluid seem to be straightforward. The cardiac output has increased, the arterial pressure has increased, and the resistance to flow of the working musculature has decreased. Furthermore, the ratio of precapillary to postcapillary resistance has been decreased, and all of these factors acting together cause an increase in capillary pressure. The increase in capillary pressure, acting through the Starling mechanism, causes fluid to filter from the capillaries into the interstitium. Therefore, the major reason for the loss of fluid from the circulation early in exercise appears to be mainly hydraulic, initiated by a functional increase in capillary pressure. Another factor which has been proposed is the osmotic pull caused by the rapid increase in concentration of osmotically active particles in the interstitium, which is characteristic during the initiation of exercise.[92,93] This osmotic pull may be important during the early seconds of exercise, but since most of the compounds liberated during exercise have relatively low reflection coefficients,[95] the osmotic imbalance is presumably soon corrected. It is difficult to see how this effect could be prolonged more than a few minutes.

While the causes for this initial loss of fluid from the circulation may be reasonably well understood, the mechanisms by which the loss can be prevented after 15 min of exercise are less well understood. Lundvall et al.[93] have shown that during exercise on a bicycle ergometer, the loss of fluid into both legs may reach 1100 ml. They further showed that the decrease in plasma volume during this period may be only 600 ml. Therefore, it is obvious that, while fluid is leaving the circulation in the exercising muscle, fluid must also be entering the circulation from other sites. Their work indicates that during leg exercise, approximately 500 ml of fluid must enter the circulation from areas other than exercising muscle. They list two reasons for this inward accumulation of fluid. (1) During the early phases of exercise, the osmolality of the blood may increase by 30 or 40 mOsm due to an inward flux of osmotically active particles from working muscle. This exposes the nonworking muscle to a tremendous osmotic pull from the cells. They have shown that intra-arterial injection of hyperosmotic fluids does indeed pull tissue fluid into the circulation.[93] Because of the rapid diffusibility of most of these substances, the imbalance presumably should be rapidly corrected.[95] It is well known that the arterial resistance to blood flow in nonworking muscles is greatly increased during exercise.[8] This effect supposedly increases the pre- to postcapillary resistance ratio so that capillary pressure is reduced and fluid is pulled into the microcirculation through the Starling mechanism. Lundvall assigns equal power to these two mechanisms during exercise.[93]

These two mechanisms, the osmotic and hydraulic pull of fluid into the circulation, cannot act to prevent the continued leak of fluid from the circulation into the exercising muscle, but rather, merely serve to retard the decrease in plasma volume. If other mechanisms did not exist to prevent further loss of fluid into the working musculature, then no true steady state could exist, and fluid would simply be transferred from non-working muscle to working muscle, and the loss of plasma volume would continue. Therefore, the final equilibrium that is reached must be determined by other mechanisms.

One of the other factors which has been mentioned is a functional decrease in capillary pressure.[42] The arguments for this basically center around the constriction of veins during muscular contraction and the decrease in venous pressure that occurs upon release of the constriction.[68,69] The theory is based upon the finding that the venous system is valved and that any increase in external pressure on the veins contained within the working muscles would propel the fluid away from the capillaries toward the central circulation. When the muscle relaxes, the decrease in venous pressure caused by expansion of the vein supposedly occurs more rapidly than blood flow would tend to fill it; therefore, capillary pressure would tend to fall during relaxation. It is difficult to envision how this might retard fluid loss from the capillary circulation, since this effect begins to appear immediately upon initiation of exercise when fluid loss is at its greatest. Furthermore, for this effect to be important during equilibrium, fluid would have to rapidly enter the capillary during the relaxation phase in an amount equal to the fluid lost during the contraction phase. An analysis of the forces involved does not indicate that this occurs. Starling's law of the capillaries states that for an equilibrium to occur between the outward and inward flux at the capillary level, all of the factors that determine filtration at the capillary level must be in balance. These factors are the capillary hydrostatic pressure, the plasma colloid osmotic pressure, tissue colloid osmotic pressure, and the interstitial fluid pressure. In the control state, there is a slight imbalance in these forces tending to favor outward flux of fluid from the capillary to the interstitial fluid spaces.[95-98] This fluid is removed by the lymphatic vessels. As discussed in the previous section, there is a large increase in capillary hydrostatic pressure during exercise. Therefore, according to the Starling capillary equilibrium, the other forces must be altered in such a manner as to oppose the increase in capillary hydrostatic pressure if an equilibrium in fluxes is to occur. The most probable force that is changed during exercise to oppose the elevated capillary pressure is the interstitial fluid pressure. As fluid leaves the circulation, an increase in interstitial fluid volume occurs, and this causes an increase in the interstitial fluid pressure of that tissue.[97] Secondly, as the muscle contracts, there is a large instantaneous increase in the total tissue pressure of that muscle, which in turn is transmitted to the interstitial fluid and to the interstitial fluid pressure.[97] Studies have shown that if interstitial fluid pressure is less than zero, approximately three-fourths of the increase in total pressure is transmitted directly to the interstitial fluid pressure. If, however, tissue pressure is greater than zero, as occurs during exercise, then the entire increase in total tissue pressure can be transmitted to the interstitial fluid pressure. Therefore, during muscular contraction, the increase in total tissue pressure is transmitted to the interstitial fluid pressure and acts to oppose the effects of an increase in capillary pressure.

With these considerations in mind, it should now be possible to construct a sequence of events that occurs in relation to the loss of plasma volume during the first 15 min of exercise. As exercise commences, the mean arterial pressure increases. The resistance to flow in the muscle decreases; thus, capillary pressure is increased. Fluid is now forced from the capillary by the increase in capillary hydrostatic pressure. Interstitial fluid pressure begins to rise as a result of the increase in interstitial fluid volume and the increase in total tissue pressure caused by muscular contraction. The increased interstitial fluid pressure then begins to oppose the outward flux of fluid from the capillary. Any fluid continuing to filter outward is removed by the lymphatic drainage system. Now an equilibrium in plasma volume can be achieved. The increased interstitial fluid pressure results in a decrease in the capillary-to-interstitium pressure gradient, and the fluid that does filter out as a result of the remaining gradient is returned to the plasma by the lymph vessels.

Cardiovascular Drift Phase

If the exercise level is above the endurance level, then no true steady state can really exist for very long. A gradual increase in heart rate will be seen until maximal heart rate levels are reached.[82] The slope of the increase in heart rate with time will be proportional to the difference between the actual work level and the endurance level. The gradual increase in heart rate is indicative of an increase in intensity of sympathetic activation seen during this phase of exercise, which has been termed the "cardiovascular drift" phase.[2,74] The term "drift"

has been used mainly because of the gradual changes seen in several cardiovascular parameters, despite the fact that oxygen consumption remains constant and there is little, if any, increase in arteriovenous oxygen difference. The drift phase is characterized by a gradual increase in heart rate, a gradual decrease in central venous pressure, stroke volume, and arterial pressure, but relatively constant cardiac output. The possible physiologic explanations for this drift phase have been (1) decrease in blood volume, (2) cardiac fatigue, and (3) peripheral factors.

Blood Volume Depletion

While it is true that plasma volume does decrease 10%-15%[90,93,94] during exercise, this decrease occurs mainly within the first few minutes. No further decrease has been noted in most cases. Therefore, since the cardiovascular drift occurs at a time when the blood volume has been found to be relatively constant, decreased circulating blood volume is not a likely explanation.

Cardiac Fatigue

Since the heart is a muscle that performs heavy levels of work for long periods of time during exercise, it is attractive to hypothesize that a gradual decrease in cardiac pumping ability (cardiac fatigue) occurs during prolonged exercise.[99,100] As exercise continues, the heart becomes increasingly unable to respond to the demands placed upon it by exercise; thus, the cardiovascular drift. However, available data do not substantiate a decrease in cardiac function in normal people. For example, despite muscle fatigue, cardiac output remains constant without any increase in right atrial pressure.[99] If cardiac fatigue were occurring at a constant cardiac output, an increase in right atrial pressure would be expected. However, the opposite is usually found; the right atrial pressure decreases.

The endurance of the heart as an effective pump can be seen in marathon runners who have been noted to run in excess of 2 hr with calculated cardiac outputs of 75%-80% of the maximum.[101] Furthermore, in isolated heart studies, Sugimoto et al.[102] have shown that the heart is capable, in some instances, of pumping a maximum cardiac output in excess of 2 hr with no measurable evidence of damage. Furthermore, they showed that once the cardiac output begins to decline because of myocardial fatigue, the damage is apparently irreversible. It is well known that after an exhaustive period of exercise interspersed with a rest period, humans are able once again to perform for short periods of time at maximum oxygen uptake.[99] Therefore, there appears to be no clear physiologic basis for implicating myocardial fatigue into the cardiovascular drift phenomenon.

Peripheral Factors

The decreased stroke volume and central venous pressure that occur despite a constant cardiac output indicate a decreased tendency for venous return and implicate the peripheral circulation as the most likely site for an explanation of cardiovascular drift. In any satisfactory explanation of cardiovascular drift, one must conform to the data that show that venous return and cardiac output remain unchanged, but stroke volume, central venous pressure, and arterial pressure tend to decrease.[2] Keeping these factors in mind, a workable hypothesis may be advanced, based upon competition within the cardiovascular system between flow regulation to working muscle and the cardiovascular demands for the elimination of an increased heat load. As discussed in a previous section, one of the effects of the sympathetic activation incurred during the initiation of exercise is constriction of the skin vasculature.[8] Thus there are two mechanisms which tend to increase body heat content during the initial phases of exercise: (1) decreased heat loss potential as a result of the skin vasoconstriction; (2) increased heat production as a by-product of work performed by the musculature. This results in a situation whereby the circulation is faced with two competing demands for blood flow. The working musculature needs the increased blood flow to continue work at its elevated level, and the skin needs increased blood flow to eliminate the increasing heat load. It would appear from the studies of Rowell[2] that if cardiac output is not near maximum, then as body temperature increases, the thermoregulatory centers elicit sympathetic vasodilatation of skin vessels and increase the sympathetic vasoconstrictor outflow to the visceral vasculature. In other words, blood volume and flow may be transferred from the kidneys, intestine, and liver to the skin, thus increasing heat elimination without decreasing blood flow to the working muscles. These studies indicate an inverse relationship between cardiac output and blood flow to the splanchnic areas during exercise.[31] Furthermore, Rowell

demonstrated that if cardiac output is near maximum, then blood flow to the splanchnic area will be minimal. Therefore, under conditions of near maximal cardiac output, any increase in skin blood flow must be subtracted from muscle blood flow, and work cannot continue at the maximal rate. Indeed, indirect evidence of this latter effect is seen when one examines race times at international class level as a function of ambient temperature. It can be seen that most of the records set in the longer distances are done so at temperatures near 40°F. As ambient temperatures increase, racing speeds decrease. This can probably be explained by the fact that as ambient temperature increases, a larger per cent of cardiac output must be shifted to the skin for cooling purposes and is no longer available to the working musculature.[84] Therefore work rate, and in this case, race speed must be reduced until a proper equilibrium is reached.

Mechanisms of Drift

While the above mechanisms appear to be reasonably straightforward, how do they explain cardiovascular drift? The thermoregulatory system incorporates, as an effector pathway, portions of the sympathetic nervous system. As body temperature increases, the thermoregulatory center increases its input to the sympathetic centers—which centers in turn increase sympathetic constrictor outflow and, in particular, sympathetic vasodilatory outflow to the skin. A competition exists in the working musculature between this sympathetic outflow and local vasodilatation. However if the work load is heavy, the increased sympathetic stimulation has little effect on the resistance of the vasculature in working muscle. The visceral area, if not already maximally vasoconstricted, will respond to sympathetic stimulation with increased arterial resistance and decreased venous compliance. This serves to expel blood from these areas to the central circulation. The skin vessels respond to the vasodilator outflow by increasing their compliance. Thus, flow and volume are shifted from the visceral area to the skin area. Furthermore, the increase in general sympathetic outflow results in an increase in heart rate. The decrease in stroke volume can be explained since the heart rate increases through this mechanism and venous return does not. As blood is shifted to the dilated skin vasculature, the capacity of the peripheral circulation increases while blood volume remains constant. Therefore, there is a decrease in central venous pressure and in mean circulatory pressure. In addition, the vasodilatation of the skin vasculature and the shift of blood from the visceral to the peripheral circulation probably results in a decrease in the resistance to venous return. As discussed in the introductory section, venous return is proportional to mean circulatory pressure divided by the resistance to venous return. The decrease in mean circulatory pressure would tend to diminish venous return, while the decrease in resistance to venous return would tend to increase venous return. The relative magnitude of these two changes is such that during this phase venous return remains constant.

In the early stages of the cardiovascular drift phase, arterial pressure may remain unchanged. However, as the heat load generated by muscular work increases, total peripheral resistance decreases. If cardiac output is maximal or if alterations in the peripheral circulation do not result in increased venous return, then no further increase in cardiac output can occur as a result of the decrease in total peripheral resistance, and arterial pressure must fall. A decrease in arterial pressure is seen in human beings late in the cardiovascular drift phase.

CONCLUSION

A review of the schema proposed in Fig. 1 may be consulted for a synopsis of the cardiovascular interactions during exercise. Before exertion begins, cortical signals may excite the vasomotor center, resulting in increased heart rate, vasomotor tone, cardiac output and arterial pressure. Simultaneous with the transmission of motor information from the cortex to the muscles, additional impulses may go from the cortex to the vasomotor center to initiate a cardiovascular response pattern. Immediately upon initiation of muscular contraction, the local vasodilator mechanism reduces resistance to flow in the working muscle. Venous

return and cardiac output are enhanced. The muscle afferent feedback mechanism monitors the completeness with which the metabolic demands of the working muscle are being met. Any error signal results in additional sympathetic discharge to increase cardiac output and perfusion pressure. Because of the competition between sympathetic discharge and the local vasodilator mechanism, increased sympathetic outflow has little direct effect on working muscle. However, increased sympathetic outflow does redistribute blood volume and flow from the skin, viscera, kidney, and nonworking muscle to working muscle. Thus in short-term exercise, all of the increased cardiac output is directed toward working muscle.

As exercise continues and body temperature rises, skin blood flow increases as a result of sympathetic vasodilatation. Blood volume and flow are directed to the skin from the visceral and nonworking muscle area. When flow to these areas approaches minimal values and cardiac output is maximal, flow to working muscle is reduced.

This report was not designed to be an exhaustive consideration of every response of individual segments of the circulation to exercise. Rather, we have attempted to present the interrelationships between individual segments of the circulation and the manner in which they interact to produce an over-all circulatory response to exercise. The most basic facet of our discussion—indeed, of the circulatory response to exercise—has been the very important effect of the large decrease in vascular resistance that occurs in exercising muscle. Proceeding from this, we have attempted to show the manner in which resistances in other areas, capacitances, local volumes, and the performance of the heart are manipulated to maintain an arterial perfusion pressure sufficient to supply the needs of the exercising muscle. Additionally, if exercise continues, the competing demands on the circulation of thermal regulatory demands must also enter upon consideration.

REFERENCES

1. Bevegard BS, Shepherd JT: Regulation of the circulation during exercise in man. Physiol. Rev. 47:178–232, 1967

2. Rowell LB: Human cardiovascular adjustments to exercise and thermal stress. Physiol Rev 54:75–159, 1974

3. Wyndham CH: The physiology of exercise under heat stress. Ann Rev Physiol 35:193–220, 1973

4. Guyton AC, Jones CE, Coleman TG: Circulatory

Physiology: Cardiac Output and Its Regulation. Philadelphia, WB Saunders & Co, 1973

5. Sagawa K, Kumada M, Schramn LP: Nervous control of the circulation, in Guyton AC, Jones CE (eds): Cardiovascular Physiology. London, Butterworths, 1974, pp 197–232

6. Rushmer RF, Smith O, Franklin D: Mechanisms of cardiac control in exercise. Circ Res 7:602–627, 1959

7. Barcroft H, Swan HJC: Sympathetic Control of Human Blood Vessels. London, Edward Arnold & Co, 1953

8. Shepherd JT: Behavior of resistance and capacitance vessels in human limbs during exercise. Circ Res 20:70–81, 1967

9. Bassenge E, Holtz J, Restorff W, et al: Effect of chemical sympathectomy on coronary flow and cardiovascular adjustment to exercise in dogs. Pflueg Arch 341:285–296, 1973

10. Bassenge E, Kucharczyk M, Holta J, et al: Treadmill exercise in dogs under adrenergic blockade adaptation of coronary and systemic hemodynamics. Pflueg Arch 332:40–55, 1972

11. Ehrlich W, Schrijen FV, Krausman DT, et al: The effect of beta-blockade on coronary and systemic circulation in dogs at rest and during adaptation to exercise. Arch Int Pharmacodyn Ther 204:213–270, 1973

12. Ekelund LG, Holmgren A: Central hemodynamics during exercise. Circ Res 20:33–43, 1967

13. Hermansen L: Oxygen transport during exercise in human subjects. Acta Physiol Scand [Suppl] 399:1–104, 1973

14. Mellander S: Tissue osmolality as a mediator of exercise hyperemia. Scand J Clin Lab Invest 29:139–144, 1974

15. Mohrman DE, Sparks HV: Resistance and venous oxygen dynamics during sinusoidal exercise of dog skeletal muscle. Circ Res 33:337–345, 1973

16. Skinner NS Jr, Powell WJ: Regulation of skeletal muscle blood flow during exercise. Circ Res 20:59–67, 1967

17. Burch GE, Murtadha J: A study of venomotor tone in a short intact venous segment of the forearm of man. Am Heart J 51:807–828, 1956

18. Freyschauss U: Cardiovascular adjustment to somatomotor activation. Acta Physiol Scand [Suppl] 342:5–63, 1970

19. Merritt FL, Weissler AM: Reflex venomotor alterations during exercise and hyperventilation. Am Heart J 58:382–387, 1959

20. Rushmer RF: Constancy of stroke volume in ventricular response to exertion. Am J Physiol 196:745–750, 1959

21. Braunwald E, Sonnenblick EH, Ross J Jr, et al: An analysis of the cardiac response to exercise. Circ Res 20:44–58, 1967

22. Cowley AW Jr, Guyton AC: Heart rate as a determinant of cardiac output in dogs with arteriovenous fistula. Am J Cardiol 28:321–325, 1971

23. Guyton AC: Determination of cardiac output by equating venous return curves with cardiac response curves. Physiol Rev 35:123–129, 1955

24. Sarnoff SJ: Myocardial contractility as described by ventricular function curves. Physiol Rev 35:107–122, 1955

25. Franklin PL, Ellis RM, Rushmer FR: Aortic blood flow in dogs during treadmill exercise. J Appl Physiol 14:809–812, 1959

26. Horwitz LD, Atkins JM, Leshin SJ: Role of the Frank-Starling mechanism in exercise. Circ Res 31:868–875, 1972

27. Dentry JW, Wiss CR, Rowell LB: Increased forearm venous compliance during exercise with nitroglycerine. Acta Cardiol 29:31–43, 1974

28. Duggan JJ, Love VL, Lyons RH: A study of reflex venomotor reactions in man. Circulation 7:869–873, 1953

29. Mark AL, Kioschos JM, Abboud FM, et al: Abnormal vascular responses to exercise in patients with aortic stenosis. J Clin Invest 52:1138–1146, 1973

30. Merrit FL, Weissler AM: Reflex venomotor alterations during exercise and hyperventilation. Am Heart J 58:382–387, 1959

31. Rowell LB: Regulation of splanchnic blood flow in man. Physiologist 16:127–142, 1973

32. Seaman RG, Wiley RL, Zechman FW, et al: Venous reactivity during static exercise (handgrip) in man. J Appl Physiol 33:858–860, 1973

33. Tonnesen KH, Uhrenholdt A: Skin vasomotor response to exercise in normal subjects and patients with valvular heart disease. Scand J Clin Lab Invest [Suppl 31] 128:51–52, 1973

34. Donald DE: Myocardial performance after excision of the extrinsic cardiac nerves in the dog. Circ Res 34:417–424, 1967

35. Donald DE, Ferguson DA, Milburn SE: Effect of beta-adrenergic receptor blockade on racing performance of greyhounds with normal and with denervated hearts. Circ Res 22:127–134, 1968

36. Mellander S: Comparative studies on the adrenergic neuro-humoral control of resistance and capacitance blood vessels in the cat. Acta Physiol Scand [Suppl 50] 176:1–86, 1960

37. Guyton AC, Douglas BH, Langston JB, et al: Instantaneous increase in mean circulatory pressure and cardiac output at onset of muscular activity. Circ Res 11:431–441, 1962

38. Granger HJ, Guyton AC: Autoregulation of the total systemic circulation following destruction of the central nervous system in the dog. Circ Res 25:379–388, 1969

39. Shepherd AP, Granger HJ, Smith EE, et al: Local control of tissue oxygen delivery and its contribution to the regulation of cardiac output. Am J Physiol 225:747–755, 1973

40. Rushmer RF, Smith DA: Cardiac control. Physiol Rev 39:41–68, 1959

41. Goodwin GM, McCloskey DI, Mitchell JH: Cardiovascular and respiratory responses to changes in central command during isometric exercise at constant muscle tension. J Physiol 219:40–41, 1971

42. Folkow B, Neil E: Circulation. Oxford, Oxford University Press, 1971

43. Krahl VE: The glomus pulmonale: its location and microscopic anatomy. in DeReuch A, O'Connor M. (eds): CIBA Foundation Symposium on Pulmonary Structure and Function. London, Churchill, pp 53–69, 1962

44. Cunningham DJC: Regulation of breathing in exercise. Circ Res 20:122–131, 1967

45. Nielsen M, Asmussen E: Humoral and nervous control of breathing in exercise, in Cunningham DJC, Lloyd BB (eds): The Regulation of Human Respiration. Oxford, Blackwell, pp 503-513, 1963

46. Warner H, Cox A: A mathematical model of heart rate control by sympathetic and vagal efferent information. J Appl Physiol 17:349-355, 1962

47. Warner H: The role of peripheral resistance in controlling cardiac output during exercise. Ann NY Acad Sci 115:669-679, 1964

48. Holmgren A: Circulatory changes during muscular work in man. Scand J Clin Lab Invest [Suppl 24] 8:1-97, 1956

49. Stegemann J, Busert A, Brock D: Influence of fitness on the blood pressure control system in man. Aerospace Med 45:45-48, 1974

50. Delius W, Wallin G, Hagbarth KE: Role of sympathetic nerve impulses in regulation of peripheral circulation. Scand J Clin Lab Invest [Suppl 31] 128:47-50, 1973

51. Coote JH, Hilton SM, Perez-Gonzalez JE: The reflex nature of the pressor response to muscular exercise. J Physiol (Lond) 215:789-804, 1971

52. Kao FR, Ray LH: Respiratory and circulatory responses of anesthetized dogs to induced muscular work. Am J Physiol 179:249-254, 1954

53. Kao FR, Ray LH: Regulation of cardiac output in anesthetized dogs during induced muscular work. Am J Physiol 179:255-260, 1954

54. McCloskey DI, Mitchell JH: Reflex cardiovascular and respiratory responses originating in exercising muscle. J Physiol 224:173-186, 1972

55. Lind AR, McNicol GW, Donald KW: Circulatory adjustments to sustained (statis) muscular activity. Proc Int Symp Physical Activity in Health and Disease, Evang K, Lange Anderson K (eds). Norway, Universitetsforlaget, 1966, pp 38-63

56. Donald KW, Lind AR, McNicol GW, et al: Cardiovascular responses to sustained (statis) contractions. Circ Res 20:5-30, 1967

57. McCloskey DI, Mitchell JH: The use of differential nerve blocking techniques to show that the cardiovascular and respiratory reflexes originating in exercising muscle are not mediated by large myelinated afferents. J Physiol 222:50P-51P, 1972

58. Liang CS, Hood WB Jr: Comparison of cardiac output responses to 2,4-dinitrophenol-induced hypermetabolism and muscular work. J Clin Invest 52:2283-2292, 1973

59. Donald DE, Shepherd JT: Response to exercise in dogs with cardiac denervation. Am J Physiol 205:393-400, 1963

60. Donald DE, Shepherd JT: Initial cardiovascular adjustment to exercise in dogs with chronic cardiac denervation. Am J Physiol 207:1325-1329, 1964

61. Guyton AC, Coleman TG, Granger HJ: Circulation: overall regulation. Ann Rev Physiol 34:13-46, 1972

62. Uvnas B: Cholinergic vasodilator innervation to skeletal muscles. Circ Res 20:83-90, 1967

63. Fujihara Y, Hildebrandt JR, Hildebrandt J: Cardio-respiratory transients in exercising man. I. Tests of superposition. J Appl Physiol 35:58-67, 1973

64. Fujihara Y, Hildebrandt J, Hildebrandt JR: Cardio-respiratory transients in exercising man. II. Linear models. J Appl Physiol 35:68-76, 1973

65. Pickering TG, Davies J: Estimation of the conduction time of the baroreceptor-cardiac reflex in man. Cardiovasc Res 7:213-219, 1973

66. Stegemann J, Kenner T: A theory on heart rate control by muscular metabolic receptors. Archiv Kreiseaufforschung 64:187-214, 1971

67. Wigertz O: Dynamics of respiratory and circulatory adaptation to muscular exercise in man. A systems analysis approach. Acta Physiol Scand [Suppl] 363:1-32, 1971

68. Folkow B, Haglund U, Jodal M, et al: Blood flow in the calf muscle of man during heavy rhythmic exercise. Acta Physiol Scand 81:157-163, 1971

69. Folkow G, Gaskell P, Waaler BA: Blood flow through limb muscles during heavy rhythmic exercise. Acta Physiol Scand 80:61-72, 1970

70. Ceretelli P: Kinetics of adaptation of cardiac output in exercise. Proc Int Symp Phys Activ 1966, pp 64-73

71. Kramer K, Obal F, Quensel W: Untersuchungen ufer der Muskelstoffwechsel des Warmebluters: III. Mitteilung. Die Sauresoffaufrrohme des Muskels wahrend Rhythmischer tatigkeit. Pfluegers Arch 241:717-729, 1939

72. Clausen JP, Klausen K, Rasmussen B, et al: Central and peripheral circulatory changes after training of the arms or legs. Am J Physiol 225:675-682, 1973

73. Clausen JP, Trap-Jensen J: Arteriohepatic venous oxygen difference and heart rate during initial phases of exercise. J Appl Physiol 37:716-719, 1974

74. Detry JM, Gerin MG, Charlier AA, et al: Hemodynamic and thermal aspects of prolonged intermittent exercise. Int Z Angew Physiol 30:171-185, 1972

75. Higgins CB, Vatner SF, Franklin D, et al: Effects of experimentally produced heart failure on the peripheral vascular response to severe exercise in conscious dogs. Circ Res 31:186-194, 1972

76. Millard RW, Higgins CB, Franklin D, et al: Regulation of the renal circulation during severe exercise in normal dogs and dogs with experimental heart failure. Circ Res 31:881-888, 1972

77. Marx HJ, Rowell LB, Conn RD, et al: Maintenance of aortic pressure and total peripheral resistance during exercise in heat. J Appl Physiol 22:519-525, 1967

78. Bruce RA, Gey GE Jr, Cooper MN, et al: Seattle heart watch. Initial clinical, circulatory and electrocardiograph response to maximal exercise. Am J Cardiol 33:459-469, 1974

79. Smulyan H, Cuddy RP, Vincent WA, et al: Initial hemodynamic responses to mild exercise in trained dogs. J Appl Physiol 20:437-442, 1965

80. Bruce RA, Cobb LA, Katsura K, et al: Exertional hypotension in cardiac patients. Circulation 19:543-551, 1959

81. Vatner SF, Franklin D, Higgins CB, et al: Left ventricular response to severe exertion in untethered dogs. J Clin Invest 51:3052-3060, 1972

82. Astrand PO, Cuddy TE, Saltin B, et al: Cardiac output during submaximal and maximal work. J Appl Physiol 19:268-274, 1964

83. Mueller EA: Die Physische Ermudüng In Handbuch der gesamtem Arfeitsmeoizen, vol 1. Munich, 1961

84. Astrand PO: Aerobic work capacity during maximal performance under various conditions. Circ Res 20:202-210, 1967

85. Astrand PO, Rodahl K: Textbook of Work Physiology. New York, McGraw-Hill, 1970

86. Anderson KL: The cardiovascular system in exercise, in Falls HB (ed): Exercise Physiology. Academic Press, New York, 1968, pp 79-128

87. Coleman TG, Manning RD Jr, Norman RA Jr, et al: Control of cardiac output by regional blood flow distribution. Ann Biomed Eng 2:149-163, 1974

88. Cade JR, Free HJ, De Quesada AN, et al: Changes in body fluid composition and volume during vigorous exercise by athletes. J Sports Med Phys Fitness 2:172-178, 1971

89. Costill DL, Sparks KE: Rapid fluid replacement following thermal dehydration. J Appl Physiol 34:299-303, 1973

90. Costil DL, Finks WJ: Plasma volume changes following exercise and thermal dehydration. J Appl Physiol 37:521-525, 1974

91. Gill DB, Costil DL: Calculation of percentage changes in volumes of blood, and red cells in dehydration. J Appl Physiol 37:247-248, 1973

92. Lundvall J, Mellander S, Westling H, et al: Dynamics of fluid transfer between the intra- and extravascular compartments during exercise. Acta Physiol Scand 80:31A-32A, 1970

93. Lundvall J, Mellander S, Westling H, et al: Fluid transfer between blood and tissues during exercise. Acta Physiol Scand 85:258-269, 1972

94. Astrand PO, and Saltin B: Plasma and red cell volume after prolonged severe exercise. J Appl Physiol 19:829-832, 1964

95. De Lanne R, Barnes JR, Brouha L: Changes in osmotic pressure and ionic concentrations during muscular work and recovery. J Appl Physiol 14:804-808, 1959

96. Guyton AC, Prather JW, Scheel K, et al: Interstitial fluid pressure: IV. Its effect on fluid movement through the capillary wall. Circ Res 19:1022-1030, 1966

97. Guyton AC, Coleman TG: Regulation of interstitial fluid volume and pressure. Ann NY Acad Sci. 150:537-547, 1968

98. Guyton AC, Granger HJ, Taylor AE: Interstitial fluid pressure. Physiol Rev 51:527-563, 1971

99. Saltin B, Stenberg J: Circulatory response to prolonged severe exercise. J Appl Physiol 19:833-838, 1964

100. Ekelund LG, Holmgren A, Ovenfoss CO: Heart volume during prolonged exercise in the supine and sitting position. Acta Physiol Scand 70:88-98, 1967

101. Fox EL, Costill DL: Estimated cardiorespiratory response during marathon running. Arch Environ Health 24:316-324, 1972

102. Sugimoto T, Allison JL, Guyton AC: Effect of maximal work load on cardiac function. Jap Heart J 14:146-153, 1973

Adaptations of Muscular Tissue to Training

John O. Holloszy

EXERCISE-TRAINING, if sufficiently vigorous, brings about adaptive increases in performance capacity. The nature of the adaptive response varies with the type of exercise stimulus. The term "exercise" includes three different types of stimulus, each with its own specific pattern of response.

One type of exercise involves the learning of movement patterns and results in the development of skill, with an increase in coordination and agility. This type of exercise is exemplified by activities such as fencing, the various ball games, driving a car, or playing a musical instrument. The primary adaptive changes take place in the central nervous system and must involve a programming process initiated by repeated performance of a movement pattern until it becomes a conditioned reflex.

A second type is strength exercise, which involves relatively few, very forceful muscle contractions and is exemplified by weight lifting. It results in hypertrophy of the muscle cells with an increase in strength. The increase in muscle cell proteins responsible for this hypertrophy appears to be due to both an increase in protein synthesis and a decrease in the rate of protein degradation.[1]

The third type is endurance exercise, which is exemplified by activities such as long-distance running, swimming, or bicycling. It results in increases in endurance and in the maximum capacity to utilize O_2 made possible by adaptations in the skeletal muscles, in the cardiovascular system, and in the autonomic nervous system. In contrast to strength exercise, endurance exercise does not result in muscle hypertrophy or an increase in strength. Instead, it brings about an increase in the capacity for aerobic metabolism.

Considerable information is now available regarding the long-term adaptations that occur in muscle tissue in response to endurance exercise. The purpose of this article is to review these adaptations and to evaluate their significance in relation to data from applied physiologic studies and in the context of the regulatory mechanisms that control the energy transfer pathways in muscle cells.

It is well known from comparative studies that there is a good correlation between the activity of a muscle and its content of mitochondria.[2,3] Within the same animal, the most active muscles have the highest respiratory capacity.[2,3] Similarly, comparisons of the same muscle groups in different species have shown that the most active animals have the highest skeletal muscle respiratory capacity. For example, the breast muscles of mallards and pigeons, birds which spend long periods in flight, are rich in mitochondria, and have ten times as great a respiratory capacity as the breast muscles of domestic chickens[2]; and the psoas muscle of the wild hare has cytochrome oxidase and succinate dehydrogenase activities three times as high as those found in the sedentary laboratory rabbit.[3] Although these differences may, in large part, be genetically determined, it now appears that adaptation to a habitually high level of physical activity also plays an important role.

EXERCISE-INDUCED INCREASE IN SKELETAL MUSCLE MYOGLOBIN

Myoglobin content generally closely parallels respiratory capacity in skeletal muscles of land mammals; skeletal muscles that are dark red in color are rich in both mitochondria and myoglobin, while white muscles have a low respiratory capacity and contain little myoglobin. Almost 50 yr ago, Whipple[4] found that the muscles of an active hunting dog had a higher content of myoglobin than did the muscles of more sedentary dogs, and suggested that exercise might increase myoglobin concentration. More recently, it has been shown under controlled experimental conditions that exercise can increase muscle myoglobin.[5,6] In rats subjected to a strenuous program of treadmill running for 14 wk, myoglobin increased approximately 80% in the hind-limb muscles.[6] Only muscles directly involved in the running showed an increase in myoglobin.[6] It has

From the Department of Preventive Medicine, Washington University School of Medicine, St. Louis, Mo.

Supported by NIH Grand HD 01613.

Reprint requests should be addressed to John O. Holloszy, M.D., Department of Preventive Medicine, Washington University, School of Medicine, 4566 Scott Avenue, St. Louis, Mo. 63110.

been shown that myoglobin increases the rate of oxygen diffusion through a fluid layer.[7,8] It seems likely that myoglobin may also facilitate oxygen utilization in muscle by increasing the rate of its diffusion through the cytoplasm to the mitochondria.

RESPONSE OF MITOCHONDRIAL OXIDATIVE ENZYMES IN SKELETAL MUSCLE

The response of skeletal muscle mitochondria to exercise-training has been studied most extensively in rats, although considerable information has more recently been obtained on humans. In rats subjected to strenuous treadmill running for 5 days/wk, up to 2 hr/day, for 14 wk or longer, an approximately twofold increase occurs in the levels of the mitochondrial respiratory chain enzymes involved in the oxidation of NADH and succinate in the leg muscles.[9] Mitochondrial ATPase (coupling factor 1), which is closely associated with the respiratory chain in the mitochondrial cristae and catalyzes the oxidative phosphorylation of ADP to ATP coupled to electron transport, is increased in parallel with the components of the respiratory chain.[10] A number of investigators working with rodents[11,12] and with humans[13-15] have confirmed that endurance exercise results in an increase in mitochondrial respiratory enzyme levels in skeletal muscles. In the studies on humans, enzyme activities were measured in muscle obtained by biopsy from the same individual so that the effects of training could be separated from interindividual genetic differences.[13-15] The levels of activity of the mitochondrial citric acid cycle enzymes also increase in muscle in response to endurance exercise.[16,17] The levels of activity of citrate synthase,[16,18] aconitase,[19] DPN-specific isocitrate dehydrogenase,[16] and succinate dehydrogenase[9,16] increase approximately two-fold in response to the exercise program mentioned above. In contrast, the levels of α-ketoglutarate dehydrogenase and malate dehydrogenase increase only about 50%–60%, while the citrate-cycle-related enzyme glutamate dehydrogenase increases approximately 35%, providing evidence for a change in mitochondrial composition.[16] The response of the enzymes involved in fatty acid catabolism to the running program mentioned above has also been examined. ATP-dependent palmityl CoA synthetase, carnitine palmityl transferase, and palmityl CoA dehydrogenase,

which are involved in the activation, transport, and catabolism of long chain fatty acids, all increased approximately twofold in gastrocnemius and quadriceps muscles of the trained rats.[19,20] Significant increases also occurred in β-hydroxybutyrate dehydrogenase, 3-ketoacid CoA-transferase, and acetoacetyl-CoA thiolase, the enzymes involved in ketone utilization in leg muscles of rats subjected to the running program.[21] The increases in mitochondrial enzyme levels are apparently due to an increase in enzyme protein, as evidenced by a doubling of the concentration of cytochrome c and an increase of approximately 60% in the protein content of the mitochondrial fraction of skeletal muscle.[9,10] Electronmicroscopic studies on biopsy specimens of human[13,22] and rat[23] skeletal muscle have provided evidence that increases in both the size and number of mitochondria are responsible for the increase in total mitochondrial protein.

CAPACITY OF SKELETAL MUSCLE TO OXIDIZE SUBSTRATES

Not surprisingly, in view of the increases in mitochondrial oxidative enzymes, endurance exercise-training increases the capacity of skeletal muscle to oxidize carbohydrate, fat, and ketones. It has been shown in rodents[9,19] and humans[13] that the capacity of muscle to oxidize pyruvate increases in response to training. The capacity of skeletal muscle to oxidize palmitate, oleate, linoleate, and palmityl CoA is also increased.[20] This increase is approximately twofold, expressed per gram of muscle, for both pyruvate and fatty acids in animals subjected to the exercise program mentioned earlier, when respiration by the mitochondrial fraction, or by a whole homogenate, of muscle is measured in the presence of nonlimiting amounts of substrate, ADP, and inorganic phosphate.[9,19,20] The mitochondria obtained from the exercised animals' muscles exhibit a high level of respiratory control and tightly coupled oxidative phosphorylation with either pyruvate or fatty acids as substrate.[9,20] This provides evidence that the increase in the capacity to oxidize fat and carbohydrate is accompanied by a parallel rise in the capacity to generate ATP via oxidative phosphorylation. It was also recently found that homogenates of gastrocnemius muscles from rats subjected to the running program oxidize β-hydroxybutyrate two to three times as rapidly as sedentary controls.[24]

Table 1. Levels of Activity of the Enzymes of the α-Glycerophosphate and Malate-Asparatate Shuttles, and of Alanine Transaminase in Gastrocnemius Muscle

Group	Fraction	α-Glycerophosphate Dehydrogenase*	Aspartate Transaminase	Malate Dehydrogenase	Alanine Transaminase†
Runners	Mitochondrial	2.27 ± 0.23	94 ± 4	452 ± 21	20.2 ± 1.4
	Cytoplasmic	33.3 ± 3.1	77 ± 5	301 ± 13	18.3 ± 0.9
Sedentary	Mitochondrial	2.38 ± 0.25	48 ± 3	279 ± 18	11.3 ± 0.8
	Cytoplasmic	35.6 ± 3.2	51 ± 5	223 ± 12	12.5 ± 0.6

Values are means ± SE. Enzyme activity is expressed as μmoles of substrate utilized per minute per gram wet weight of muscle.

*Data from Holloszy and Oscai.[27]

†Data from Molé, Baldwin, Terjung, et al.[29]

RESPONSES OF CERTAIN OTHER MITOCHONDRIAL AND RELATED ENZYMES

Mitochondria from normal mammalian tissues are impermeable to NADH. A number of mechanisms have been proposed to explain how NADH formed during glycolysis is oxidized.[25] The best documented of these are the malate-aspartate shuttle and the α-glycerophosphate shuttle, which appear to function in a number of mammalian tissues.[25] Since muscles of trained individuals appear to produce less lactate than those of untrained individuals, even at comparable rates of glycolysis,[26] it was of interest to determine whether an adaptive increase in the capacity to transfer reducing equivalents to the respiratory chain from cytoplasmic NADH occurs in response to endurance exercise. Mitochondrial α-glycerophosphate dehydrogenase, expressed per gram of gastrocnemius muscle, is unaffected by exercise.[27] In contrast, the enzymes of the malate-asparate shuttle are increased in both the mitochondria and cytoplasm of leg muscles of rats subjected to the running program mentioned earlier (Table 1). Mitochondrial aspartate transaminase activity increased twofold, while mitochondrial malate dehydrogenase activity increased 60% in gastrocnemius and soleus muscles. The cytoplasmic forms of these enzymes also increased significantly, but only one-half as much as the mitochondrial enzymes.

An alternative pathway of pyruvate removal in muscle is conversion to alanine via the alanine transaminase reaction. The quantitative importance of this pathway has been demonstrated by Felig and Wahren.[28] Increases in alanine transaminase activity of approximately 80% in the mitochondrial, and 50% in the cytoplasmic forms occurred in gastrocnemius muscles of rats subjected to the running program.[29] It seems possible that this adaptation could result in conversion of a greater proportion of the pyruvate formed in muscle during exercise to alanine and less to lactate by increasing the capacity of alanine transaminase to compete with lactate dehydrogenase for pyruvate. An increase in the rate of alanine production with a proportional decrease in lactate formation could protect against the development of acidosis in muscle during strenuous exercise.

As described earlier in this review, the levels of activity of a number of mitochondrial enzymes and the concentration of cytochrome c increase approximately twofold in hind-limb muscles of rats in response to a program of running; yet mitochondrial protein concentration increases only 60%. This difference is probably due to a change in mitochondrial composition. Although some mitochondrial enzymes increase twofold, others increase only 35%–60%, while still others do not increase at all. In addition to α-glycerophosphate dehydrogenase,[27] creatine phosphokinase and adenylate kinase[10] are among the mitochondrial enzymes that do increase in response to endurance exercise. The activities of these enzymes are unchanged when expressed per g of muscle; however, as a result of the increase in mitochondrial protein, the specific activities of these enzymes are decreased when expressed per milligram of mitochondrial protein,[10,27] Since the major feature of the adaptation in skeletal muscle is an increase in the capacity for aerobic metabolism, it is not very surprising that mitochondrial α-glycerophosphate dehydrogenase, adenylate kinase, and creatine phosphokinase do not increase in response to endurance exercise. It has been shown that the capacity of a muscle to oxidize α-glycerophosphate parallels its glycolytic capacity and is inversely related to its capacity for aerobic metabolism.[30]

Table 2. Adaptive Responses of Various Mitochondrial Enzymes in Fast-Twitch Red, Slow-Twitch Red, and Fast-Twitch White Types of Muscle to Exercise-Training

Muscle Type	Citrate Synthase*		Carnitine Palmityltransferase†		β-Hydroxybutyrate Dehydrogenase*		Cytochrome Oxidase†	
	Sedentary	Runners	Sedentary	Runners	Sedentary	Runners	Sedentary	Runners
White	7 ± 1	13 ± 1	0.11 ± 0.01	0.20 ± 0.02	ND	0.03 ± 0.01	15 ± 1	30 ± 2
Fast-red	41 ± 3	77 ± 4	0.72 ± 0.06	1.20 ± 0.09	0.14 ± 0.02	0.80 ± 0.05	74 ± 7	182 ± 6
Slow-red	27 ± 1	55 ± 2	0.63 ± 0.07	1.20 ± 0.05	0.34 ± 0.03	0.88 ± 0.07	55 ± 4	120 ± 9

Values are means ± SE. Enzyme activity is expressed as μmoles of substrate utilized per minute per gram wet weight of muscle.

*Data from Winder, Baldwin, and Holloszy.[21]

†Data from Baldwin, Klinkerfuss, Terjung, et al.[18]

White muscle, which has a high glycogenolytic capacity and a low capacity for aerobic metabolism, has high levels of α-glycerophosphate dehydrogenase, adenylate kinase, and creatine phosphokinase relative to cardiac muscle, which has a very high capacity for oxidative metabolism and a relatively low glycogenolytic capacity.[30-33] It thus appears that when skeletal muscle adapts to endurance exercise, it becomes more like cardiac muscle, in that its content of mitochondria and its capacity to generate ATP from oxidation of pyruvate and fatty acids increases. As a result of the decrease in the specific activities of creatine phosphokinase, adenylate kinase and α-glycerophosphate dehydrogenase expressed per mg of mitochondrial protein, skeletal muscle mitochondria also become more like heart mitochondria in their enzyme pattern.

ADAPTIVE RESPONSES OF MITOCHONDRIAL ENZYMES IN DIFFERENT TYPES OF SKELETAL MUSCLE

Mixed skeletal muscles, such as the gastrocnemius and quadriceps on which the initial studies of the response to exercise-training were conducted, are a mixture of different fiber types. In rodents, these are the fast-twitch white fibers that have a low respiratory capacity, a high glycogenolytic capacity, and high myosin ATPase activity; the slow-twitch red fibers that have a moderately high respiratory capacity, a low glycogenolytic capacity, and low myosin ATPase activity; and the fast-twitch red muscle fibers that have a high respiratory capacity, a high glycolytic capacity, and high myosin ATPase activity.[18,33-36] In histochemical studies employing the staining intensities of succinate dehydrogenase, DPNH diaphorase, or malate dehydrogenase to distinguish

the fiber types, it was found that the percentage of fibers with the staining characteristics of white muscle decreased, while the percentage of red-appearing fibers increased in mixed skeletal muscle of rodents subjected to endurance exercise.[37-39] It might appear from these results that endurance exercise brings about the conversion of some white fibers to red; however, as shown in Table 2, biochemical studies have shown that mitochondrial enzymes increase in all three fiber types, and, although the capacity of white muscle for oxidative metabolism increases, white fibers are not converted to red. The stains for the respiratory enzymes as they are generally used are relatively insensitive and are not appropriate for quantitation of enzyme activity, but serve to distinguish fibers with an oxidative capacity above some critical level that makes them appear "red," from "white" fibers with a respiratory capacity below this level. Endurance exercise apparently increases respiratory enzyme levels sufficiently in certain white fibers—perhaps those with the highest respiratory capacity initially—to reach the critical staining intensity needed to give a "red" appearance. The difference between red and white fibers is however maintained, and in the case of some enzymes, intensified.

It is of interest that the responses of some mitochondrial enzymes vary considerably among the different types of skeletal muscle. This is most evident for the enzymes involved in ketone oxidation.[21] In rats subjected to a program of treadmill running for 14 wk, β-hydroxybutyrate dehydrogenase became measurable at very low levels in white muscle, but increased 2.6-fold in slow red muscle and sixfold in fast red muscle (Table 2). There was a twofold increase in 3-ketoacid CoA-transferase in both fast red and white types of muscle, but only 26% in slow red muscle.[21] Acetoacetyl-CoA thiolase activity increased 40%–45% in all three types of skeletal muscle.[21] In contrast, citrate synthase and cytochrome c increased approximately twofold in all three types of skeletal muscle. In general, the exercise-induced adaptations tend to make skeletal muscles more like heart muscle in their mitochondrial enzyme activity patterns and levels.

There are major species differences in the characteristics of the three types of skeletal muscle fiber. In contrast to rodents, in a number of species[40-42] including man,[43] it is the slow-twitch red fibers that have the highest respiratory capacity, while the fast-twitch red fibers have a moderate or "intermediate" respiratory capacity. In rodents, it is possible to obtain relatively pure samples of the different muscle fiber types for biochemical analysis. In man, the different fiber types are intermingled so that biopsies obtained from muscles such as the vastus lateralis are mixtures of the three fiber types. As a result, no biochemical studies of the effects of exercise-training on the different muscle fiber types have been performed as yet. Another complicating factor in evaluating the effects of exercise on human muscle is that there appear to be major interindividual differences in the relative proportions of the different fiber types in muscles such as the quadriceps. These differences are probably genetically determined and may play a role in determining an individual's ability in different types of athletic activity. In a study in which the histochemical characteristics of skeletal muscle from competitive athletes in different athletic events were compared with each other and with untrained subjects, it was found that endurance athletes tended to have a higher percentage of slow-twitch red fibers than weightlifters, sprinters, and nonathletes.[44] On the other hand, no change in the relative percentages of slow-twitch and fast-twitch fibers occurred in the vastus lateralis muscles of untrained men subjected to a strenuous training program on a bicycle erogometer for 1 hr/day, 4 days/wk for 5 mo.[15] This program resulted in a twofold increase in succinate dehydrogenase activity, which was used as a mitochondrial marker in the mixed muscle. In this study, the oxidative capacity of the fast-twitch and slow-twitch muscle fibers was evaluated histochemically, using the intensity of staining for DPNH diaphorase; it was found that DPNH-diaphorase activity increased in both slow-twitch

and fast-twitch fibers.[15] The fast-twitch red and fast-twitch white fibers were not distinguished from each other, so the relative magnitudes of the adaptive responses to endurance exercise of these two muscle fiber types in man are not known.

ADAPTIVE RESPONSES OF THE GLYCOLYTIC ENZYMES IN SKELETAL MUSCLE TO ENDURANCE EXERCISE

A number of studies have shown that exercise results in an increase in hexokinase activity in skeletal muscle.[33,45-48] In rats subjected to a strenuous program of running, hexokinase activity increased approximately 170% in fast-twitch red muscle, 52% in slow-twitch red muscle, and only 30% in white muscle, which has the lowest initial level of hexokinase of the three types of muscle.[33] It is of interest that insulin, like exercise, affects hexokinase activity in skeletal muscle; insulin deprivation results in a decrease of hexokinase activity, while insulin administration can increase hexokinase activity to supernormal levels.[49] Katzen et al. have suggested that the effect of insulin may be mediated by increased entry of glucose into muscle cells.[49] The effect of exercise on hexokinase activity seems compatible with this hypothesis, because repeated muscle contractions have a marked "insulin-like" effect on glucose transport into muscle.[50-52] In contrast to the adaptive increases in mitochondrial enzymes that are brought about only by prolonged bouts of exercise during many weeks, adaptive increases in hexokinase activity occur in response to single bouts of prolonged exercise[47] or a few brief bouts of exercise.[45]

The other glycolytic enzymes in the fast-twitch red and slow-twitch red types of muscle undergo rather small changes in response to endurance exercise in the rat. In fast-twitch red muscle, which has a high glycolytic capacity, a decrease of approximately 20% occurred in the levels of glycogen phosphorylase, phosphofructokinase, glyceraldehyde-3-phosphate dehydrogenase, pyruvate kinase, lactate dehydrogenase, and cytoplasmic α-glycerophosphate dehydrogenase in response to the running program mentioned earlier.[33] Slow-twitch red muscle, which has a low glycogenolytic capacity in contrast to fast-twitch red muscle, underwent a 50% increase in cytoplasmic α-glycerophosphate dehydrogenase activity, and 18%–35% increases in

Table 3. Comparison of Fast-Twitch Red and Slow-Twitch Red Types of Skeletal Muscle, Before and After Exercise-Training, With Heart Muscle

Muscle	Group	Citrate Synthase*	Cytochrome Oxidase†	Hexokinase‡	Phosphofructokinase‡
Fast-red	Sedentary	41 ± 3	74 ± 7	1.50 ± 0.05	72 ± 3
	Runners	77 ± 4	182 ± 6	4.10 ± 0.29	59 ± 3
Heart		145 ± 8	297 ± 18	7.13 ± 0.54	30 ± 1
Slow-red	Runners	55 ± 2	120 ± 9	2.39 ± 0.18	24 ± 1
	Sedentary	27 ± 1	55 ± 4	1.57 ± 0.13	20 ± 1

Values are means ± SE. Enzyme activity is expressed as μmoles of substrate utilized per minute per gram wet weight of muscle.

*Data from Winder, Baldwin, and Holloszy.[21]

†Data from Baldwin, Klinkerfuss, Terjung, et al.[18]

‡Data from Baldwin, Winder, Terjung, et al.[33]

the levels of phosphorylase, phosphofructokinase, glyceraldehyde-3-phosphate dehydrogenase, and pyruvate kinase.[33] In white muscle, the only change found in the levels of the glycolytic enzymes other than hexokinase was a 15% decrease in lactate dehydrogenase.[33] In studies on mixed muscles, such as the gastrocnemius and quadriceps, the exercise-induced decreases in the glyolytic enzymes in fast-twitch red muscle are obscured by the increased enzyme levels in slow-twitch red fibers and the unchanged glycolytic enzyme levels in the white fibers.[33,46]

In a carefully controlled study on the effects of endurance exercise on human quadriceps muscle, no significant changes were found in the levels of a number of glycolytic enzymes.[13] Similarly, comparisons of levels of phosphofructokinase activity in biopsy specimens of quadriceps muscles from competitive athletes of various types and from untrained individuals showed no obvious differences between endurance athletes and strength athletes or untrained individuals.[44]

Except for the large increase in hexokinase activity in fast-twitch red muscle, the exercise-induced changes in the levels of the glycolytic enzymes in fast-twitch and slow-twitch red fibers are small, and their physiologic significance is not clear. However, it does seem reasonable that some relationship that is optimal for the aerobic metabolism of carbohydrate must exist between the glycolytic and respiratory capacities of muscle. Such a relationship appears to exist in normal heart muscle, which obtains its energy from aerobic metabolism, taking up lactate rather than forming it, even during catecholamine stress[53] and strenuous work.[54] At the other extreme, white muscle, which has a poor blood supply and appears to function for short bursts of very strenuous activity, obtains most of its energy from anaerobic metabolism with rapid glycogen depletion and production of large amounts of lactate.[55,56] Fast-twitch red skeletal muscle has a high capacity for glycolysis and glycogenolysis, but in addition, has approximately five times as great a respiratory capacity as white muscle.[18,33] When fast-twitch red muscle adapts to endurance exercise, it becomes more like heart muscle in its enzyme pattern as a result of the adaptive increases in respiratory capacity and hexokinase activity and the decreases in the levels of the enzymes involved in the conversion of glycogen to lactate (Table 3). Slow-twitch red skeletal muscle, like heart muscle, appears to obtain most of its energy from aerobic metabolism;[55,56] however, its capacities for glycolysis and for respiration are lower than those of heart muscle. Slow-twitch red muscle also becomes more like cardiac muscle when it adapts to endurance exercise as a result of increases in both its respiratory and glycolytic capacities (Table 3).

DIFFERENCES IN THE MAGNITUDE OF THE ADAPTIVE RESPONSES TO ENDURANCE EXERCISE IN THE DIFFERENT MUSCLE FIBER TYPES

Data from cross-innervation studies suggest that skeletal muscle fibers may have the potential for conversion from one type to another.[57,58] However, as previously reviewed, normal exercise, while bringing about major biochemical adaptations in muscle, does not result in conversion of one fiber type to another.[18,33] The white fibers have the lowest respiratory capacity, hexokinase activity, and the highest glycogenolytic capacity, and therefore have the greatest potential for exercise-induced adaptive change and undergo the smallest increases in respiratory capacity and hexokinase activity and little or no change in glycogenolytic enzyme activity. On the other hand, the fast-twitch red fibers, which have the highest respiratory capacity and hexokinase activity, somewhat surprisingly undergo the largest absolute increases in oxidative capacity and hexokinase.

Since the extent of an adaptive response is usually related to the magnitude of the inducing stimulus, the small changes in enzyme levels in white muscle relative to similar changes in red muscle could reflect a lesser participation in endurance exercise. This possibility has been investigated using muscle glycogen depletion as an indicator of prior contractile activity. In rats subjected to the 2-hr-long program of running used in some of the training studies described earlier, glycogen concentration decreased approximately 5.6 mg/g of muscle in fast-twitch red muscle, 2.7 mg/g in slow-twitch red muscle, and only 0.3 mg/g in white muscle.[59] Similarly, muscle biopsy studies on humans have shown that exercise of an intensity that can be maintained continuously for prolonged periods results in glycogen depletion primarily in the red fibers, with little involvement of the white fibers.[60] It seems reasonable to assume that a positive relationship exists between the magnitude of an inducing stimulus—in this case, the habitual level of contractile activity—and the extent of the adaptive response. The finding that white muscle is minimally involved in endurance exercise thus helps to explain why the absolute increases in respiratory capacity and hexokinase activity are so much smaller in white muscle than in red.

ADAPTIVE RESPONSE OF CARDIAC MUSCLE

Heart muscle does not undergo an adaptive increase in respiratory capacity such as is seen in skeletal muscle in response to endurance exercise.[62,63] The levels of activity of a variety of mitochondrial marker enzymes and the concentrations of cytochrome c and mitochondrial protein per gram of heart are unchanged in the hearts of trained animals.[62,63] Also, in contrast to skeletal muscle, the heart hypertrophies in response to strenuous endurance exercise, so that trained individuals have heavier hearts than sedentary controls of the same body weight. In normal individuals, this increase in the size of the heart relative to the

body could play an important role in the increase in work capacity brought about by training. In the absence of cardiovascular pathology, there appears to be a good correlation between heart size and maximum cardiac output.[64] An increase in the ratio of heart weight to body weight should, therefore, result in an increase in the maximum capacity to deliver blood to the working muscles. As a consequence, the hypertrophied trained heart should be able to supply oxygen to a larger mass of muscle during exercise.

There is evidence suggesting that myocardial contractility is enhanced by endurance exercise training.[65,66] It has been reported that the specific activities of actomyosin and myosin ATPase are increased in hearts of rats subjected to programs of swimming;[67,68] this adaptation could play a role in increasing myocardial contractility. Endurance exercise also appears to protect the heart against hypoxia, so that the trained heart's function deteriorates more slowly than that of the untrained heart under hypoxic conditions.[69] The biochemical basis for this protective effect is unknown.

PHYSIOLOGIC MANIFESTATIONS OF THE ADAPTATIONS TO ENDURANCE EXERCISE

Endurance exercise training results in an increase in maximum O_2 uptake capacity ($\dot{V}_{O_2 max}$). The magnitude of this increase depends on the individual's initial level of training and on the intensity, frequency, and duration of the exercise. In the majority of studies the increase has been in the range of 10%–20% after 3–6 mo of training. However, increases in the range of 37%–44% have been reported if training is sufficiently prolonged and intense.[70,71] Generally, the increase in $\dot{V}_{O_2 max}$ results equally from an increase in cardiac output secondary to a higher stroke volume and an increase in arteriovenous O_2 difference.[70-73] Thus, increased extraction of O_2 by the working muscles appears to play as important a role as increased cardiac output in bringing about the increase in $\dot{V}_{O_2 max}$ seen with endurance-exercise training.

Major effects of training are also demonstrable during submaximal exercise; that is, work requiring less than the $\dot{V}_{O_2 max}$. It has been shown with serial muscle biopsies that during submaximal exercise of the same intensity (i.e., at the same rate of O_2 consumption), individuals deplete their muscle glycogen stores more slowly when they are trained than when they are untrained.[74,75] This is in keeping with the observation that during sub-maximal exercise, individuals who have adapted to endurance exercise derive a greater percentage of their energy from oxidation of fatty acids and less from carbohydrate than do untrained individuals.[74-77] This is reflected in a lower RQ[74-76] and an increased rate of conversion of ^{14}C-labeled long-chain fatty acids to CO_2.[77] Trained men have lower RQs than untrained men, even during work of the same relative intensity (i.e., at the same per-centage of their $\dot{V}_{O_2 max}$).[74,75]

It is well established that, during submaximal exercise, physically trained individuals have lower blood[26,72,74,75,78,79] and muscle[26,75] lactate levels than untrained individuals. This appears to be true not only at the same absolute work level and O_2 uptake,[26,72,78,79] but even at the same relative O_2 uptake[26,74,75] when the trained individual is exer-cising at a higher work level than the untrained individual. It was for a long time generally believed that lactate production by working muscles re-flects muscle hypoxia even during relatively mild exercise. In this context, it was thought that the lower lactage levels and greater endurance seen in trained individuals during submaximal exercise re-sulted from improved delivery of oxygen to the working muscles made possible by the well docu-mented, exercise-induced cardiovascular adapta-tions. However, Jobsis and Stainsby[80] have used reflectance fluorometry to measure the steady-state oxidation-reduction level of mitochondrial NAD, and found that dog gastrocnemius muscle, stimulated to contract in situ, was well oxygenated when contracting at a frequency that resulted in an outpouring of lactate. They interpreted this finding to indicate that the lactate production was not the result of hypoxic stimulation of anaerobic glycol-ysis, but rather, of an imbalance between the rate of glycolysis and the rate of pyruvate utilization in the citrate cycle.[80] While this finding demonstrates that lactate production during exercise is not nec-essarily evidence of muscle hypoxia, it does not rule out the possibility that the working muscles may become hypoxic during strenuous exercise. However, if untrained muscles were hypoxic during submaximal exercise, and if trained muscles pro-duced less lactate because of a better oxygen sup-ply, then one would expect the trained individual to have a higher O_2 consumption than the un-trained individual at the same submaximal exercise level. For if a tissue were hypoxic, one would ex-pect its O_2 consumption to rise if its oxygen supply were increased. It is, however, well documented that O_2 consumption is the same in the trained and untrained states at the same submaximal work level if efficiency of movement is unchanged.[70,75,81] Furthermore, a number of investigators have shown, using the ^{133}Xe clearance method, that blood flow per kg of working muscle is ac-tually lower, not higher, in trained individuals than in untrained at the same, absolute, submaximal work level.[14,81,82] The working muscles compen-sate for the lower blood flow in the trained state by extracting more O_2; this is reflected in a greater arteriovenous O_2 difference during submaximal exercise.[70,72]

MECHANISMS BY WHICH THE BIOCHEMICAL ADAPTATIONS IN MUSCLE HELP TO EXPLAIN THE PHYSIOLOGIC DIFFERENCES BETWEEN TRAINED AND UNTRAINED INDIVIDUALS

The rate at which muscle cells consume oxygen during work is primarily a function of the fre-quency of contraction when load is held constant; the O_2 consumption of muscle cells can be varied over a wide range by varying the work rate.[83,84] The mechanism by which O_2 consumption is geared to work rate relates to the tight coupling of oxidative phosphorylation to electron transport. When O_2 and substrate are not rate limiting, the rate of respiration appears to be an inverse function of the ratio $ATP/(ADP + P_i)$.[85-88] In resting muscle, ADP and P_i concentrations and the rate of O_2 consumption are low. When muscle contracts, ATP and creatine phosphate are split and the intra-mitochondrial levels of ADP, P_i, and creatine rise, and the rate of respiration increases. The increase in mitochondrial ADP concentration appears to follow a saturation curve; the steady-state level of ADP attained in the mitochondria is a function of the frequency of muscle contraction,[89] and—when substrate and O_2 are not limiting—determines the rate of O_2 consumption.

During work at a rate that results in a submaxi-mal rate of O_2 consumption, once steady-state levels of mitochondrial ADP and of O_2 consump-tion are attained in a muscle cell, the rate of ATP formation via oxidative phosphorylation during and between muscle contractions must be suffi-ciently great to balance the rate of ATP splitting during the contraction. In the period between the beginning of work and the attainment of the steady-state level of O_2 consumption, before ATP hydrolysis is balanced by oxidative phosphorylation, the concentrations of creatine phosphate and ATP fall in muscle until the steady state is attained.[90-92] Simultaneously, the concentrations of ADP and P_i rise in the mitochondria until electron transport, O_2 consumption, and oxidative phosphorylation increase sufficiently to balance ATP breakdown. Oxygen consumption is the same in the trained and untrained states at the same submaximal work rate.[70,75,81] Since skeletal muscle that has adapted to endurance exercise has up to twice as many mitochondrial cristae per gram as untrained muscle, the steady-state levels of intramitochondrial ADP and P_i required to attain the same submaximal rate of O_2 consumption at a given work rate must be lower in trained muscle than in untrained muscle. This is so because with more mitochondrial respiratory chains, the rate of electron transport and O_2 consumption per respiratory chain must be lower to attain the same total O_2 consumption. In other words, the greater the number of mitochondria per gram of muscle, the lower the O_2 uptake per mitochondrion must be to maintain a given submaximal level of O_2 uptake per gram of muscle. In this context, it seems reasonable that in the process of attaining a given steady-state level of O_2 consumption, creatine phosphate (CP) and ATP levels must decrease less, and ADP, P_i, creatine, and, perhaps, AMP and ammonia levels must increase to a lesser extent in muscles of trained individuals as compared to the muscles of untrained individuals. (The high levels of adenylate kinase present in muscle result in conversion of some of the ADP that is formed to AMP, some of which is deaminated in turn by the action of AMP deaminase, resulting in the formation of ammonia.)

The intracellular levels of ATP, CP, P_i, AMP, ADP, and ammonia play major roles in controlling the rate of glycolysis in muscle.[93-97] ATP and creatine phosphate inhibit phosphofructokinase, and this inhibition is counteracted by P_i, ADP, AMP, and ammonia.[93-97] Therefore, because of higher steady-state levels of ATP and CP and lower levels of P_i, ADP, and, possibly, AMP and ammonia, glycolysis should occur at a slower rate in muscle that has adapted to endurance exercise than in untrained muscle at a given submaximal rate of work and O_2 utilization. This could in part explain the slower rates of muscle glycogen depletion and lactate formation seen during submaximal exercise in the trained state as compared to the untrained state. Experimental evidence supporting this line of reasoning has come from muscle biopsy studies on exercising humans.[26] At the same submaximal level of work and O_2 consumption, the decreases in the steady-state concentrations of CP and ATP, the rate of glycogen depletion, and the increase in lactate in quadriceps muscle were all lower when individuals were retested after they had adapted to a program of endurance exercise.[26]

Another factor that helps to account for the decreased rates of glycogen depletion and lactate production is the shift in the carbon source of the citric acid cycle. As discussed earlier, during submaximal exercise, the trained individual derives a greater percentage of his energy from fat oxidation than the untrained individual. It seems reasonable to ask why this should be, since endurance exercise induces comparable increases in the capacities of skeletal muscle to oxidize fat and carbohydrate.[9,18,20] The answer probably lies in certain of the control mechanisms that regulate carbohydrate metabolism. Among these is the rate of fatty acid oxidation. High rates of fat oxidation inhibit glycolysis and pyruvate oxidation.[98-100] At a given metabolic rate, the rate of fatty acid oxidation by a tissue appears to be determined by two factors: the concentration of fatty acids (i.e., substrate availability), and the capacity of the tissue to oxidize fat. When the metabolic rate is constant, at rest or during steady-state exercise, the rate of fat oxidation increases linearly with fatty acid concentration.[101,102] Saturating concentrations of free fatty acids do not appear to have been attained in the in vivo experiments reported in the literature. Thus, the availability of fatty acids to the mitochondria is probably the rate-limiting factor for fatty acid oxidation at any given respiratory rate, in vivo. However, at any given concentration of fatty acids, the rate of fatty acid oxidation will be highest in those tissues that have the greatest capacity to oxidize fat. For example, at the same concentration of fatty acids, the heart will oxidize fatty acids more rapidly than skeletal muscle, and red muscle will oxidize fat more rapidly than white muscle. Since the rate at which a substrate is utilized is a function of the level of enzyme activity regardless of whether or not substrate concentration is at a saturating level, the muscles of trained individuals, with their greater capacity for fat oxidation, could be expected to oxidize more fat at the same fatty acid concentration than those of untrained individuals. An increase in the oxidation of fatty acids results in a decrease in carbohydrate utilization,[98,99] brought about, in part, by a reduction in the rate of glycolysis,[99] which may be mediated by an increase in the concentration of citrate, an inhibitor of phosphofructokinase.[100]

One factor that has been implicated in the development of muscle fatigue during prolonged exercise, is depletion of muscle glycogen stores.[103,104] The adaptations induced in skeletal muscle by endurance exercise could, by the mechanisms discussed above, be responsible for postponing depletion of muscle glycogen and the fatigue associated with it. It has been suggested that another factor that can result in the development of fatigue during more strenuous exercise is the accumulation of high concentrations of lactate in muscle.[91,105] It is well documented that, at the same submaximal work rate, lactic acid concentrations are lower in skeletal muscle and blood in the trained state as compared to the untrained state. This difference may be explained by a decrease in the rate of glycolysis by the mechanisms discussed previously, and perhaps by the increases in the capacities of alanine transaminase and of the malate-aspartate shuttle to compete with lactate dehydrogenase for pyruvate and NADH, respectively. A third factor which may limit endurance during prolonged exercise is the development of hypoglycemia.[106,107] Increased oxidation of fatty acids appears to decrease glucose uptake[108] and could, through this mechanism, protect physically trained individuals against hypoglycemia during prolonged exercise.

MAXIMUM CAPACITY TO CONSUME O_2

An adaptive increase in maximum cardiac output occurs in response to endurance exercise.[70-73] This implies an increase in the maximum capacity to supply O_2 to the working muscles. However, studies using the ^{133}Xe clearance method have shown that maximum blood flow to the working muscles, expressed as ml per g of muscle per min, is not increased in the trained state.[82] It would, therefore, appear that any increase in $\dot{V}_{O_2max}$ brought about by an increase in maximum cardiac output is the result of delivery of O_2 to a larger mass of working muscle, rather than to delivery of more O_2 to the individual muscle cells. Although

considerable variability in response has been noted among individuals, on the average, an increase in maximum cardiac output appears to account for approximately 50% of the rise in $\dot{V}_{O_2max}$ that occurs in response to training.[70-73] The other 50% of the increase is accounted for by increased extraction of O_2 by the working muscles; this is reflected in an increased arteriovenous O_2 difference and a lower O_2 tension in venous blood.[70-73] There is no experimental information regarding the mechanism by which trained muscle cells extract more O_2 from the blood. However, if delivery of O_2 to the muscle cells during maximal exercise is the same in the trained and untrained states, as suggested by the ^{133}Xe clearance data, it seems reasonable that O_2 tension in the muscle cells and secondarily in the capillaries must be lower in the trained state as a result of the greater number of muscle mitochondria and the higher work rate required to attain $\dot{V}_{O_2max}$.

SUMMARY AND CONCLUSIONS

Skeletal muscle adapts to endurance exercise, such as long distance running, with an increase in the capacity for aerobic metabolism. This is reflected in an increase in the capacities of whole homogenates and of the mitochondrial fraction of muscle to oxidize pyruvate and long-chain fatty acids. Underlying this increase in the ability to obtain energy by respiration is an increase in the levels of a number of mitochondrial enzymes. These include the enzymes involved in fatty acid oxidation, the enzymes of the citrate cycle, the components of the respiratory chain that link the oxidation of succinate and NADH to oxygen, and coupling factor 1. These increases in mitochondrial enzyme activity appear to be due to an increase in enzyme protein, as evidenced by a doubling of the concentration of cytochrome c and a 60% increase in the protein content of the mitochondrial fraction of skeletal muscle. Electron-microscopic studies suggest that increases in both the size and number of mitochondria are responsible for the increase in mitochondrial protein. All three types of skeletal muscle, fast-twitch red, slow-twitch red, and fast-twitch white, but not heart muscle, participate in this increase in respiratory capacity. However, white muscle appears to be minimally involved in endurance exercise, and its adaptive responses are very small compared to those seen in red muscle. Major alterations in composition of skeletal muscle mitochondria also occur in response to endurance exercise training. As a result of these and other endurance-exercise-induced biochemical adaptations, fast-twitch red and slow-twitch red skeletal muscle fibers become more like heart muscle in their enzyme patterns. The endurance-exercise-induced adaptations in muscle tissue described in this review help to explain the biochemical and physiologic phenomena responsible for the lower lactate levels, the slower glycogen depletion, the lower RQ and the greater endurance during submaximal exercise, as well as the greater $\dot{V}_{O_2max}$ seen in the trained state as compared to the untrained state.

Now that the adaptive responses of muscle to endurance exercise have, to a large extent, been characterized, it seems likely that the main emphasis of future research in this area will be to determine the mechanisms by which these adaptations are brought about.

ACKNOWLEDGMENT

The secretarial assistance of Ms. Sara Watson in the preparation of this manuscript is gratefully acknowledged.

REFERENCES

1. Goldberg AL: Protein turnover in skeletal muscle I. Protein catabolism during work-induced hypertrophy and growth induced with growth hormone. J Biol Chem 244: 3217-3223, 1969

2. Paul MH, Sperling E: Cyclophorase system XXIII. Correlation of cyclophorase activity and mitochondrial density in striated muscle. Proc Soc Exp Biol Med 79: 352-354, 1952

3. Lawrie RA: The activity of the cytochrome system in muscle and its relation to myoglobin. Biochem J 55: 298-305, 1953

4. Whipple GH: The hemoglobin of striated muscle I. Variations due to age and exercise. Am J Physiol 76:693-707, 1926

5. Lawrie RA: Effect of enforced exercise on myoglobin concentration in muscle. Nature (London) 171:1069-1070, 1953

6. Pattengale PK, Holloszy JO: Augmentation of skeletal muscle myoglobin by a program of treadmill running. Am J Physiol 213:783-785, 1967

7. Hemmingsen EA: Enhancement of oxygen transport by myoglobin. Comp Biochem Physiol 10:239-244, 1963

8. Scholander PF: Oxygen transport through hemoglobin solutions. Science 131:585-590, 1960

9. Holloszy JO: Biochemical adaptations in muscle. Effects of exercise on mitochondrial oxygen uptake and respiratory enzyme activity in skeletal muscle. J Biol Chem 242:2278-2282, 1967

10. Oscai LB, Holloszy JO: Biochemical adaptations in muscle II. Response of mitochondrial adenosine triphosphatase, creatine phosphokinase, and adenylate kinase activities in skeletal muscle to exercise. J Biol Chem 246: 6968-6972, 1971

11. Barnard RJ, Peter JB: Effect of exercise on skeletal muscle III. Cytochrome changes. Am J Physiol 31:904-908, 1971

12. Gollnick PD, Ianuzzo CD: Hormoanl deficiencies and the metabolic adaptations of rats to training. Am J Physiol 223:278-282, 1972

13. Morgan TE, Cobb LA, Short FA, et al: Effect of long-term exercise on human muscle mitochondria, in Pernow B, Saltin B (eds): Muscle Metabolism During Exercise. New York, Plenum, 1971, pp 87-95

14. Varnauskas E, Björntorp P, Fahlén M, et al: Effects of physical training on exercise blood flow and enzymatic activity in skeletal muscle. Cardiovasc Res 4:418-422, 1970

15. Gollnick PD, Armstrong RB, Saltin B, et al: Effect of training on enzyme activity and fiber composition of human skeletal muscle. J Appl Physiol 34:107-111, 1973

16. Holloszy JO, Oscai LB, Don IJ, et al: Mitochondrial citric acid cycle and related enzymes: adaptive response to exercise. Biochem Biophys Res Commun 40:1368-1373, 1970

17. Dohm GL, Huston RL, Askew EW, et al: Effects of exercise, training and diet on muscle citric acid cycle enzyme activity. Can J Biochem 51:849-854, 1973

18. Baldwin KM, Klinkerfuss GH, Terjung RL, et al: Respiratory capacity of white, red and intermediate muscle: adaptive response to exercise. Am J Physiol 222:373-378, 1972

19. Holloszy JO, Molé PA, Baldwin KM, et al: Exercise induced enzymatic adaptations in muscle, in Keul J (ed): Limiting Factors of Physical Performance, Stuttgart, Georg Thieme, 1973

20. Molé PA, Oscai LB, Holloszy JO: Adaptation of muscle to exercise. Increase in levels of palmityl CoA synthetase, carnitine palmityltransferase, and palmityl CoA dehydrogenase and in the capacity to oxidize fatty acids. J Clin Invest 50:2323-2330, 1971

21. Winder WW, Baldwin KM, Holloszy JO: Enzymes involved in ketone utilization in different types of muscle: adaptation to exercise. Eur J Biochem 47:461-467, 1974

22. Hoppeler H, Lüthi P, Claassen H, et al: The ultrastructure of normal human skeletal muscle. A morphometric analysis of untrained men, women and well-trained orienteers. Pfluegers Arch 344:217-232, 1973

23. Gollnick PD, King DW: Effect of exercise and training on mitochondria of rat skeletal muscle. Am J Physiol 216:1502-1509, 1969

24. Winder WW, Baldwin KM, Holloszy JO: Exercise induced adaptive increase in rate of oxidation of β-hydroxybutyrate by skeletal muscle. Proc Soc Exp Biol Med 143: 753-755, 1973

25. Van Dam K, Meyer AJ: Oxidation and energy conservation by mitochondria. Ann Rev Biochem 40:115-160, 1971

26. Saltin B, Karlsson J: Muscle ATP, CP and lactate during exercise after physical conditioning, in Pernow B, Saltin B (eds): Muscle Metabolism During Exercise. New York, Plenum, 1971, pp 395–399

27. Holloszy JO, Oscai LB: Effect of exercise on α-glycerophosphate dehydrogenase activity in skeletal muscle. Arch Biochem Biophys 130:653–656, 1969

28. Felig P, Wahren J: Amino acid metabolism in exercising man. J Clin Invest 50:2703–2714, 1971

29. Molé PA, Baldwin KM, Terjung RL, et al: Enzymatic pathways of pyruvate metabolism in skeletal muscle: adaptations to exercise. Am J Physiol 224:50–54, 1973

30. Pette D: Mitochondrial enzyme activities, in Tager JM, Papa S, Quagliariello E, Slater EC (eds): Regulation of metabolic processes in mitochondria. Amsterdam, Elsevier, 1966, pp 28–49

31. Dart CH, Holloszy JO: Hypertrophied non-failing rat heart: Partial biochemical characterization. Circ Res 25:245–253, 1969

32. Shonk EE, Boxer GE: Enzyme patterns in human tissues. I. Methods for the determination of glycolytic enzymes. Cancer Res 24:709–721, 1964

33. Baldwin KM, Winder WW, Terjung RL, et al: Glycolytic enzymes in different types of skeletal muscle: adaptation to exercise. Am J Physiol 225:962–966, 1973

34. Barnard RJ, Edgerton VR, Furukawa T, et al: Histochemical, biochemical and contractile properties of red, white and intermediate fibers. Am J Physiol 220:410–415, 1971

35. Edgerton VR, Simpson DR: The intermediate muscle fiber of rats and guinea pigs. J Histochem Cytochem 17:828–838, 1969

36. Peter JB, Barnard RJ, Edgerton VR, et al: Metabolic profiles of three fiber types of skeletal muscle in guinea pigs and rabbits. Biochemistry 14:2627–2633, 1972

37. Barnard RJ, Edgerton VR, Peter JB: Effect of exercise on skeletal muscle I. Biochemical and histochemical properties. J Appl Physiol 28:762–766, 1970

38. Edgerton VR, Gerchman L, Carrow R: Histochemical changes in rat skeletal muscle after exercise. Exp Neurol 24:110–123, 1969

39. Faulkner JA, Maxwell LC, Brook DA, et al: Adaptation of guinea pig plantaris muscle fibers to endurance training. Am J Physiol 221:291–297, 1971

40. Burke RE, Levine DN, Zajac FE, et al: Mammalian motor units: Physiological-histochemical correlation in three types in cat gastrocnemius. Science 174:709–712, 1971

41. Davies AS, Gunn HM: Histochemical fiber types in the mammalian diaphragm. J Anat 112:41–60, 1972

42. Fitts RH, Nagle FJ, Cassens RG: Characteristics of skeletal muscle fiber types in the miniature pig and the effect of training. Can J Physiol Pharmacol 51:825–831, 1973

43. Dubowitz V, Brooke MH: Muscle biopsy: a modern approach. London, Saunders, 1973, pp 50–60

44. Gollnick PD, Armstrong RB, Saubert CW, et al: Enzyme activity and fiber composition in skeletal muscle of untrained and trained men. J Appl Physiol 33:312–319, 1972

45. Barnard RJ, Peter JB: Effect of training and exhaustion on hexokinase activity of skeletal muscle. J Appl Physiol 27:691–695, 1969

46. Holloszy JO, Oscai LB, Molé PA, et al: Biochemical adaptations to endurance exercise in skeletal muscle, in Pernow B, Saltin B (eds): Muscle Metabolism During Exercise. New York, Plenum, 1971, pp 51–61

47. Lamb DR, Peter JB, Jeffress RN, et al: Glycogen, hexokinase, and glycogen synthetase adaptations to exercise. Am J Physiol 217:1628–1632, 1969

48. Peter JB, Jeffress RN, Lamb DR: Exercise: effects on hexokinase activity in red and white skeletal muscle. Science 160:200–201, 1968

49. Katzen HM, Soderman DD, Wiley CE: Multiple forms of hexokinase: activities associated with subcellular particulate and soluble fractions of normal and streptozotocin diabetic rat tissues. J Biol Chem 255:4081–4096, 1970

50. Helmreich E, Cori CF: Studies of tissue permeability II. The distribution of pentoses between plasma and muscle. J Biol Chem 224:663–679, 1957

51. Holloszy JO, Narahara HT: Studies of tissue permeability X. Changes in permeability to 3-methylglucose associated with contraction of isolated frog muscle. J Biol Chem 240:3493–3500, 1965

52. Holloszy JO, Narahara HT: Enhanced permeability to sugar associated with muscle contraction: studies of the role of Ca^{++}. J Gen Physiol 50:551–562, 1967

53. Herman MV, Elliot WC, Gorlin R: An electrocardiographic, anatomic, and metabolic study of zonal myocardial ischemia in coronary heart disease. Circulation 35:834–846, 1967

54. Keul J, Keppler D, Doll E: Lactate-pyruvate ratio and its relation to oxygen pressure in arterial, coronar venous and femoral venous blood. Arch Int Physiol Biochim 75:573–578, 1967

55. Baldwin KM, Tipton CM: Work and metabolic patterns of fast and slow twitch skeletal muscle contracting in situ. Pfluegers Arch 334:345–356, 1972

56. Edstrom L, Kugelberg E: Histochemical composition, distribution of fibers and fatiguability of single motor units: anterior tibial muscle of the rat. J Neurol Neurosurg Psychiatry 31:424–433, 1968

57. Bárány M, Close RL: The transformation of myosin in cross-innervated rat muscles. J Physiol 213:455–474, 1971

58. Romanul FCA, Van Der Meulen JP: Slow and fast muscles after cross innervation. Enzymatic and physiological changes. Arch Neurol 17:387–402, 1967

59. Baldwin KM, Reitman JS, Terjung RL, et al: Substrate depletion in different types of muscle and in liver during prolonged running. Am J Physiol 225:1045–1050, 1973

60. Gollnick PD, Armstrong RB, Saubert CW, et al: Glycogen depletion patterns in human skeletal muscle fibers during prolonged work. Pfluegers Arch 344:1–12, 1973

61. Terjung RL, Winder WW, Baldwin KM, et al: Effect of exercise on turnover of cytochrome c in skeletal muscle. J Biol Chem 248:7404–7406, 1973

62. Oscai LB, Molé PA, Brei B, et al: Cardiac growth and respiratory enzyme levels in male rats subjected to a running program. Am J Physiol 220:1238-1241, 1971

63. Oscai LB, Molé PA, Holloszy JO: Effects of exercise on cardiac weight and mitochondria in male and female rats. Am J Physiol 220:1944-1948, 1971

64. Grande F, Taylor HL: Adaptive changes in the heart, vessels, and patterns of control under chronically high loads, in Handbook of Physiology, Circulation, vol 3. Washington DC, American Physiological Society, 1965, sect 2, p 2615

65. Crews J, Aldinger EE: Effect of chronic exercise on myocardial function. Am Heart J 74:536-542, 1967

66. Penpargkul S, Scheuer J: The effect of physical training upon the mechanical and metabolic performance of the rat heart. J Clin Invest 49:1859-1868, 1970

67. Bhan AK, Scheuer J: Effects of physical training on cardiac actomyosin adenosine triphosphatase activity. Am J Physiol 223:1486-1490, 1972

68. Wilkerson JE, Evonuk E: Changes in cardiac and skeletal muscle myosin ATPase activities after exercise. J Appl Physiol 30:328-330, 1971

69. Scheuer J, Stezoski SW: Effect of physical training on the mechanical and metabolic responses of the rat heart to hypoxia. Circ Res 30:418-429, 1972

70. Saltin B, Blomquist G, Mitchell JH, et al: Response to exercise after bed rest and after training. Circulation 38 (Suppl 7):1-78, 1968

71. Ekblom B: Effect of physical training on oxygen transport system in man. Acta Physiol Scand [Suppl] 328:1-45, 1969

72. Ekblom B, Astrand P-O, Saltin B, et al: Effect of training on circulatory response to exercise. J Appl Physiol 24:518-528, 1968

73. Rowell LB: Cardiovascular limitations to work capacity, in Simonson E (ed): Physiology of Work Capacity and Fatigue. Springfield, Thomas, 1971, pp 132-169

74. Hermansen L, Hultman E, Saltin B: Muscle glycogen during prolonged severe exercise. Acta Physiol Scand 71:129-139, 1967

75. Saltin B, Karlsson J: Muscle glycogen utilization during work of different intensities, in Pernow B, Saltin B (eds): Muscle Metabolism During Exercise. New York, Plenum, 1971, pp 289-299

76. Christensen EH, Hansen O: Respiratorischen Quotient und O_2-Aufnahme. Skand Arch Physiol 81:180-189, 1939

77. Issekutz B, Miller HI, Rodahl K: Lipid and carbohydrate metabolism during exercise. Fed Proc 25:1415-1420, 1966

78. Cobb LA, Johnson WP: Hemodynamic relationships of anaerobic metabolism and plasma free fatty acids during prolonged strenuous exercise in trained and untrained subjects. J Clin Invest 42:800-810, 1963

79. Robinson S, Harmon PM: The lactic acid mechanism and certain properties of the blood in relation to training. Am J Physiol 132:757-769, 1941

80. Jobsis FF, Stainsby WN: Oxidation of NADH during contractions of circulated mammalian skeletal muscle. Resp Physiol 4:292-300, 1968

81. Clausen JP, Larsen OA, Trap-Jensen J: Physical-training in the management of coronary artery disease. Circulation 40:143-154, 1969

82. Grimby G, Häggendal E, Saltin B: Local xenon-133 clearance from the quadriceps muscle during exercise. J Appl Physiol 22:305-310, 1967

83. Chapler CK, Stainsby WN: Carbohydrate metabolism in contracting dog skeletal muscle in situ. Am J Physiol 215:995-1004, 1968

84. Folkow B, Halicka DH: A comparison between "red" and "white" muscle with respect to blood supply, capillary surface area and oxygen uptake during rest and exercise. Microvasc Res 1:1-14, 1968

85. Chance B: The response of mitochondria to muscular contraction. Ann NY Acad Sci 81:477-489, 1959

86. Lardy HA, Wellman H: The catalytic effect of 2,4-dinitrophenol on adenosine triphosphate hydrolysis by cell particles and soluble enzymes. J Biol Chem 201:357-370, 1953

87. Chance B, Williams GR: The respiratory chain and oxidative phosphorylation. Adv Enzymol 17:65-134, 1956

88. Klingenberg M, Von Hafen H: Hydrogen pathway in mitochondria. I. Hydrogen transfer from succinate to acetoacetate. Biochem Z 337:120-145, 1963

89. Jöbsis FF, Duffield JC: Oxidative and glycolytic recovery metabolism in muscle: fluorometric observations on their relative contributions. J Gen Physiol 50:1009-1047, 1967

90. Hultman E, Bergstrom J, McLennan Anderson N: Breakdown and resynthesis of phosphorylcreatine and adenosine triphosphate in connection with muscular work in man. Scand J Clin Lab Invest 19:56-66, 1967

91. Karlsson J, Saltin B: Lactate, ATP, and CP in working muscles during exhaustive exercise in man. J Appl Physiol 29:598-602, 1970

92. Piiper J, Di Prampero PE, Cerretelli P: O_2 consumption, O_2 debt, and high-energy phosphates in the gastrocnemius muscle of the dog. Am J Physiol 215:523-531, 1968

93. Wu R, Racker E: Regulatory mechanisms in carbohydrate metabolism. III. Limiting factors in glycolysis of ascites tumor cells. J Biol Chem 234:1029-1035, 1959

94. Passonneau JV, Lowry OH: P-fructokinase and control of the citric acid cycle. Biochem Biophys Res Commun 13:372-379, 1963

95. Uyeda K, Racker E: Regulatory mechanisms in carbohydrate metabolism. VII. Hexokinase and phosphofructokinase. J Biol Chem 240:4682-4688, 1965

96. Williamson JR: Glycolytic control mechanisms. II. Kinetics of intermediate changes during aerobic-anoxic transition in perfused rat heart. J Biol Chem 241:5026-5036, 1966

97. Krzanowski J, Matschinsky FM: Regulation of phosphofructokinase by phosphocreatine and phosphorylated glycolytic intermediates. Biochem Biophys Res Commun 34:816-823, 1969

98. Paul P, Issekutz B, Miller HI: Interrelationship of free fatty acids and glucose metabolism in the dog. Am J Physiol 211:1313-1320, 1966

99. Newsholme EA, Randle PJ: Regulation of glucose uptake by muscle. 7. Effects of fatty acids, ketone bodies and pyruvate, and of alloxan-diabetes, starvation, hypo-

physectomy and adrenalectomy on the concentrations of hexose phosphates, nucleotides and inorganic phosphate in perfused rat heart. Biochem J 93:641-651, 1964

100. Parmeggiani A, Bowman RH: Regulation of phosphofructokinase activity by citrate in normal and diabetic muscle. Biochem Biophys Res Commun 12:268-273, 1963

101. Paul P: FFA metabolism of normal dogs during steady-state exercise at different work loads. J Appl Physiol 28:127-132, 1970

102. Paul P, Issekutz B: Role of extramuscular energy sources in the metabolism of the exercising dog. J Appl Physiol 22:615-622, 1967

103. Ahlborg B, Bergstrom J, Ekelund LG, et al: Muscle glycogen and muscle electrolytes during prolonged physical exercise. Acta Physiol Scand 70:129-142, 1967

104. Bergstrom J, Hermansen L, Hultman E, Saltin B: Diet, muscle glycogen and physical performance. Acta Physiol Scand 71:140-150, 1967

105. Hill AV, Kupalov P: Anaerobic and aerobic activity in isolated muscle. Proc Roy Soc (Series B) 105: 313-328, 1929

106. Christensen EH, Hansen O: Hypoglykämie, Arbeitsfähigkeit und Ermüdung. Skand Arch Physiol 81: 172-179, 1939

107. Pruett EDR: Glucose and insulin during prolonged work stress in men living on different diets. J Appl Physiol 28:199-208, 1970

108. Randle PJ, Newsholme EA, Garland PB: Regulation of glucose uptake by muscle. 8. Effects of fatty acids, ketone bodies and pyruvate, and of alloxan diabetes and starvation, on the metabolic rate of glucose in rat heart and diaphragm muscle. Biochem J 93:652-665, 1964

Circulatory Adjustments to Dynamic Exercise and Effect of Physical Training in Normal Subjects and in Patients With Coronary Artery Disease

Jan Praetorius Clausen

DURING the past decade, exercise tests and physical training programs have been used with increasing frequency in the diagnosis and management of coronary artery disease (CAD). Even though severe restrictions in physical activity were previously recommended to such patients, training studies have demonstrated that properly executed training programs effectively improve the exercise tolerance in the majority of CAD patients[1-13] while incurring only small risks.[12,14] Furthermore, exercise tests performed according to a suitable protocol provide valuable diagnostic information about the functional capacity of the cardiovascular system and form a rational basis for recommendations on physical activity in these patients.[15]

Studies of the cardiovascular adjustments to exercise and training have mainly been concerned with central circulatory parameters. Prerequisite to a high level of endurance performance is a great capacity of the oxygen transport system. For example, maximal oxygen uptake has been correlated to heart volume, blood volume, and the total amount of hemoglobin.[16,17] Moreover, the cardiac stroke volume (SV) appears to be a functional circulatory parameter that most clearly separates well trained athletes from sedentary subjects.[18] The finding that SV increases in response to training[19,20] has focused attention on the importance of the heart as a pump. The opinion that improved circulatory adjustment to submaximal exercise and increased maximal aerobic capacity are both related to primary central cardiovascular adaptations has thus prevailed.

Recent evidence however, suggests this cause and effect concept may not be valid, and it is now recognized that the effects of training are not limited to the central circulation.[21] In this context,

studies performed on patients with CAD and impaired cardiac function have been important in drawing attention to previously unnoticed peripheral effects of training.[2,3,6,13]

The present paper focuses upon the importance of peripheral circulatory alterations during adjustments to exercise and training. Although training results in central circulatory adaptations and may also improve left ventricular function, the prime importance of such adaptations as regards the circulatory and metabolic response to training will be questioned. The thesis that increased maximal exercise capacity can at least in part be attributed to local alterations in the trained muscles will be presented and analyzed. While it is accepted that maximal oxygen uptake is limited by the blood oxygen transport capacity,[22] it will be postulated that the primary event normally responsible for an enhanced oxygen supply after training is an increased ability to reduce resistance to blood flow in exercising muscles rather than improved performance of the central pump.

Although athletes may regularly perform exercise of an intensity and duration requiring maximal oxygen uptake, the beneficial effects normal subjects and patients with CAD obtain from physical training are related to a more optimal circulatory regulation during submaximal exercise; consequently, the focus of this presentation will be related to submaximal exercise.

CIRCULATORY ADJUSTMENTS TO EXERCISE IN NORMAL SUBJECTS

The following survey of the normal cardiovascular adjustment to exercise is limited to factors pertinent to physical training of patients with CAD. More detailed accounts of the normal response to exercise can be found in recent books or reviews.[17,22-27]

In connection with training of patients with CAD, only one type of muscular work is of interest; namely, rhythmic or dynamic exercise, in which a considerable part of the skeletal muscle mass is active. This applies to naturally occurring physical activities as walking, running, swimming,

From the Departments of Clinical Physiology of Frederiksberg Hospital and Bispebjerg Hospital, Copenhagen, Denmark.

Reprint requests should be addressed to Dr. Jan Praetorius Clausen, Department of Clinical Physiology, Frederiksberg Hospital, 2000 Copenhagen F, Denmark.

bicycling, and rowing. Only these types of activity will be referred to and only at work intensities that can be continued for 3–5 min or more.

Muscle Metabolism and Perfusion

Dynamic muscular exercise is characterized by a high metabolic rate in the muscle cells with the skeletal muscle functioning in a manner similar to the myocardium, with regularly alternating contraction and relaxation phases. The mechanical energy expended is grossly proportional to the force and the frequency of contraction, and it is derived from the breakdown of adenosine triphosphate (ATP) and creatine phosphate (CP).[28]

Only a limited number of a muscle's fibers, and thus, of its maximal contractile power, can be used in dynamic work continuing for several minutes. During maximal exercise on a bicycle ergometer with a pedaling frequency of 60 rpm, about 15%–20% of the maximal isometric strength of the quadriceps muscle is mobilized. This is thought related to the fact that skeletal muscle, in contrast to myocardium, is composed of several types of fibers with different enzymatic characteristics.[29] Some fibers are similar to cardiac muscle being rich in oxidative intramitochondrial enzymes connected to the citric acid cycle, the fatty acid cycle, and the respiratory chain. These are the classical "red" muscle fibers.[30] At the other end of a continuous spectrum is the typical "white" muscle fiber, with a high content of enzymes necessary for anaerobic glycolysis, but containing few mitochondria. Due to their great capability for aerobic metabolism, red fibers sustain rhythmic contractions for long periods of time, whereas the anaerobic white fibers require longer restitution phases even after short periods of activity.[31,32]

At lower levels of force development, only red fibers are activated, but with increasing force, an augmented number of motorunits containing an anaerobic enzymatic profile is recruited.[33] This presumably explains the progressive lactate release from muscles that is characteristic of increased work loads rather than muscle hypoxia, as previously thought.[34]

Despite an increasing contribution of anaerobic metabolic processes at heavier exercise levels, the major portion of the energy expended during dynamic work lasting several minutes results from aerobic metabolism of glucose and free fatty acids.[17] Under such situations, local O_2 consumption in the muscle may be augmented by a factor of one hundred. Oxygen extraction per milliliter of blood perfusing the muscle may increase three- to fourfold, and the enhanced muscle blood flow (MBF) is responsible for the remainder of the augmented oxygen uptake. In human muscle, maximal MBF is in the order of 70–100 ml $\times$ 100 g^{-1} $\times$ min^{-1} against a resting value of 2–5 ml $\times$ 100 g^{-1} $\times$ min^{-1}.[35,36] The increase in MBF is locally controlled by release of vasodilator metabolites and thereby closely geared to the metabolic demands.[37,38] Muscle blood flow per unit weight of muscle is closely related to the relative work load; i.e., percentage of maximal work load (Fig. 1).[36,39,40] The metabolites responsible for the exercise-induced vasodilation and hyperemia in muscle are not yet conclusively identified. The finding that both MBF[36,39,40] and ATP–CP depletion[41] are related to the relative work load supports the speculation that split products from high energy phosphates may be involved.[37]

Total Body Oxygen Uptake and Cardiac Output

During strenuous exercise, $\dot{V}O_2$ can attain individually varying maximal values, typically ranging from 2.0 to 6.0 l O_2/min.[17] The maximal oxygen consumption ($\dot{V}O_{2max}$) is a highly reproducible measure of a given subject's capability to perform this type of exercise, and it constitutes a useful physiologic reference standard.[22] The conditions required to obtain $\dot{V}O_{2max}$ and its physiologic implications have recently been reviewed in detail by Rowell[22] and by Hermansen.[42] The $\dot{V}O_{2max}$ for a given type of work is normally achieved at a work intensity that can be sustained for at least 3 min, but will cause complete exhaustion within 5–10 min. At this intensity of exercise, the cardiovascular functional capacity with respect to increase in cardiac output ($\dot{Q}$), widening of systemic arteriovenous oxygen difference (AVDO$_2$), and elevation of heart rate (HR) will be challenged maximally for the given type of exercise. However, the relative contribution of $\dot{Q}$ and AVDO$_2$ to the augmented oxygen supply varies according to the time the exercise is performed. The same $\dot{V}O_{2max}$ is measured at exhaustive exercise, which can be tolerated for 3–4 min and 6–9 min, respectively, but $\dot{Q}$ may be about 3 l/min lower during the shortest maximal effort.[43] At any submaximal $\dot{V}O_2$, the extent of the change in circulatory parameters will depend primarily on the relative work load; i.e., the percentage of $\dot{V}O_{2max}$ required.

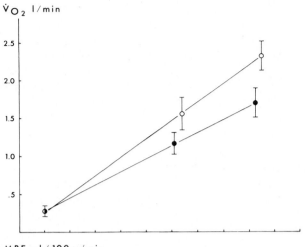

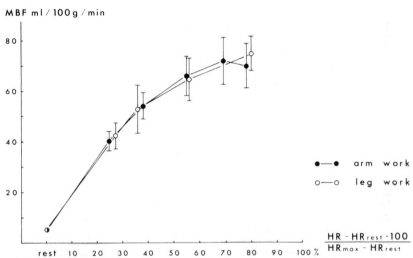

Fig. 1. Oxygen uptake ($\dot{V}O_2$) (upper panel) and muscle blood flow (MBF) (lower panel) measured by the ^{133}Xe-clearance method in m. biceps brachii during arm exercise (arm-cranking) and in m. vastus lateralis during leg exercise (bicycling). Both $\dot{V}O_2$ and MBF are related to the relative work load expressed as heart rate (HR) in per cent of the total range between resting and maximal HR. It should be noted that MBF per unit tissue is the same during arm exercise as during leg exercise at the same relative work load, whereas absolute $\dot{V}O_2$ is higher during leg exercise (from Clausen[36] with permission).

Figure 2 summarizes the changes in $\dot{Q}$ and its regional distribution in relation to $\dot{V}O_2$ with progressive increases in work load, together with the concomitant response of HR, stroke volume, and blood pressures. In order to underline the significance of the size of the active muscle mass and the relative work load, two different types of work are shown: Leg exercise performed on a bicycle ergometer, and arm cranking performed on a similar ergometer. During the latter type of work, the highest $\dot{V}O_2$ that can be obtained is normally about 70% of $\dot{V}O_{2max}$ during leg exercise.[44]

$\dot{Q}$ increases almost rectilinearly with $\dot{V}O_2$, and the rate of increase at submaximal levels is the same during exercise with small muscle groups (arm exercise) as during exercise with great muscle groups (leg exercise).[21,45,46] The relation between the increase in $\dot{Q}$ and the increase in $\dot{V}O_2$ during exercise—which is about 6 l blood flow/l O_2 uptake/min—shows only minor interindividual varia-

tions in healthy subjects, whereas the intercept with the y axis—i.e., resting $\dot{Q}$—may vary with body posture, sex, and age.[47]

Regional Distribution of Cardiac Output

The relative constancy of the increase in $\dot{Q}$ with increasing $\dot{V}O_2$ is due to the fact that total MBF—which is grossly predictable from the relative work load and the size of the active muscle mass (Fig. 1)—constitutes the prime determinant for the increase in $\dot{Q}$. Blood flow to nonexercising tissues also behaves in a predictable manner in relation to the increase in $\dot{V}O_2$ during exercise. Among the major regional circuits in nonexercising tissues, the cerebral blood flow (CBF) probably remains constant or increases slightly during exercise.[48] In contrast, the blood flow to most other parallel-coupled circuits is reduced due to constriction of resistance vessels mediated by the sympathetic nervous system.[22,25,49] Quantitatively most important

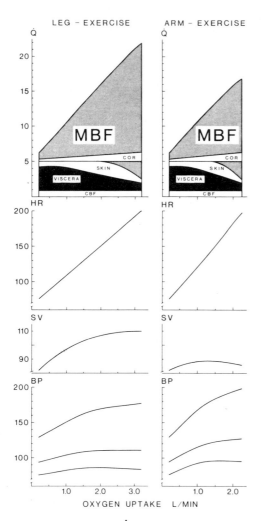

Fig. 2. Cardiac output (Q̇) in l/min and estimates of its regional distribution in relation to the oxygen uptake (V̇O₂) at rest and during submaximal and maximal leg exercise (bicycling) and arm exercise (arm cranking). At any V̇O₂, values apply to the situation after 5-7 min of exercise when V̇O₂ and Q̇ have reached a steady state. In the diagrams below, corresponding values are shown for heart rate (HR) in beats/min, for stroke volume (SV) in ml, and for aortic pressures (BP): systolic, mean, and diastolic in mm Hg. Based on data from Clausen et al.,[21] Rowell,[22] Kitamura et al.,[61] and Wade and Bishop.[25] It should be noted that during maximal exercise as well as at any relative V̇O₂, the perfusion of nonworking tissues and the heart can be assumed to be the same during arm exercise as during leg exercise and at any absolute V̇O₂, Q̇ is the same for the two types of exercise.

in this context are the vascular beds in the abdominal viscera (splanchnic-hepatic-blood flow (SBF) and renal blood flow (RBF)), in noncontracting muscles, and in the skin. In man it has been demonstrated that the reduction of SBF and RBF during exercise is a function of the relative work load. [21,22,50,51] For example, in normal subjects, the reduction in SBF is the same during arm exercise

as during leg exercise at a given relative V̇O₂, and a maximal reduction to 30% of the resting SBF could be predicted for both types of exercise.[21] In other words, the degree of flow reduction at a given absolute submaximal V̇O₂ was more pronounced during exercise with smaller muscle groups (Fig. 2). Muscle blood flow in noncontracting muscles also decreases in proportion to the work intensity.[52]

Skin blood flow in response to exercise is complicated, because two different mechanisms tend to change flow in opposite directions. Skin is supplied by sympathetic vasoconstrictor nerves mediating flow reduction during exercise. On the other hand, reflexes related to body thermoregulation tend to cause vasodilation to facilitate heat dissipation.[22] As a net result, during exercise in neutral environments, skin flow decreases during the first 5 min, but subsequently increases above resting values, provided the work load requires less than 50%-60% of V̇O₂max. At still higher V̇O₂, skin flow again decreases, and at maximal levels, skin vasoconstricts even in hot environment.[22]

Relation Between HR and SV During Exercise

Figure 2 shows that the increase in V̇O₂ is accompanied by a near linear rise in HR, and the increase in HR over the resting value is—like the degree of visceral vasoconstriction—a function of the relative work intensity. Thus HR at a given submaximal V̇O₂ is lower the larger the active muscle mass: at the same V̇O₂, HR is lower during bicycling than during arm cranking.[21,44,53] Heart rate is also lower during running than during bicycling, [42,54] and lower during walking with ski sticks ("skiwalking") than during running.[42]

Since the relation between Q̇ and V̇O₂ is the same for all types of exercise, the lower HR during exercise with large muscle groups implies a larger stroke volume (SV). Figure 2 shows that in the same person, SV is greater during leg exercise than during arm exercise at all absolute and relative work levels.

Relation Between HR and Visceral Blood Flow During Exercise

As discussed previously the increase in HR and degree of visceral vasoconstriction are both functions of the relative work intensity. Consequently, HR and SBF (or RBF) are closely related to each other during steady-state exercise.[21,22,51] This relationship is practically the same during arm exer-

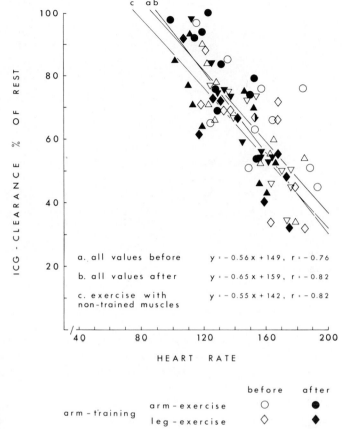

Fig. 3. Reductions in splanchnic-hepatic blood flow (SBF) expressed as per cent of resting indocyanine green (ICG) clearance during arm exercise and leg exercise. Values are from ten healthy young male subjects before and after training of either the arms or the legs. For both types of exercise, there is a close and significant relation between SBF% and HR that is maintained after training, even though HR is reduced considerably (from Clausen et al.,[21] with permission).

cise and leg exercise (Fig. 3).[21] An intimate connection between the HR and SBF response has been further documented[55] during the first 3–4 min of exercise: in this study, HR increased steeply and SBF decreased steeply, but the changes in the two parameters followed a common time course. At any time, the relative change in HR equaled that of SBF. This affords strong support to Rowell's conclusion that "increased sympathetic nervous outflow to the heart to increase its rate is accompanied by a proportional increase in sympathetic vasomotor outflow to visceral organs."[22]

Relation Between Arterial Blood Pressure and Blood Flow During Exercise

Although arterial blood pressures increases during exercise,[47] the pressure increase for a given increase in $\dot{Q}$ is greater during exercise with small muscle groups (arms) than during exercise with larger muscle groups (legs)[21,45,46,56] (Fig. 2). Total peripheral resistance (TPR) must therefore be

higher during arm, as compared to leg exercise. In order to analyze this phenomenon, it is convenient to use reciprocals of resistances; i.e., conductances. Expressed in this manner, the regional flow impediments can simply be added up to give that of the total organism. In the hypothetical example analyzed in Fig. 4, normal subjects worked at a submaximal $\dot{V}O_2$ of $1.5 \, l \times min^{-1}$, corresponding to a $\dot{Q}$ of $14.2 \, l \times min^{-1}$ at both arm and leg work. Mean blood pressure, (MBP) was 107 mm Hg during leg exercise and 122 mm Hg during arm exercise and total conductance, calculated as $\dot{Q}/MBP$, showed a proportional difference between the two types of exercise. Regional conductances were calculated as estimated regional flows* divided by

---

*Estimates of regional flows in normal subjects were obtained as follows: Myocardial blood flow (cor), CBF, SBF, and RBF at rest and during exercise were read from Fig. 2. The rest of $\dot{Q}$ was distributed on arms, legs, and truncus using axillary and femoral $AVDO_2$, remaining

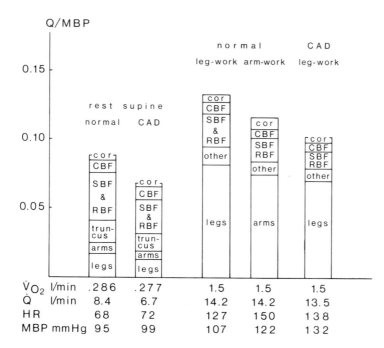

	normal	CAD			
			leg-work	arm-work	leg-work
$\dot{V}O_2$ l/min	.286	.277	1.5	1.5	1.5
$\dot{Q}$ l/min	8.4	6.7	14.2	14.2	13.5
HR	68	72	127	150	138
MBP mmHg	95	99	107	122	132

Fig. 4. Total and regional conductance ($\dot{Q}$/MBP); i. e., the flow in l/min/mm Hg of driving pressure. Estimates for normal young male subjects at rest and during submaximal arm and leg exercise and for patients with CAD at rest and during submaximal leg exercise. Below the columns, corresponding values for oxygen uptake ($\dot{V}O_2$), cardiac output ($\dot{Q}$), heart rate (HR), and arterial mean blood pressure (MBP) are shown. At the same $\dot{V}O_2$ (1.5 l/min), total conductance is lower during arm exercise than during leg exercise due to lower conductance both in nonexercising tissues and in exercising extremities. At rest, total conductance is lower in patients with CAD than in young subjects, but the regional distribution is the same. During exercise, conductance in both nonexercising tissues and exercising extremities are lower in CAD patients as compared to the healthy subjects (estimates based on data from Clausen et al.[21] and Clausen and Trap-Jensen[3]).

MBP. According to these calculations, about 50% of the difference in total conductance between arm and leg exercise can be related to a more pronounced vasoconstriction in nonexercising tissues during arm exercise. A $\dot{V}O_2$ of $1.5 \, l \, O_2 \times min^{-1}$ is a greater relative load for the arm muscles than for the leg muscles, and SBF was reduced to 65% of the resting value during arm work at $1.5 \, l \, O_2 \times min^{-1}$, but only to 75% during leg work.[21] The remaining difference in total conductance between arm and leg exercise is placed in the exercising muscles. Although total MBF seems to be almost the same at the given $\dot{V}O_2$ during the two types of work, the conductance in the active muscles during arm work is less than the conductance in the active muscles during leg work.

Several explanations can be proposed for this phenomenon. A greater proportion of the muscles engaged in arm work may perform isometric contractions in order to stabilize the body. The mechanical efficiency (relation between mechanical work and oxygen consumption) is 7%–8% lower during isolated arm exercise than during leg exercise.[45] Furthermore, it is conceivable that a more efficient muscle pump, in connection with more optimal hydrostatic conditions, contributes to a relatively greater decrease in the resistance of the leg muscles during upright exercise.[57,58] However, it cannot be excluded that for some reason, arm muscles require higher driving pressures to achieve a given muscle blood flow.

Myocardial Perfusion and Oxygen Uptake

Myocardial blood flow is adapted to local O_2 requirements through metabolically controlled vasodilation.[37] Myocardial O_2 uptake ($M\dot{V}O_2$) is in analogy to that of skeletal muscles, determined by the force of contraction and the frequency of contraction (HR). The force of contraction or the tension development depends on the intraventricular pressures, the initial length of myocardial fibers (end-diastolic volume), the ventricular wall thickness, and the contractile state of the myocardial fibers.[59] A close relationship has been demonstrated between coronary blood flow (and/or $M\dot{V}O_2$) and the rate pressure product (RPP), which is HR $\times$ systolic blood pressure, or between $M\dot{V}O_2$ and HR alone.[60–62]

$\dot{V}O_2$, and the relation between arm and leg volumes. During exercise, $\dot{V}O_2$ in nonexercising tissues was assumed to be unchanged, compared to the resting value and flow to exercising extremities as assessed to total $\dot{V}O_2 - \dot{V}O_2$ in nonexercising tissues divided by the regional $AVDO_2$. In patients with CAD, axillary and femoral $AVDO_2$ was not measured, but it was assumed that flow in the arms, legs, and truncus at rest made up similar fractions of the remaining $\dot{Q}$ as in young healthy subjects, and that flow to nonworking tissues changes in parallel with SBF. The analysis was based on data from Clausen et al.[21] and Clausen and Trap-Jensen.[3]

This probably reflects that the size of the heart normally changes little during exercise,[63] and that contractility, expressed by the rate of rise in left ventricular pressure (dP/dt/P), changes in parallel with HR and RPP.[64] The finding that beta-receptor blockade, which markedly reduces contractility as well as HR and systolic pressure, does not change the relation between RPP and $M\dot{V}O_2$ during exercise can be interpreted as confirming this fact.[62]

The correlation of myocardial blood flow with HR and systolic blood pressure means that both myocardial flow and oxygen consumption are functions of total body $\dot{V}O_2$ in per cent of $\dot{V}O_{2max}$ and not directly related to the external work load the subject performs. At a given submaximal pulmonary $\dot{V}O_2$, $M\dot{V}O_2$ is lower the higher $\dot{V}O_{2max}$ is. The relationship between $M\dot{V}O_2$ and the relative work load plays an important role for the exercise capacity of patients with CAD and the effect of training thereon.

Integrated Circulatory Regulation During Exercise

Precise integration of the cardiovascular adaptations to exercise depends upon the coordination and interaction of a multiplicity of nervous reflexes and intrinsic circulatory mechanisms. The vasodilation in muscle that is locally adjusted to the work load may be considered the fundamental determinant of $\dot{Q}$ during exercise. This postulate is supported by evidence from experiments performed on dogs with denervated hearts, where local vasodilation in active muscles in connection with the Frank-Starling mechanism of the heart insured a normal relation between $\dot{Q}$ and $\dot{V}O_2$ during submaximal exercise, even when performed at strenuous levels.[65] Moreover, experiments involving spontaneous exercise after destruction of the total sympathetic system[66] or electrically induced contractions after destruction of the entire nervous system[67] have shown that nervous control of circulation during exercise regulates arterial blood pressure to a greater extent than it does the regulation of $\dot{Q}$. Hence, an as yet unidentified chemical mechanism that mediates exercise hyperemia in skeletal muscles is directly responsible for the increase in $\dot{Q}$ during exercise, rather than nervous circulatory control.

However, this does not mean that the nervous reflexes are unimportant for the integrated circulatory regulation during exercise. Maintenance of arterial blood pressure by peripheral vasoconstriction is necessary for the intrinsic adjustment of $\dot{Q}$ to metabolic demands at higher work loads.[66] Moreover, nervous stimulation of the heart augments contractility and insures rapid adjustment of $\dot{Q}$ to a given $\dot{V}O_2$,[68] and enables the heart to deliver an increased $\dot{Q}$ with essentially unchanged stroke volume (SV) and only minor changes in filling pressures and volumes.[63]

As discussed below, the increased sympathetic stimulation of the heart during steady-state exercise may be partly or entirely mediated by afferent nervous impulses originating in the active muscles, and this may be the main reason why HR correlates so closely to $\dot{V}O_2$.[69] If it can be demonstrated that muscle metabolic rate controls both $\dot{Q}$ and HR during exercise, then an independent control of SV seems to be excluded. This interpretation agrees with that of Bevegård and Sphepherd,[24] who described the heart as a force-fed pump designed to discharge whatever volume it receives. Due to the great adaptability of the heart as regards SV, this can be done over a wide range of HR.

The above model for circulatory regulation during exercise is mainly based on results from animal experiments, but it seems to be valid also in man. Younger patients with congenital complete atrioventricular block have a much impaired HR increase during exercise, but a normal $\dot{Q}$ in relation to $\dot{V}O_2$ at submaximal levels.[70,71] Conversely, in normal subjects, abrupt exclusion of blood flow in the legs during treadmill walking by inflation of pneumatic cuffs around the thighs to pressures exceeding systolic arterial pressure results in a marked decrease in muscle-blood-flow controlled $\dot{Q}$, whereas the relation between neurogenically controlled HR and the work intensity is unchanged.[72]

The ability to adapt, during exercise with variation in SV if the HR response is impaired has certain limitations that become especially important in the diseased myocardium. In patients with acquired AV block and reduced left ventricular function, the compensatory enlargement of SV frequently insufficient, both at rest and during exercise, to insure a normal $\dot{Q}$ and BP.[73] When a fall in BP occurs in patients with AV block, a steep rise in auricular rate reveals that the nervous control system makes a vain effort to compensate.[70]

Situations where vasomotor function is affected indicate that in man, a major purpose of sympathetic vasoconstriction is maintenance of MBP. If peripheral vasoconstriction is prevented by vasodilator drugs or due to dysfunction of the sympathetic vasoconstrictor system, a marked decrease in MBP occurs during mild supine exercise, even in the presence of a normal increase in $\dot{Q}$ with $\dot{V}O_2$.[24,72]

Apart from maintaining MBP, vasoconstriction causes a redistribution of blood flow and blood volume. At maximal exercise, a total flow of about 3 l/min can be directed to active muscles instead of to nonexercising tissues (Fig. 2). The total release of blood volume from nonworking tissues has not been quantitatively assessed in man or animals. In one young male subject, the reduction in splanchnic-hepatic blood volume during upright bicycling was directly proportional to the decrease in SBF and amounted to 170 and 360 ml at work loads which increased HR to 132 and 149, respectively.[55] During submaximal exercise in environments that are thermally neutral, changes in regional flow and volume of this order of magnitude would not appear absolutely necessary to insure a sufficient oxygen supply to exercising muscles. In contrast, during maximal exercise, especially if $\dot{Q}_{max}$ and $\dot{V}O_{2max}$ are low, this redistribution of blood flow and blood volume represents an appreciable contribution to maximal O_2 transport.[22]

Summary

The above description of the normal central and peripheral circulatory adjustment to exercise can be recapitulated as follows:

During dynamic exercise, $\dot{Q}$ increases in direct proportion to the augmentation of $\dot{V}O_2$. The increase in $\dot{Q}$ is directed to exercising skeletal muscles, to the myocardium and—if exercise is continued for more than approximately 5 min—also to the skin. Blood flow to most "nonexercising" tissues (SBF, RBF, and noncontracting muscles) is reduced due to a general sympathetic vasoconstriction. At submaximal levels, muscle blood flow per unit tissue, the degree of peripheral vasoconstriction, the acceleration of HR, and in consequence, the increase in myocardial blood flow and oxygen consumption are all functions of the relative $\dot{V}O_2$; i.e., the actual $\dot{V}O_2$ expressed as a percentage of the highest achievable $\dot{V}O_2$ for the given type of exercise.

Arguments can be advanced to show that during exercise, the increase in $\dot{Q}$ (mainly going to active skeletal muscles) in proportion to increase in $\dot{V}O_2$ (mainly taking place in skeletal muscle mitochon-

dria) is locally regulated at the level of contracting skeletal muscles by metabolically controlled vasodilation. Also, since the increase in HR is regulated in proportion to muscle $\dot{V}O_2$, the stroke volume (SV) can be considered a secondary variable.

This model may seem oversimplified. For instance, important circulatory reflexes arising from vascular baro- and volume receptors are not taken into account, nor are cardiac reflexes elicited from the heart itself. However, the significance of such reflexes for the circulatory regulation during exercise is still not clear, and it is the author's opinion that even with this omission, the above description of the normal circulation during exercise serves as a background for a description of circulation in patients with CAD. As far as the adaptation of total blood flow to skeletal muscle oxygen requirements is concerned, emphasis is on peripheral mechanisms. In agreement with this hypothesis is the observation that patients with CAD who suffer from a primary affection of the central pump often preserve a sufficient oxygen supply to exercising muscles despite abnormal cardiac function during exercise.

CIRCULATORY ADJUSTMENTS TO EXERCISE IN PATIENTS WITH CAD

Central and Peripheral Circulation

Most patients with CAD who have been included in exercise and training studies have had healed myocardial infarction and/or stable angina pectoris and have been between 35 and 65 years of age. Both the aging process and myocardial lesions contribute to the modification of the circulatory response to exercise in this group, as compared to healthy young people.

In advanced age—especially after 60 years—the circulation tends to become hypokinetic; i.e., $\dot{Q}/\dot{V}O_2$ is reduced.[74-76] The decline of $\dot{Q}$ in l/min is almost the same during submaximal exercise as at rest, and thus the increase in $\dot{Q}$ with $\dot{V}O_2$ is essentially the same in older as in younger subjects. Stroke volume is lower at a given $\dot{V}O_2$, while arterial blood pressures are higher; $\dot{Q}_{max}$, HR_{max} and $\dot{V}O_{2max}$ decline with aging.[75-77]

In general, CAD subtracts further from physical working capacity, but depending on the premorbid level and the severity of the disease, a wide range of impairment in cardiovascular adjustment to exercise may be seen among patients with CAD. Some patients can hardly be distinguished from healthy subjects, but the majority are likely to have lower than normal $\dot{Q}_{max}$ and $\dot{V}O_{2max}$.[6,78] Patients with angina pectoris tend to have lower $\dot{V}O_{2max}$ than patients with uncomplicated healed myocardial infarction.[78] The reduced $\dot{V}O_{2max}$ in patients with CAD is associated with subnormal HR_{max} and SV_{max}, whereas $AVDO_{2max}$ is within normal limits. The maximal BP response can be elevated, normal, or reduced; the latter especially in patients with angina pectoris.[78]

$\dot{Q}/\dot{V}O_2$ during submaximal exercise is most often the same as in healthy subjects of the same age, but it may tend to decline with increasing severity of CAD.[78] With very severe impairment, but without decompensation at rest, the increase in HR during exercise occurs without any rise in $\dot{Q}$. This implies a reduction in SV counterbalancing the HR increase.[3] Even though $\dot{Q}/\dot{V}O_2$ is often normal at submaximal loads, SV is usually reduced and HR, relatively elevated. In contrast to the normal response, SV in patients with CAD regularly decreases markedly at work loads requiring more than about 60%–70% of $\dot{V}O_{2max}$.[3,6,78,79] The fall in SV may be relatively greater than the increase in HR and thus prevent further increase in $\dot{Q}$ with increasing work load. Widening of $AVDO_2$ permits some additional increase of $\dot{V}O_2$.[3,6,78,79]

The phenomenon described above may be taken to indicate impaired left ventricular function in these patients at high relative work loads. Left ventricular function in patients with CAD during exercise has almost exclusively been studied with the patient lying on the catheterization table, and most often, only during mild exercise. In this situation, indices of left ventricular contractility such as mean systolic ejection rate and the rate of rise of pressure at a given pressure (dP/dt/P) are reduced in patients with CAD as compared to normal subjects.[64,80,81] Moreover, pulmonary capillary wedge pressure (PCW) and left ventricular end-diastolic pressure ($LVED_p$) are elevated in many patients.[82–86] The elevation of $LVED_p$ correlates positively to the severity of CAD expressed by the number of coronary vessels involved with more than 75% obstruction.[86]

The impaired left ventricular response to exercise can be due to either permanent myocardial lesions—scar and fibrosis—or to transient ischemia caused by increased myocardial O_2 requirements during exercise. It seems reasonable to assume that reversible ischemia, rather than irreversible lesions, is responsible when left ventricular function is normal at rest, and the increase in PCW or $LVED_p$ can be prevented or attenuated by administration of nitroglycerin or digitalis prior to exercise.[82–85,87] It should be noted that development of such reversible left ventricular failure is not dependent on whether the patient experiences angina pectoris or not.[84,86]

In patients with CAD, exercise performed in the supine position, as in the studies cited above, is much more stressful to the heart than exercise performed in the more natural upright position.[54,88] Bygdeman and Wahren[88] found considerably less pronounced elevation of PCW in patients with angina pectoris when they exercised in the upright position than when they exercised in the supine position. Accordingly, patients with CAD can exercise to significantly higher levels in the upright position than they can in supine position.[54,88] Although an exercise test performed in the supine position may be more sensitive in disclosing potential left ventricular failure than exercise performed in the upright position, the latter will provide more information about the patients' tolerance to daily life activities.

Peripheral circulatory regulation in patients with CAD is in principle similar to that seen in young healthy subjects. It was noted, however, that MBF measured by the ^{133}Xe-clearance technique increased less in relation to the work load, and that maximal MBF was lower as compared to young healthy subjects: 37 ml $\times$ 100 g^{-1} $\times$ min^{-1} versus 60–70 ml $\times$ 100 g^{-1} $\times$ min^{-1}.[3,35,36,39] This difference seems overly large, since leg blood flow measured by indicator dilution techniques is lower in middle-aged, well trained subjects than in young normal subjects,[89] but not so much lower that it could account for a difference of 20–30 ml $\times$ 100 g^{-1} $\times$ min^{-1}. It is possible that a higher perivascular fat content in the leg muscles of middle-aged patients with CAD reduces the clearance rate of the lipophilic tracer ^{133}Xe.[3,35]

Clausen and Trap-Jensen[3] showed that the increase in MBF with increased work load in patients with CAD is associated with a graded reduction in SBF, similar to that of normal subjects. Splanchnic-hepatic blood flow at rest is somewhat low in patients with CAD, as compared to the values normally seen in young healthy subjects (1380 ml/min

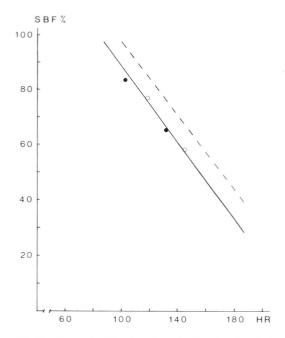

Fig. 5. Regression line for the reduction in splanchnic-hepatic flow in per cent of resting value (SBF%) in relation to heart rate (HR) in patients with CAD (Clausen and Trap-Jensen[3]). Group mean values (N = 6) measured before training (○) and after training (●). Broken line is the SBF%/HR regression from normal young subjects (Clausen et al.,[21] Rowell[22]).

versus 1500 ml/min), but the SBF%/HR relation during exercise has the same slope as in normal young subjects (Fig. 5). Since HR_{max} declines with age and CAD, the unchanged SBF%/HR relation in middle-aged patients with CAD implies that the reduction in SBF during maximal exercise is less pronounced than in young subjects. These patients with CAD had HR_{max} values between 145–150 beats/min. In Fig. 5, this corresponds to a maximal reduction of SBF to about 55% of the value at rest. Young normal subjects with HR_{max} values between 190 and 200 reduce SBF during maximal exercise to 20%–30% of the resting value.[21,22] This finding indicates that maximal sympathetic vasoconstriction may, in a manner similar to HR_{max}, decline with aging (and CAD). This agrees with the fact that even well trained, middle-aged subjects have relatively low systemic $AVDO_2$,[90] despite the fact that $AVDO_{2max}$ over the exercising legs is higher than in young subjects.[89]

Although the maximal flow reduction is less pronounced, the total peripheral resistance (TPR) is higher at all work levels in patients with CAD[3,78] and in normal middle-aged subjects,[74−76] as com-

pared to normal young subjects.[21] This can be related to the fact that TPR is higher during supine rest. While TPR during exercise falls the same amount of units in relation to $\dot{V}O_2$, it does not reach the same low values as in young subjects at any absolute and relative $\dot{V}O_2$.

Figure 4 includes an estimation of total and regional conductances in patients with CAD at rest and during exercise at $\dot{V}O_2$ of $1.5\,1 \times min^{-1}$. These can be compared to corresponding estimates from healthy young subjects at rest and during arm or leg exercise at the same $\dot{V}O_2$. While $\dot{Q}$ in the patients with CAD during leg exercise amounted to 95% of that seen in young healthy subjects, the total conductance was only 77%. Two thirds of this difference is accounted for by nonworking tissues. The higher resistance in nonworking tissues is partly explained by a higher value at rest and partly by a more pronounced vasoconstriction during exercise because the relative work load was higher. At the $\dot{V}O_2$ of $1.5\,1 \times min^{-1}$, SBF was 58% of the resting value in the patients with CAD. At the same $\dot{V}O_2$, the corresponding values for young normal subjects were 65% and 75%, respectively, for arm and leg exercise (Fig. 4).

The remaining one third of the difference in conductance between the patients and the normal subjects must be due to a greater resistance in the exercising muscles of the patients. After subtraction of estimated flow values to nonworking tissues from $\dot{Q}$, about 9 l/min remain to the active muscles in patients with CAD as well as in the normal subjects during leg and arm exercise. This agrees with the finding that the increase of $\dot{Q}$ in excess of the resting value is almost the same in the three situations. However, these 9 l of blood/min are forwarded by a much higher driving pressure in the patients with CAD.

Younger patients with essential hypertension have a similar pattern for regional conductance as do patients with CAD.[91] Although absolute values for regional and total conductance are lower in the hypertensive patients, the regional distribution is the same. These patients have subnormal values for leg blood flow, despite elevated driving pressures. Depression of the driving pressure obtained by a beta-receptor blocking drug (propranolol) causes further reduction in leg blood flow. Thus in these patients, a reduction in driving pressure is not compensated by further vasodilation in muscle. Although this may be due to vascular changes inherent to hypertension, we find it most likely that patients with CAD have a similar fixed, although less pronounced resistance in their muscular vascular bed, as well as in other vascular beds. (Further support to this hypopthesis can be derived from the information given later in Fig. 13.)

Angina Pectoris on Exertion

Although patients with angina pectoris often exhibit a more profound impairment of left ventricular function and of working capacity than patients with CAD without angina, there seems not to be any specific differences in their central or peripheral circulatory response to exercise. Accordingly, the abnormalities in hemodynamic adaptations in a patient with angina pectoris are present also at work loads that do not provoke angina pectoris.[92]

From the point of view of an exercise physiologist, the patient with angina pectoris is peculiar in that his capacity for dynamic work is not limited by his total body $\dot{V}O_{2max}$, but by $\dot{V}O_{2max}$ in myocardial regions supplied by narrowed coronary arteries. If pain is prevented by prophylactic administration of nitroglycerin, a patient with angina pectoris can exercise longer at a given work load or achieve higher work loads and thus obtain a higher $\dot{V}O_{2max}$.[93]

Robinson[94] demonstrated that when pain is provoked in patients with angina pectoris, this occurs at an individually fairly constant threshold value for the rate pressure product (RPP). This relationship between the onset of angina and the pressure work of the heart has later been confirmed and further elucidated by other investigators.[11,12,88,95–99] It has been demonstrated that angina occurs at the same individual RPP value even when provocation of pain is facilitated by elevated or by reduced environmental temperature, emotional stress, cigarette smoking, and in the postprandial period.[95] It appears that all these situations per se increase HR and/or SBP, and that this increase is added to that caused by exercise stress. It has further been shown that the constancy of the RPP threshold, originally found in the laboratory setting, also applies to the unrestricted patient during daily life activity.[99] For detailed analysis of the relation between the onset of anginal pain and the cardiac pressure work, it is however, most convenient to use exercise tests performed on a bicycle ergometer or treadmill.

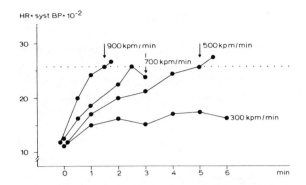

Fig. 6. Values for the product of systolic blood pressure (SBP) and heart rate (HR) measured at short intervals from continuous recordings of intra-arterial blood pressure in a patient with typical exertional angina pectoris performing repeated bouts of exercise on bicycle ergometer at 300, 500, 700, and 900 kpm/min (corresponding approximately to 50, 82, 115, and 150 watts, respectively). At the three highest work loads, the patient experienced chest pain. Onset of anginal pain is indicated by arrows. Note that pain was provoked at essentially the same product of HR and SBP on the different work loads. Between the exercise periods, the patient rested until at least 5-10 min after pain had disappeared (from Trap-Jensen and Clausen,[194] with permission).

Figure 6 shows a continuous registration of RPP in a patient with angina pectoris performing successive periods of leg exercise (bicycling). Independent of the external work load, pain is experienced when his critical value for RPP is reached. In 29 patients with typical exertional angina pectoris who performed a total of 119 leg exercise periods according to the schedule shown in Fig. 6, the individual RPP threshold was reproducible with a coefficient of variation of on average 6.2% ± SD 3.3.[97]

The angina threshold for HR or SBP considered separately shows a similar reproducibility as RPP, with the coefficients of variation being 6.2% ± SD 2.7 and 4.9% ± SD 3.0%, respectively.[97] The use of other indices of myocardial pressure work and $M\dot{V}O_2$ which, besides HR and SBP, also incorporate the ejection time (such as the tension time index and the triple product) does not improve the accuracy with which the angina threshold can be assessed.[96] This agrees with the finding in normal subjects that such indices are not better correlated to $M\dot{V}O_2$ during exercise than RPP or HR alone.[61]

The close relationship between the onset of angina and RPP or HR indicates that other determinants of $M\dot{V}O_2$ are normally unchanged or vary in proportion to RPP and HR in patients with CAD.

However, it is possible to show that end-diastolic heart volume has an independent significance for the appearance of angina during exercise. Angina pectoris is provoked at a lower HR and SBP, and thus a lower RPP, when exercise is performed in the supine position as compared to the upright position.[88] In normal subjects, heart volume is generally larger during supine exercise than during exercise in the upright position.[100] An increased end-diastolic volume will, according to the La Place relationship, augment ventricular wall tension for a given intraventricular pressure and thereby raise $M\dot{V}O_2$.[59] At the same time, the increased wall tension probably reduces myocardial blood flow by decreasing the pressure gradient between coronary arteries and the smaller intramural vessels.[101] Thus, $M\dot{V}O_2$ at a given RPP can be expected to be higher in the recumbent position than in the sitting position and the maximal myocardial perfusion, probably lower, both contributing to reduce the RPP anginal threshold during supine exercise.

A difference in ventricular volume also probably explains why patients with angina pectoris tolerate higher RPP values during upright arm exercise than during upright leg exercise. In 11 patients with typical angina at exertion, the RPP pain threshold was, on the average, 260 during arm exercise versus 204 during leg exercise.[97] The difference (21%) was highly significant ($p < 0.001$) and was due both to a higher HR (136 versus 122, Δ 10.3%) and a higher SBP (191 versus 169, Δ 11.5%). The absolute work loads, which were lower during arm exercise, were chosen so that the time to onset of pain was approximately the same for the two types of work. Thus, the most likely explanation for the higher RPP during arm exercise seems to be that the smaller SV is attended by decreased ventricular diastolic filling and a lowered end-diastolic pressure. Our results are in disagreement with the findings of Wahren and Bygdemann,[98] who reported almost identical RPP thresholds for angina during arm and leg exercise. The experimental design in the two studies does not offer any obvious explanation for the discrepancy between the results obtained.

Summary

The circulatory adjustment to exercise in patients with CAD typically differs from that of normal subjects in that the maximal values for $\dot{Q}$ (and thus for $\dot{V}O_2$), for HR, and for blood pressures are lower. During submaximal exercise, the relation between $\dot{Q}$ and $\dot{V}O_2$ tends to be reduced. Moreover, most of the patients with CAD exhibit signs of left ventricular failure during exercise, including a decrease in SV at higher work loads, reduced myocardial contractility, and increased LVEDp. Nonetheless, the peripheral circulatory regulation in patients with CAD corresponds in principle to that seen in healthy subjects of the same age. Patients with angina pectoris do not differ from other patients with CAD in any specific manner with respect to circulatory regulation during exercise. However, maximal performance in patients with angina pectoris is limited by a subnormal maximal myocardial oxygen uptake and not by total body $\dot{V}O_{2max}$. A given patient with angina pectoris has a reproducible pain threshold value for easily obtainable indices of myocardial oxygen consumption, like HR or the product of HR and systolic blood pressure (RPP). When an increase in HR and systolic blood pressure is elicited by exercise and/or by changes in environmental temperature, by emotional upset and in connection with smoking or in the postprandial period, pain is experienced if an individual critical RPP value is reached. However, in a given patient, the RPP threshold may vary in situations where left ventricular volume is changed, because RPP does not take this important determinant of myocardial oxygen consumption into account. Thus, with reference to upright leg exercise, angina pectoris is provoked at a lower RPP value during supine exercise associated with a large heart volume, whereas the RPP pain threshold is higher during arm exercise, where heart volume presumably is smaller.

EFFECTS OF TRAINING ON CIRCULATORY ADJUSTMENT AT REST AND DURING EXERCISE IN NORMAL SUBJECTS AND IN PATIENTS WITH CAD

Effect of Training on Circulation at Rest

It is well known that trained athletes have a lower HR at rest than normal sedentary people and that a reduction in resting HR is fairly constantly observed in response to a period of physical training.[16,20,21,102] The mechanism underlying the sinus bradycardia at rest induced by training has not been clarified. There can be little doubt that training changes the balance between sympathetic and parasympathetic activity in the heart towards greater dominance of the parasympathetic component both in animals and man,[102-105] but whether intra- or extracardiac factors are responsible for this change has not been decided. Several different explanations have been proposed, such as cardiac hypertrophy,[19] increased blood volume,[106] and reduced stimulation from peripheral receptors,[69] but these have not been substantiated by conclusive evidence. In a group of healthy young subjects, we found that the reduction in resting HR obtained by training of the leg muscles is significantly greater than that seen after training of the arm muscles.[21] This finding suggests that some factors related to the total muscle mass engaged in the training or the absolute $\dot{V}O_2$, $\dot{Q}$, or SV attained during the training sessions are important in producing the bradycardia at rest.

In cardiac patients, the fall in resting HR is usually less pronounced than in younger subjects.[2,3,13,97,107,108] Only Detry et al.[6] report a fall in resting HR in patients with CAD, which, in beats/min, corresponds to that seen in healthy young subjects.

Apart from the bradycardia, training causes no consistent circulatory changes at rest. Resting $\dot{Q}$ in normal subjects as well as in patients with CAD has been found to decrease[20,21,109] or to show only small and statistically insignificant changes after training.[2,3,76,107,108,110] Peripheral circulatory parameters at rest have only been assessed in few studies. In patients with CAD, SBF was unchanged after a training period,[3] and so was indocyanine green (ICG) clearance rate in healthy young subjects[21]; $AVDO_2$ from the arms and legs at rest increased in two studies performed on healthy young subjects. In both studies, $\dot{Q}$ was lower at rest after training.[20,21]

Effect of Training on Circulation During Submaximal Exercise

Central Circulation

Training causes a decrease in HR attended by an increase in SV during submaximal exercise. If only $\dot{Q}$, HR, and $\dot{V}O_2$ are measured during one type of exercise, this may be the only appreciable circulatory effect training produces in healthy young subjects at a given submaximal $\dot{V}O_2$.[20,21,110,111] In only one study among those in which $\dot{Q}$ was measured with dye-dilution or direct Fick technique, training caused a significant decrease in $\dot{Q}/\dot{V}O_2$.[112] In consequence, it has been assumed by many investigators that the reduction in HR is secondary to the larger SV, which in turn is attributed to myocardial hypertrophy[19] or an increase in blood volume.[106]

However, an increase in SV is not a prerequisite for the fall in HR induced by training. Investigations performed in patients with CAD have clearly demonstrated that the reduction in HR at submaximal $\dot{V}O_2$ can occur without concomitant augmentation of SV.[3,6,13,109] The general validity of an explanation for the HR deceleration at submaximal work based exclusively on central circulatory adaptations was contested by Müller[113] as far back as 1943. In an 18-year-old male subject who performed two subsequent training periods, the first with leg muscles and the second with arm muscles, Müller observed that the decrease in HR obtained by training of the arms did not carry over to leg exercise. Thus, he concluded that the fall in HR at a given $\dot{V}O_2$ was caused by adaptations in the trained muscles rather than by a direct effect on the heart. This observation has not received appropriate attention.

We have recently performed a series of studies on healthy young subjects in which the circulatory response to arm and leg exercise was assessed after a period of training of either the arms or the legs.[21,114] The change in HR after arm training was essentially in agreement with Müller's conclusions. As shown in Fig. 7 and in Fig. 8A and B, arm training causes a very marked reduction in HR during exercise with trained arm muscles. This reduction is most pronounced at the heaviest of two submaximal loads. During exercise with the nontrained leg muscles, a much less pronounced decrease in HR is seen, a deceleration, which in beats/min corresponds to that seen at rest. If only the increase in HR in excess of the resting value (ΔHR) is considered, no training effect whatsoever occurs during exercise with nontrained muscles. These findings could be taken to indicate that two different components contribute to the training bradycardia: one that is present both at rest and during exercise and another that is confined to exercise performed with the trained muscles. While the former could be caused by cardiac as well as extracardiac changes, the latter somehow appears to be related to adaptations in the trained muscles.

The HR response to leg training is, in a qualitative sense, the same as that seen after arm training. However, after this type of training, the decrease in HR at rest and during exercise with nontrained

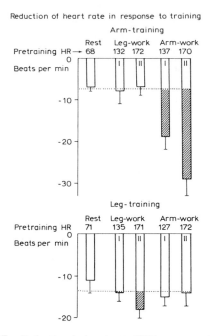

Reduction of heart rate in response to training

Fig. 7. Reduction in heart rate (HR) at rest and during submaximal leg work and arm work after arm training (above) and leg training (below). Values are from 13 healthy young subjects (Clausen et al.[21]). Hatched areas indicate the fall in HR in excess of the reduction at rest and during exercise with nontrained extremities. Pretraining absolute values for HR are shown above each column (figure from Clausen,[195] with permission).

muscles (i.e., the arms) is much more pronounced, and the difference in HR reduction between work with trained and nontrained muscles is smaller. A significant pre- to posttraining change in ΔHR is only seen during heavy exercise with trained legs (Fig. 7). Furthermore this is only valid for HR counted between the sixth and seventh minute of exercise corresponding to the time for the determination of $\dot{Q}$ in this study. At the end of the 15 min of exercise, the reduction in HR during exercise with nontrained arm muscles is equal to or greater than that seen during exercise with trained leg muscles (Fig. 8B). Also, after leg training, the reduction in HR during exercise with trained muscles is most pronounced at the heaviest of the two submaximal loads (Fig. 7).

The finding that the reduction in HR during exercise with trained muscles becomes more pronounced the higher the work load, while the opposite is seen during exercise with nontrained muscles may have implications as to the mechanism behind the HR deceleration in the two different situations. Experiments involving selective blockade of the parasympathetic and sympathetic stimulation of

the heart by atropine and/or beta-receptor blocking agents have shown that both withdrawal of the vagal tonus on the sinus node and increased sympathetic stimulation participate in accelerating HR during exercise and that the relative contribution of these two mechanisms depends on the relative work load.[115,116] At moderate work loads, i.e., up to about 50% of $\dot{V}O_{2max}$, the increase in HR is mediated predominantly by withdrawal of the parasympathetic activity; above this level, increased sympathetic stimulation becomes progressively more important. This relationship between the relative $\dot{V}O_2$ and the relative contribution of vagal withdrawal and sympathetic stimulation to HR acceleration is not affected by leg training as far as leg exercise is concerned.[102]

After arm training, the pre- to posttraining difference in HR during arm exercise is most pronounced at the heaviest of two submaximal loads (Figs. 7 and 8A)—an effect on HR which could have been obtained by a large dose of a beta-blocking drug. In contrast, when calculated as paired observations, the post- to pretraining HR difference during exercise with nontrained legs is most pronounced at the lowest of two submaximal loads (Fig. 8A), and this difference, together with the fall in resting HR, could be abolished by a fairly small dose of atropine. Using the same analogy for leg training, the dose of atropine needed to raise HR at rest and during arm work to the pretraining levels should have been greater. On the other hand, the dose of beta-receptor blocker sufficient to accomplish the decrease seen during submaximal leg exercise would have been smaller. In other words, it might be suggested that the fall in HR at rest and during exercise with nontrained muscles is caused predominantly by increased vagal tone on the heart, while the reduction in HR during exercise with trained muscles results, to a greater extent, from a decrease in sympathetic drive.

By which mechanisms does training change the autonomic stimulation of the heart during exercise? As stated above, part of the HR reduction is related to changes in the trained muscles. Possible explanations for this effect are discussed below. However, the reduction in HR during exercise with nontrained muscles may depend on different mechanisms, which at the same time may account for the training bradycardia at rest. The two most often cited hypotheses relate the training bradycardia to augmentation of blood volume and of heart

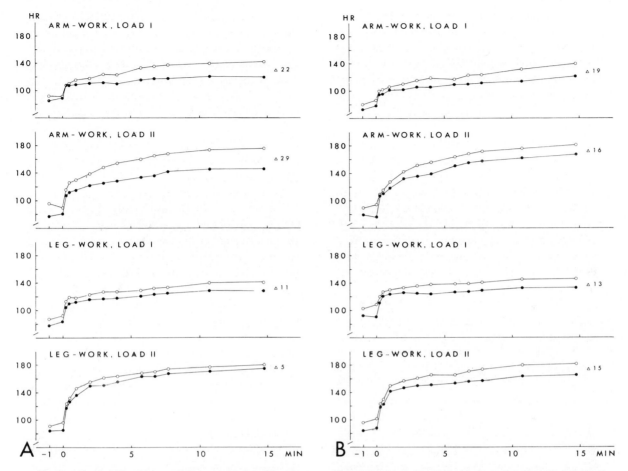

Fig. 8. (A and B) Heart rate (HR) measured at short intervals from continuous ECG recordings during 15-min periods of submaximal arm work and leg work before (unfilled circles) and after (filled circles) arm training (N = 5) (Fig. 8A) and leg training (N = 5) (Fig. 8B) Pre- to posttraining differences in beats/min at the fifteenth minute of exercise are shown after each pair of curves (based on data from Clausen et al.[21]).

volume, respectively. Heart rate at rest has been shown to vary in parallel with changes in blood volume,[106] and a decrease in HR during submaximal leg exercise has been observed with acute expansion of blood volume by transfusions.[117–119] However, it is still not definitively proven that the 6%–10% increase in blood volume seen after training[106,120] directly influences HR during exercise. The significance of variations in anatomic dimensions of the heart as they relate to changes in HR is also unsettled. Endurance athletes have greater heart volumes and lower HR than nontrained people.[16] However, training programs do not consistently increase heart volume[121]; further, the heart volume as assessed by x-ray is partly related to the level of sympathetic stimulation of the heart.[122] Variations in myocardial functional properties may finally be considered. As will be dis-

cussed subsequently, training probably increases intrinsic myocardial contractility. It seems reasonable to assume that an increased contractile force may elicit baroreceptor or "cardiac-cardiac" reflexes tending to decelerate HR. However, experimental evidence that such mechanisms contribute to the training bradycardia has not been provided.

$\dot{Q}/\dot{V}O_2$ is essentially unchanged during exercise with trained muscles, after both arm and leg training and during exercise with nontrained legs.[21] However, during heavy exercise with nontrained arms, $\dot{Q}$ and arterial MBP are significantly increased by almost 2 l/min and 12 mm Hg. As HR decreases, at the same time, an impressive augmentation in SV is observed (+20 ml = 22%).[21] Thus in this peculiar situation (arm work after leg training), the heart produces an increased $\dot{Q}$ against an increased afterload. Since we have no reason to believe that the sympathetic stimulation of the heart is increased during exercise with the nontrained muscles, this may indicate an enhanced intrinsic contractility of myocardial fibers induced by training. This assumption is consonant with the finding that training increases myocardial contractility in animals, presumably due to an increased ATPase activity.[123]

The reason why $\dot{Q}$ and MBP do not show a similar increase in response to training during submaximal exercise with trained muscles is probably that the intrinsic potentiality for enhanced myocardial contractility is offset by reduced extrinsic sympathetic stimulation of the heart and reduced peripheral resistance (see below). According to Wink and Roskamm,[64] top-trained athletes have reduced dP/dt/P values in comparison with untrained persons at all relative work loads.

In the majority of patients with CAD in whom $\dot{Q}$ has been measured during submaximal exercise in the upright position before and after training, $\dot{Q}/\dot{V}O_2$ decreased—the change in $\dot{Q}$ ranging from 10% to 14%.[3,6,13,109] In two groups no significant change in $\dot{Q}/\dot{V}O_2$ occurred.[2,4] Accordingly, changes in SV during submaximal exercise varying from an increase of 18% to a decrease of 6% have been seen in patients with CAD. Whether a change of $\dot{Q}/\dot{V}O_2$ occurs in patients with CAD or not seems not to depend on initial $\dot{Q}/\dot{V}O_2$ values. Decreased $\dot{Q}/\dot{V}O_2$ after training has been observed in groups of patients with CAD with average hypokinetic,[13] normokinetic,[6] and hyperkinetic circulation.[3]

During exercise with trained arm muscles, healthy young subjects have lower arterial blood pressures after training,[21] whereas these pressures after leg training remain essentially unchanged during leg exercise.[20,21,112] In contrast after training healthy, middle-aged subjects, patients with essential hypertension as well as patients with CAD often show a relative decrease in MBP at a given $\dot{V}O_2$ of about 10%.[2-4,6,10,11,76,110,124,125]

Regional Blood Flow

Nonworking tissues. From the finding that the reduction in blood flow to abdominal viscera (SBF and RBF) is closely related to relative $\dot{V}O_2$ and varies in proportion to HR during submaximal exercise,[21,22,50,51] it could be anticipated that the reduction in these flows should be less pronounced at a given $\dot{V}O_2$ following training; i.e., with in-

creases in $\dot{V}O_{2max}$, the same submaximal $\dot{V}O_2$ constitutes a reduced relative $\dot{V}O_2$ after training. In agreement hereto, we have observed that SBF at a given submaximal $\dot{V}O_2$ is less reduced after a period of physical conditioning in normal young subjects[21] as well as in patients with CAD.[3] The change in SBF expressed as a percentage of the resting value (SBF%) is proportional to the decrease in HR, and thus the close relationship between SBF% and HR is not influenced by training (Figs. 3 and 5). This applies to leg training as well as to arm training (Fig. 3).

However, like ΔHR, SBF% only changes during exercise performed with trained muscles (Fig. 9). By further analogy to the changes in HR, the relative increase in SBF is greater during exercise with trained arm muscles than during exercise with trained leg muscles, and, for the respective types of exercise, more pronounced at the heaviest of two submaximal work loads (Fig. 9). The reduction in HR during exercise with nontrained muscles that is not attended by any significant change in SBF% causes a slight parallel displacement of the SBF%/HR relation. The change in intercept is too small, however, in comparison with the dispersion of the SBF% values to be of statistical significance (Fig. 3).

The effect of training on other regional blood flows has not been systematically studied. Data on $AVDO_2$ over nonworking extremities during submaximal exercise suggest a relatively increased perfusion to these regions also.[21] This change is, with one exception, confined to exercise with trained muscles groups. The exception concerns heavy submaximal exercise with nontrained arms where decreases of 10% are seen in $AVDO_2$ over the resting legs. However, since MBP increases by 12% in this situation, the degree of vasoconstriction in the nonexercising legs is practically unchanged.[21]

Muscle blood flow. Figure 10 depicts an estimation of the changes in $\dot{Q}$ and its distribution between nonworking tissues and active muscles in a normal young person exercising at different work intensities before and after training. $\dot{Q}_{max}$ and $\dot{V}O_{2max}$ are increased after training, but at submaximal levels, $\dot{Q}$ is unchanged. After training, the flow to nonworking tissues is relatively increased at a given submaximal $\dot{V}O_2$, whereas these flows are unaltered at rest and at maximal work. It can be inferred that the increase of $\dot{Q}$ at work levels

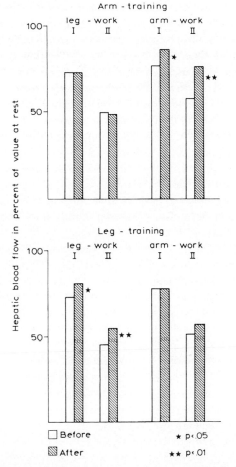

Fig. 9. Splanchnic-hepatic blood flow (ICG-clearance) in per cent of the value at rest during leg work and arm work before and after training of the arms (N = 5) (upper panel) and the legs (N = 5) (lower panel). Significant pre- to posttraining differences were only seen during exercise with trained muscle groups (data from Clausen et al.[21]; figure from Clausen,[196] with permission).

exceeding the pretraining maximum is directed to the exercising muscles. In contrast, at submaximal levels where the flow to nonworking tissues is increased as compared to the pretrained state, a smaller fraction of the unchanged $\dot{Q}$ appears to be available for exercising muscles.

In young subjects, the absolute change in flow to nonexercising tissues is too small in comparison to the accuracy of $\dot{Q}$ determinations to allow the conclusion that total MBF is decreased at a given $\dot{V}O_2$ after training. In contrast, total MBF must be reduced in the patients with CAD who, after training, showed significant reductions in $\dot{Q}$ of 10%–14%[3,6,13,109] with concomitant relative increase in SBF.[3] In a group of patients with CAD in whom

both $\dot{Q}$ and SBF were measured, training reduced $\dot{Q}$ during moderate submaximal exercise by 1.7 l/min.[3] The pre- to posttraining increase in SBF was modest (7%; Fig. 5), and thus the total increase in flow to nonworking tissues hardly exceeded 150–200 ml. This implies a total decrease in MBF of about 1.9 l/min at this work load.

Various experimental findings directly relating MBF during exercise to training support the assumption that in normal subjects as well as in patients with CAD, trained muscles extract more oxygen from the blood and thus provide the same submaximal $\dot{V}O_2$ with a reduced MBF.

Measurements of MBF per unit weight of tissue by the local ^{133}Xe-clearance method have repeatedly shown that after training, the clearance rate from the exercising vastus lateralis muscle is reduced at the same work load performed on bicycle ergometer in patients with CAD as well as in normal young and middle-aged subjects.[2,3,40,126,127]

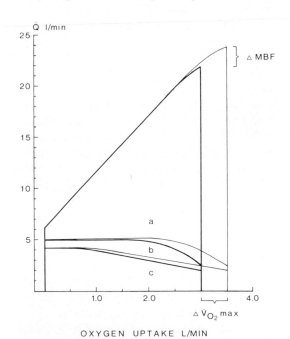

Fig. 10. Cardiac output ($\dot{Q}$) and its distribution on exercising muscles (a), skin (b), and remaining nonexercising tissues (c) in relation to oxygen uptake ($\dot{V}O_2$) during submaximal and maximal leg exercise (bicycling). Heavy lines indicate values before leg training, and thin lines indicate values after leg training. Flow in nonexercising tissues at rest, during maximal exercise, and at any relative $\dot{V}O_2$ is the same before and after training. Increases in total muscle blood flow ($\triangle$MBF) and in maximal oxygen uptake ($\triangle\dot{V}O_{2max}$) are shown (estimates based on values from Clausen et al.,[21] Rowell,[22] and Wade and Bishop[25]).

This finding is in keeping with the concept that MBF per unit weight of tissue is a function of the relative work load.[36,39,40] However, a decreased MBF per unit weight of tissue does not necessarily imply reduced total MBF, but may also conform to a distribution of unchanged flow to a greater muscle mass. Moreover, it cannot be excluded that training changes the lipid content of muscle tissue in a manner that could reduce the clearance rate of a lipophilic tracer.[128,129]

Further indications of reduced MBF following training come from measurements of the flow in the calf or in the forearm by plethysmographic techniques performed immediately after exercise. Such studies have consistently demonstrated reduced values after a given submaximal work load in response to training.[130-132] This is likely to result from a reduced blood flow also during exercise because postexercise hyperemia is proportional to, albeit not identical with, the flow during submaximal exercise.[133,134]

That trained muscles have increased O_2 extraction during submaximal work is further supported by the fact that $AVDO_2$ over the working trained extremity is increased.[20,21] The increased $AVDO_2$ is confined to the extremity used for the training work[21] and may thus be attributed to local adaptations. The widening of $AVDO_2$ is especially pronounced after arm training, as it was in the case for other changes confined to exercise with trained muscles.[21] Hypothetically, the increased $AVDO_2$ could result from decreased perfusion of other tissue components in the extremity, but this seems unlikely, since $AVDO_2$ in the nonworking extremities is smaller, suggesting an increased flow to these tissues.[21]

Speculations on the Mechanisms Behind Adaptations Confined to Exercise With Trained Muscles

According to the above, training changes the different local flows during exercise in such a way that, within the framework of an unchanged or reduced $\dot{Q}$, its regional distribution at a given submaximal work load deviates less from that seen at rest: the perfusion of nonworking tissues is relatively greater and the flow to active muscles less elevated. However, this is only valid for exercise performed with trained muscles.

Changes in several noncirculatory parameters are also confined to exercise performed with trained muscle groups. A reduced ventilatory equivalent ($\dot{V}E/\dot{V}O_2$) is only seen during exercise with trained muscles, and moreover, is more marked after arm training than after leg training.[135] The same is true for an increased mechanical efficiency, for a reduction of the respiratory quotient (RQ), for a decrease of the blood lactate concentration and of the lactate release from the exercising extremity,[136] as well as for a less pronounced acute expansion of upper arm volume after arm exercise[21] (Table 1). The fact that all these changes do not carry over to exercise performed with nontrained muscles suggests that they in one way or another depend on local adaptations in the trained muscles.

What kind of local adaptations in skeletal muscles could produce such effects? Within the last 6-8 yr, it has been shown in animals as well as in man that endurance training causes a marked augmentation in the number and/or size of muscle cell mitochondria, with a concomitant increase in the concentration and activity of the enzymes involved in aerobic metabolism.[34, Holloszy pp 445-458, this issue]. Although the precise mechanism mediating exercise hyperemia is unknown, it seems acceptable that enhanced content of oxidative enzymes enables a reduction in MBF at a given submaximal $\dot{V}O_2$. After training, due to the increased capacity for oxidative phosphorylation, ATP and CP in active muscles stabilize at a higher steady-state level.[41] At the same time glycolysis occurs at a slower rate, pH is relatively increased, and the concentration of multiple intermediate metabolic products may be lower.[34] In consequence, the intra- and intercellular biochemical milieu—concentrations of electrolytes and osmolality included—is less disturbed as compared to the conditions at rest. Whatever substance or combinations of chemical alterations cause the vasodilation, their extent of change is probably reduced at a given respiratory rate in trained muscle tissue, and the vasodilation is thus diminished. According to Holloszy,[34] the oxidative enzymatic alterations in trained muscles also yield a plausible explanation for a decreased lactate production and RQ at submaximal work loads.

It is tempting to hold the enzymatic adaptations in skeletal muscle responsible also for the changes, confined to exercise with trained muscles, in neurogenically controlled circulatory and respiratory parameters, but it must be emphasized that such a postulate is highly speculative. Although

Table 1. Systemic Effects of Training and Effects that are Confined to Exercise With Trained Muscles*

Systemic Effects	Effects Confined to Exercise With Trained Muscles
Reduction in HR at rest and during submaximal exercise with nontrained muscles	Reduction of ΔHR during submaximal exercise
Increase in $\dot{Q}$ and BP. Only seen during heavy submaximal exercise with nontrained arms after leg training	Reduction of sympathetic vasoconstriction in nonexercising tissues during submaximal exercise
Decrease in blood hemoglobin concentration	Reduction in MBF during submaximal exercise and concomitant increase of regional and/or systemic $AVDO_2$
Displacement to the right of O_2 hemoglobin dissociation curve	Reduction in $\dot{Q}/\dot{V}O_2$ during submaximal exercise. Most often seen in patients with CAD
Increase in $\dot{V}O_{2\,max}$ attended by an increase in MBP_{max}	Reduction in BP during submaximal exercise
	Decrease in $\Delta\dot{V}E/\Delta\dot{V}O_2$ during submaximal exercise
	Increase in mechanical efficiency
	Decrease in blood lactate content and lactate release from exercising extremity during submaximal exercise
	Decrease in RQ during submaximal exercise
	Increase of pH and decrease of pCO_2 in venous blood from exercising extremity
	Decrease in acute postexercise expansion of upper arm volume
	Increase in $\dot{V}O_{2\,max}$ caused by increased O_2 extraction or decrease in TPR

*Based on data from Clausen et al.,[21] Rasmussen et al.,[135] and Klausen et al.[136]

the increases in HR, peripheral vasoconstriction, and $\dot{V}E$ during exercise are the most dramatic manifestations of cardiovascular and respiratory reflexes* existing, it is still not established how they are brought about.

There are two main theories concerning the point of origin of the nervous stimulation of the cardiovascular and respiratory system during exercise. According to the first, it depends on "cortical irradiation";[138] i.e., collateral information to cardiovascular centers concomitant with the impulse traffic in descending motor tracts to active muscles. According to the second, afferent nervous impulses elicited from receptors in skeletal muscle stimulate the cardiovascular system.[23]

A cardiovascular reflex pattern similar to that seen during exercise, including HR increase, peripheral vasoconstriction, and increased ventilation can be provoked by stimulation of cortico-hypothalamic centers.[49,139] Experiments performed in man support the idea that at least part of the increase in HR, $\dot{V}E$, and BP caused by isometric muscle contractions can be attributed to a "central command."[140,141]

However, a similar cardiovascular reflex pattern can also be mediated by afferent nervous impulses originating in contracting muscles. Animal experiments have demonstrated that these impulses are conducted in nerve fibers connected to receptors sensitive to metabolic alterations.[69,142–145] None of these investigations, however, were conducted in such a way as to make the results directly applicable to the situation in spontaneous dynamic exercise. On the other hand, studies performed in man suggest that afferent nervous information plays an important role for the adjustment of HR, BP, and $\dot{V}E$ to metabolic intensity during dynamic exercise.[72,146,147] In addition, as shown in Fig. 11, both during arm and leg exercise, $\Delta\dot{V}E$ has a similar relationship to ΔHR as the percentage reduction in SBF before and after arm and leg training.[21,135] This indicates that the activation mechanisms of these three parameters have common features and are susceptible to influences from local adaptations in trained muscles.

These findings do not determine if the changes in ΔHR, SBF%, and $\Delta\dot{V}E$ after training are due to reduced need for "central command" because enzymatic adaptations have improved the muscles' performance in rhythmic exercise, or whether the cardiorespiratory alterations in the trained state

---

*It would seem superfluous today to repeat arguments that these adjustments depend on nervous mechanisms.[137]

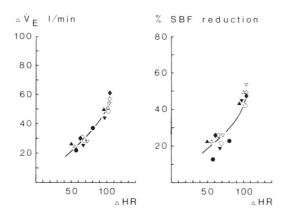

Fig. 11. Increase in pulmonary ventilation in excess of the resting value (ΔVE) (left panel) and reduction in splanchnic-hepatic blood flow in per cent of the resting value (% SBF) (right panel) in relation to the increase in heart rate (ΔHR) during submaximal exercise. Group means are for arm exercise and leg exercise before and after training of either the arms or the legs. Same symbols as in Fig. 3. Lines through symbols are fitted by eye (based on data from Clausen et al.[21] and Rasmussen et al.[135]).

result from reduced afferent impulse traffic from exercising muscles because diminished disturbance of metabolic balance means less stimulation of possible metabolic receptors.

A hypothesis including both possibilities could suggest that the "central command" is most important in assuring an instantaneous cardiorespiratory reaction at the onset of exercise.[139] Later on, the precise cardiorespiratory adjustment may depend on a feedback mechanism involving afferent nervous information about how the actual respiratory rate in contracting muscles compares to their maximal capacity for oxidative phosphorylation.

The Relative Contribution of Central and Peripheral Effects of Training to Changes in Circulatory Regulation During Submaximal Exercise

Normal Subjects

Comparison of responses to exercise with trained and nontrained muscles shows that when exercise is performed with trained muscles, the changes in circulatory regulation result from interaction between systemic circulatory changes and alterations due to local adaptations in the muscles.[21] Table 1 summarizes circulatory, respiratory, and metabolic changes induced by training that are known to belong to one of the two categories.

Local changes are most conspicuous after arm training, whereas systemic alterations are more pronounced after leg training.[21] One interpretation of this finding is that systemic changes involving central circulatory parameters occur in proportion to the muscle mass used during the training and that local changes are most likely to occur when the muscles involved are unaccustomed to heavy dynamic exercise. However, there is also the possibility that the peculiar circulatory regulation inherent to arm exercise discloses both types of training effects most clearly. Further, it could be suggested that the very pronounced circulatory and respiratory changes seen during exercise with trained arm muscles may reflect that the subjects had *learned* to exercise more economically and to minimize the "wasteful" isometric component of arm exercise. The mechanical efficiency did increase in both groups for exercise with trained muscles and most of all after arm-training (7.5% versus 4.5%), but compared to the changes in HR and SBF%, etc., these differences were relatively small.[21] Moreover, marked decreases in regional lactate release and in postexercise edema in the upper arm testified to the occurrence of considerable local adaptations in the trained arm muscles probably exceeding those in the trained leg muscles.[21,136]

With CAD Patients

In the view of the comparatively small absolute work loads which can be sustained by patients with CAD during training sessions and their presumed decreased cardiac adaptability to training, peripheral training effects could be expected to be relatively more important in these patients than in healthy young subjects. Several findings corroborate this assumption.

The increase in $\dot{Q}$ and blood pressures seen in normal young subjects during heavy arm work after leg training is probably due to improved myocardial performance.[21] Patients with angina pectoris do not increase blood pressures during heavy arm exercise after leg training.[97] The ratio between the reduction in HR at rest and that seen during exercise with trained muscles may reflect the relative contribution of systemic and peripheral changes to the HR reduction. After leg training, this ratio was 0.60–0.80 in normal subjects, [20,21,110] while it was 0.20–0.33 after arm training.[21] In patients with CAD, values of 0.20–

0.33 are most often seen during leg exercise after leg-training,[2,3,5,97] suggesting a relative contribution of peripheral factors similar to that seen after arm training in young subjects. However, it should be mentioned that factors like anxiety may influence HR at rest considerably. Thus, the ratios from other studies of patients with CAD have shown greater variations, ranging from 0.00[13] to 0.73.[6] Furthermore, low ratios may be due to aging rather than to CAD, since they have also been found in training studies involving middle-aged subjects.[76,124]

In contrast, the reduction in $\dot{Q}/\dot{V}O_2$ during submaximal exercise—which can be considered a peripheral training effect—is undoubtly seen more often in patients with CAD than in normal young and middle-aged subjects.

Effect of Training on $\dot{V}O_2$ and Circulation at Maximal Work

Training increases $\dot{V}O_{2max}$ in normal young and middle-aged subjects,[20-22,76,110-112,124,148] as well as in patients with CAD with or without angina pectoris.[4-6,8,11,12] The increase of $\dot{V}O_{2max}$ that is obtained by training depends on the pretraining level, the intensity and duration of training, and the age of the subjects.[20,76,110,148] Percentage increases in sedentary young normal subjects are usually in the range of 10% to 30%.[20-22,110-112,148] However, after a 3 wk period of bed rest, a subsequent 8 wk training period may increase $\dot{V}O_{2max}$ by almost 100%.[20] In normal middle-aged subjects, an average increase of 17%–18% in $\dot{V}O_{2max}$ has been seen.[76,124]

In patients with CAD,[4-6,8,11] $\Delta\dot{V}O_{2max}$ ranging from 16% to 56%* has been reported. The improvement in symptom-limited $\dot{V}O_{2max}$ of 32%–56% seen in patients with angina pectoris[5,6,11] exceeds the increase in "real" $\dot{V}O_{2max}$ of 16% seen in patients with CAD without angina.[5,6] However, due to the very low initial values normally found in patients with CAD, the absolute $\dot{V}O_{2max}$ in these patients is modest after training as compared to healthy subjects in the same age group.

---

*The rather great variations in $\dot{V}O_{2max}$ increase among the different studies may partly reflect that not all patients are equally "trainable," but difficulties inherent to the determination of $\dot{V}O_{2max}$ in such patients do certainly play a role.

Mechanisms by Which $\dot{V}O_{2max}$ is Increased

In the absence of lung disease, it is generally agreed that respiration imposes no limitation on $\dot{V}O_{2max}$,[149] and interest can focus on circulation. In terms of the Fick equation, $\dot{V}O_{2max}$ can thus be expressed as:

$$\dot{V}O_{2max} = HR_{max} \times SV_{max} \times AVDO_{2max}$$

Increased $\dot{V}O_{2max}$ after training can be attended by an increase in any of the factors on the right side of the equation. However, an increased HR_{max} is only seen in patients with angina pectoris who have a symptom-limited $\dot{V}O_{2max}$. In other patients with CAD and in normal subjects in whom a real $\dot{V}O_{2max}$ can be obtained, HR_{max} is unchanged or reduced after training.[20]

Increased Oxygen Transport

Apparently the perfusion of nonexercising tissues at maximum exercise is not altered by training,[21,22] and in consequence, as illustrated in Fig. 10, the increase in $\dot{Q}_{max}$ is directed to the exercising muscles. In principle, an increase in MBF_{max} can be obtained in two ways: either by an increased driving pressure or by a decreased resistance in the muscle. Both alternatives have been observed.

At least in one specific situation—namely, maximal work with nontrained arms after leg training—a primary increase in BP seems to be solely responsible for the enhancement of MBF_{max} and $\dot{V}O_{2max}$.[21] The experimental data supporting this conclusion are summarized in Fig. 12. Leg training augmented $\dot{V}O_{2max}$ during arm work by 10%. (The corresponding increase for leg work was 17%.) During maximal arm exercise, $AVDO_2$ in exercising arms as well as in nonexercising legs was unchanged compared to the pretraining value. This can be taken to indicate that blood flow to nonworking tissues was unchanged and that an increased oxygen supply to the active muscles occurred without concomitant augmentation of local oxygen extraction. Such change was not expected in the nontrained arms, since it is believed to depend on local enzymatic adaptations. Regrettably, $\dot{Q}_{max}$ and BP_{max} were not measured in this study. However, during strenuous submaximal exercise, both $\dot{Q}$ and MBP were increased by 18% and 10%, respectively. It does not seem unreasonable to assume that an increase in these

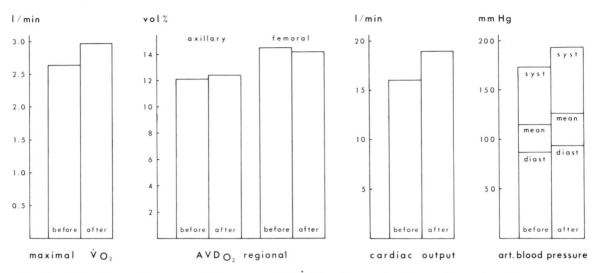

Fig. 12. Effect of leg training on maximal oxygen uptake ($\dot{V}O_2$) and maximal axillary and femoral arteriovenous oxygen differences (AVDO$_2$) during maximal arm exercise, and on cardiac output and aortic pressures during heavy submaximal arm exercise. Mean values are from three healthy young male subjects (Clausen et al.[21]). After training during exercise with nontrained arms, VO$_{2max}$ increased, whereas AVDO$_{2max}$ was unchanged both in exercising arms and resting legs. Cardiac output and aortic pressures were increased during heavy submaximal exercise.

two parameters also occurred during maximal arm exercise, which increase could account for the 10% increase in $\dot{V}O_{2max}$. If so, two conclusions can be drawn: (1) increased driving pressure can increase MBF$_{max}$ and $\dot{V}O_{2max}$; (2) local metabolic capacity in muscle does not limit $\dot{V}O_{2max}$.

Possible explanations for the increase in $\dot{Q}$ and MBP during heavy submaximal arm exercise after leg training were discussed above, and improved myocardial pump function was proposed. The above finding does not imply that an increased $\dot{Q}_{max}$ after training always results from increased contractility or otherwise improved myocardial performance. The most common way to increase $\dot{Q}_{max}$ in response to training seems to be reducing total peripheral resistance (TPR) rather than augmenting MBP. After leg training during leg exercise requiring $\dot{V}O_{2max}$, MBP$_{max}$ is normally unchanged as compared to the pretraining value.[20,76,110] Thus, the increase in $\dot{Q}_{max}$ can be related to a reduction in TPR. In one study only, MBP$_{max}$ was increased in response to training and $\dot{V}O_{2max}$ was increased without change in TPR.[112] In this study, after training, several subjects had unchanged $\dot{Q}_{max}$ concomitant with increased MBP.

That this is an unusual finding is apparent from Fig. 13, which demonstrates, $\dot{V}O_{2max}$ to be an inverse function of minimum TPR and that

changes in $\dot{V}O_{2max}$, whether they are increases caused by training[20,76,79,110,150] or decreases caused by bed rest,[20] are associated with an inversely directed change in TPR. This is also true when different types of exercise that produce different values for $\dot{V}O_{2max}$ in the same subject are examined. From data available in the literature, it can be calculated that the higher $\dot{V}O_{2max}$ values measured during leg exercise compared to arm exercise,[46] during running compared to bicycling,[42] and during bicycling in the upright position compared to bicycling in the supine position[46] are attended by a proportional difference in TPR (Fig. 13). A reduction in $\dot{V}O_{2max}$ seen in one study after beta-receptor blockade could be related to an increase in TPR$_{max}$ so that the hyperbolic $\dot{V}O_{2max}$/TPR relation is maintained.[151] In another study involving beta-receptor blockade, both $\dot{V}O_{2max}$ and TPR were unaffected[102] (Fig. 13).

Variation in TPR thus seems to be a primary factor in the main part of the change in $\dot{V}O_{2max}$. Top-trained athletes are characterized by an extreme ability to reduce resistance to flow. They produce $\dot{Q}_{max}$ values of an average 36 l/min with MBP$_{max}$ values of 116 mm Hg.[18] In this upper left part of the curve relating $\dot{V}O_{2max}$ to TPR, only minor variations in TPR correspond to rather large changes in $\dot{V}O_{2max}$.

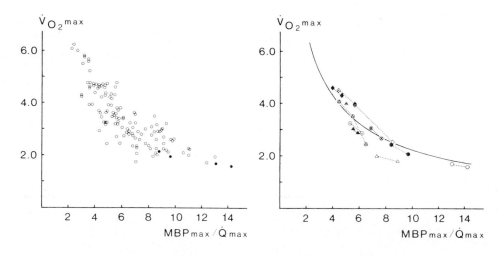

TOTAL PERIPHERAL RESISTANCE AT $V_{O_2}max$

Fig. 13. Maximal oxygen consumption ($\dot{V}_{O_2max}$) in relation to total peripheral resistance ($MBP_{max}/\dot{Q}_{max}$). Based on values on $\dot{V}_{O_2max}$, $\dot{Q}_{max}$, and MBP_{max} from the literature. Left-sided panel gives individual values (○) and, from one study,[110] group mean values (●) for top-trained young athletes,[18] well trained middle-aged athletes,[90] young and middle-aged healthy men and women,[42,46,76,110] and from patients with CAD[79] and essential hypertension[91] during maximal exercise on bicycle ergometer or treadmill and also for healthy young subjects during maximal arm cranking.[46] Top-trained athletes with highest $\dot{V}_{O_2}$ have lowest TPR values. In contrast, patients with CAD and middle-aged subjects with low $\dot{V}_{O_2max}$ have very high TPR values.

Right-sided panel gives group mean values from studies where variations of $\dot{V}_{O_2max}$ were induced by training or bed rest (circles), by beta-receptor blockade (triangles), or different types of exercise (rectangles). Read from right to left, symbols indicate ○......○ middle-aged women before and after training,[110] ●——● nontrained and trained patients with CAD,[79] ⊗——⊗ middle-aged healthy men before and after training,[76] (⊙ ------ ⊙) healthy young subjects exercising with one leg before and after training of the same leg,[150] ⊛------ ⊛ ------ ⊛ healthy young subjects after and before bed rest and after training,[20] ▲ ------ ▲ healthy subjects and △ ------ △ cardiac patients with and without beta-receptor blockade,[151] △ unchanged values with and without beta-receptor blockade,[116] ◇ ------ ◇ arm cranking and bicycling in healthy young subjects[46] ◇ ------ ◇ supine and upright bicycling in healthy young subjects,[46] and ◆ ------ ◆ bicycling and treadmill running in healthy young subjects.[42] Any intervention that changed $\dot{V}_{O_2max}$ in these groups also grossly changed TPR in accordance with the regression line $y = 11.8/x^{0.72}$, $r = 0.87$, $P < 0.001$ (full line) calculated from the 125 individual values shown on the left panel.

In contrast, middle-aged women located in the lower right part of the $\dot{V}_{O_2max}$/TPR curve provide a $\dot{Q}_{max}$ of only 11.5 l/min by a MBP of 164 mm Hg,[110] with a TPR 4.5 times greater than that of top-trained athletes. Moreover, due to the flatter slope of this part of the curve, much larger decreases in TPR are required to obtain only a moderate increase in $\dot{V}_{O_2max}$.

The above assumption that the increase in $\dot{Q}_{max}$ following training results from a decrease in TPR implies that the augmentation of SV is a secondary event, due to the fact that $\dot{Q}$ is greater at any HR after training. Since maximal vasoconstriction in nonworking tissues is probably the same during different types of exercise and is not influenced by training,[21,22] the variations in TPR responsible for the difference in $\dot{Q}_{max}$ induced by different types of work and training must be located in exercising muscles. While it is evident that exercise performed with a larger muscle mass can be at-

tended by a lower TPR as compared to exercise performed with relatively small muscle groups, no definite explanation can be given for the reduced resistance in maximally exercising trained muscles. Tentative interpretations may involve greater vasodilation or effective cross-sectional area of the vascular bed, because enzymatic adaptations allow more muscle fibers to participate in maximal dynamic exercise. A more efficient skeletal muscle pump may also contribute. Whether training increases the muscle capillary density in man is still an open question. Longitudinal training studies on normal young subjects[20] as well as comparisons of well trained athletes and untrained subjects suggest that this is not the case.[152]

Increased Oxygen Extraction

Approximately 50% of the increase in $\dot{V}_{O_2max}$ obtained by training in healthy sedentary young subjects is due to increased systemic $AVDO_{2max}$.

[20,111,112] Both after arm training[21] and leg training,[20] this change in systemic O_2 extraction can be explained by increased $AVDO_{2max}$ in exercising trained extremities, whereas $AVDO_2$ in resting extremities during maximal work is essentially unaffected by training[21] and so is probably $AVDO_2$ from abdominal viscera.

The main reason why trained muscles extract more oxygen from blood and are able to function at a lower pO_2 probably relates to the observed mitochondrial and enzymatic adaptations,[34] although this is not proven. Additive factors may be increased myoglobin content[153] and displacement to the right of the O_2-Hb dissociation curve.[135,] Holloszy pp 445–458, this issue.

Relative Contribution of Increased Oxygen Supply and Increased Oxygen Extraction to $\Delta \dot{V}O_{2max}$

From the above evidence, it seems well established that muscle tissue is able to increase its maximal respiratory rate by virtue of increased delivery of oxygen and by increasing its metabolic capacity. A certain content or activity of Krebs-cycle and respiratory chain enzymes enables a certain maximal local $\dot{V}O_2$ for a given minimal O_2 tension. An increased oxygen supply seemingly allows the same amount of mitochondria to produce a higher respiratory rate and ATP synthesis rate. Our findings of increased $\dot{V}O_{2max}$ during arm exercise after leg training[21] and experiments involving increased pO_2 in inspired air to elevate oxygen content in arterial blood confirm this.[154] An increased amount of mitochondria can, within certain limits, augment local $\dot{V}O_{2max}$ at a given maximal oxygen supply and increase respiratory rate even further if oxygen supply is increased at the same time.

In some patients with CAD, an increase in $\dot{V}O_{2max}$ seems to be achieved exclusively by an increase in $AVDO_2$ without concomitant increase in $\dot{Q}_{max}$.[6] This observation further emphasizes the importance of peripheral adaptations for improved physical performance in patients with CAD. A similar reaction to training has been observed in one group of middle-aged subjects.[124] It may seem surprising that normal middle-aged men[76] and young and middle-aged women[110] have been reported to increase $\dot{V}O_{2max}$ exclusively by augmentation of $\dot{Q}_{max}$. Since peripheral circulatory parameters were not measured in these studies, it cannot be decided whether the unchanged total

$AVDO_{2max}$ reflected failure to increase $AVDO_{2max}$ in the trained leg muscles. This would be an unexpected finding, because normal middle-aged men exhibit oxidative enzymatic adaptations and decrease of ^{133}Xe-clearance rate in trained muscles of the same order of magnitude as observed in healthy young subjects.[127] An explanation will have to await measurements of SBF and/or other regional flows in a longitudinal training study of a similar group.

Well trained athletes have comparatively small $AVDO_{2max}$ and also do not increase systemic $AVDO_{2max}$ with training.[18,20] In addition, they have relatively low hemoglobin concentrations in blood, and it is possible that a low blood viscosity plays a role for the very low TPR and large $\dot{Q}_{max}$ they achieve. Their MBF_{max} seems to be more ample in relation to tissue metabolic capacity than in untrained persons.

Summary

In healthy subjects as well as in patients with CAD, training changes the circulatory adjustment to submaximal exercise and causes an increase in $\dot{V}O_{2max}$. After training at a given submaximal $\dot{V}O_2$, the metabolically controlled vasodilation in active skeletal muscles, as well as the neurogenically controlled increase in HR (ΔHR) and peripheral vasoconstriction are less pronounced. Thus there is a reduction in total MBF and a relative increase in flow to nonexercising tissues occurring with unchanged $\dot{Q}$, or—especially in patients with CAD—with a lower $\dot{Q}$. The decrease in MBF, in ΔHR, and in peripheral vasoconstriction is confined to exercise with trained muscles and is probably mediated by oxidative enzymatic adaptations in skeletal muscle cells. Improved local aerobic metabolic capacity can also explain a reduced lactate release from trained muscles, a lower respiratory quotient (RQ), and a decreased ventilatory equivalent ($\dot{V}E/\dot{V}O_2$) at a given submaximal $\dot{V}O_2$. Systemic training effects can be shown at rest or during exercise with nontrained muscles. They include a reduction in HR and, during heavy exercise with nontrained arms after training of the legs, an increase in $\dot{Q}$ and in MBP that is probably due to improved myocardial performance. $\dot{V}O_{2max}$ is increased by an augmentation of blood supply to exercising muscles and by increased oxygen extraction. The increase in maximal total MBF is usually related to a reduced local vascular resistance, but may also be caused by an increase in driving pressure. The increase in oxygen extraction results presumably from oxidative enzymatic adaptations. In normal young subjects, the relative contribution of systemic and peripheral effects of training to the circulatory changes depends on the pretraining state of the muscles, the training intensity, and the muscle mass engaged in the training. In patients with CAD, peripheral effects always seem most important.

EFFECT OF PHYSICAL TRAINING IN PATIENTS WITH ANGINA PECTORIS

The two last sections of this review will be devoted to the mode of action of training in angina pectoris and its effectiveness in alleviating this symptom as compared to other modes of treatment. In the absence of contraindications, regular physical training can be recommended to most cardiac patients as well as to all healthy people in order to avoid the adverse effects of inactivity on cardiovascular function[20] and to improve subnormal working capacity. However, in the clinic, the use of systematic training programs has a specific indication as a means of alleviating angina pectoris on exertion. It has been documented in several studies that after a period of physical training, there is an increase in the lowest work load needed to provoke angina, an increase in the time to onset of pain on a given work load, and an increase in the highest work load the patient can sustain during a given period of time.[2,3,5,6, 10-12,96,97]

Mode of Action of Training in Angina Pectoris

Although the central and peripheral circulatory adaptations in response to training seen in patients with angina pectoris are qualitatively similar to those seen in other patients with CAD or in normal subjects, the manner in which physical working capacity is improved in patients with angina is fundamentally different. While maximal exercise capacity in subjects not limited by chest pain is augmented by an increased maximal oxygen supply and/or an enhanced extraction in active skeletal muscles, the increased exercise tolerance in patients with exertional angina pectoris is mainly due to a reduced relation between the oxygen consumption of the myocardium and that of the total body during exercise; i.e., less need

of myocardial $\dot{V}O_2$ for the same total body $\dot{V}O_2$. That the effect of training on angina depends on a reduced $M\dot{V}O_2$ at a given intensity of external work is suggested by the finding of reduced values for HR and systolic blood pressure (SBP) during submaximal exercise in patients with CAD after training.[1-4,10,13] However, of more specific interest are studies in which the pain threshold for indices of $M\dot{V}O_2$-RPP, triple product, or tension time index have been assessed during exercise at different work loads before and after training.[11,96,97]

When an exercise test like that shown in Fig. 6 is repeated in a patient with angina pectoris after a few months of physical training, lower values for HR and frequently also for SBP are seen at the respective work loads at any given time. Thus, longer time and/or higher work loads are required to reach the RPP pain threshold value after training. Furthermore, the RPP pain threshold is often increased, adding further to increased exercise tolerance. In some instances, it is not possible to provoke pain after training, since these patients are now limited by fatigue instead of angina pectoris.

When measured at the time of onset of pain in the pretraining exercise test, RPP, triple product, or tension time index at a given work load are reduced by 8%-18% after training.[11,96,97] Although the reduction in RPP or other indices of $M\dot{V}O_2$ have been reported to be attended by a fall in both HR and SBP,[11,96] the reduction in HR is the most constant finding, the SBP change being more variable. Compilation of the data from 90 pair of pre- to posttraining bicycle exercise periods in 25 patients with angina pectoris showed an average decrease in RPP at the time of onset of pain of 10% due to a significant reduction in HR, but with no significant change in SBP.[97] All but two patients had lower HR at all work loads, but SBP was only reduced at all work loads in six patients.

Although practically all patients who are able to accomplish a conditioning program also show a training effect in terms of HR reduction at a given work load, exercise tolerance cannot be improved by training in all patients. In three of the 25 patients investigated by us, the time to onset of pain on a given work load was unchanged or even reduced. All three patients had a training effect on HR at the same work load, but angina was experienced at a lower RPP, suggesting a progression in heart disease during the training period in these three patients.

The fall in HR and blood pressure at the same work load after training, which can be assumed to reduce $M\dot{V}O_2$, is mediated by the same mechanisms as in patients with CAD without angina and in healthy subjects. In the previously mentioned 25 patients with angina pectoris, the ratio between the decrease in HR at rest and the decrease during exercise was, on the average, 0.41, indicating that peripheral factors play a major role in reducing HR in these middle-aged patients. The main part of the training effect in angina pectoris is probably due to local adaptations in the trained muscles rather than to an effect on heart itself. Nonetheless, the findings that most trained patients tolerate a greater RPP before pain is provoked and that some patients (in our material, six of 25) are completely free from angina could suggest a direct effect of training on the heart.

Patients who improve from training but in whom pain can still be provoked augment the RPP pain threshold by 13%–22%.[6,11,12,96] In principle, there can be two explanations why angina is provoked at a higher product of HR and SBP after training. Either a decrease in one or more of the other determinants of $M\dot{V}O_2$ allows higher values for HR and SBP to be achieved at the same $M\dot{V}O_2$, or there is a higher $M\dot{V}O_{2\,max}$ due to improved O_2 supply to the region of the myocardium from which ischemic pain is provoked.

The three main determinants of $M\dot{V}O_2$ not encompassed by RPP are myocardial contractility, left ventricular enddiastolic volume ($LVED_{vol}$), and left ventricular wall thickness. Changes in contractility in response to training may occur in parallel to changes in HR,[64] but this has not been directly demonstrated in patients with angina pectoris. As an indicator of left ventricular filling pressure (and possibly also of volume), PCW has been measured before and after training in patients with CAD, but only during exercise in the supine position.[107,108] Whether or not elevated before training, these pressures did not change in response to training. It is an open question what happens to $LVED_{vol}$ during upright exercise after a period of training. It would not seem unlikely, especially in cases in which $\dot{Q}/\dot{V}O_2$ is reduced, that $LVED_{vol}$ increased less and that this was the explanation for the higher RPP threshold.

In one investigation of patients with CAD, left ventricular diastolic wall thickness was assessed by an ultrasonic technique and was reported to increase after training.[155] Even if such a change were a constant finding, its significance as to the economizing effect on $M\dot{V}O_2$ is difficult to evaluate.

The alternative explanation that the higher RPP pain threshold after training results from increased $M\dot{V}O_{2\,max}$ has also not been documented thus far. Both increased coronary oxygen supply and increased oxygen extraction could contribute.

Although stenotic changes in coronary arteries per se are known to enhance the development of collateral vessels in the myocardial vasculature in man,[156] further improvement of collateral circulation in response to training has only been shown in animal experiments involving artificial narrowing of coronary vessels.[157,158] Moreover, it is questionable if such a change, even if it occurs, could be documented in man. Probably the caliber of newly formed collateral vessel would be of an order of magnitude which could not be visualized and quantitated by coronary angiography.[158] Measurement of total coronary blood flow does not give information about the regional perfusion, and methods permitting evaluation of regional myocardial perfusion[159] are not practicable in man during upright exercise.

Increased oxygen extraction from coronary blood could result from an increased content of mitochondrial enzymes, but demonstration of such changes has not been accomplished in man. Moreover, coronary $AVDO_2$ is already high in patients with CAD as compared to normal subjects.[60]

If training displaces the O_2Hb-dissociation curve to the right in patients with angina pectoris as is the case in normal young subjects,[135] this could facilitate oxygen transfer from blood to myocardial tissue. However, this effect has also not been assessed in patients with angina pectoris.

A last hypothetical means of improving O_2 supply to ischemic regions could include a change in "proximal steal";[160] i.e., a reduction of the flow to regions supplied by stenotic vessels because vasodilation in parallel coupled regions reduces the driving pressure. Dynamic studies performed with gamma camera technique have suggested the occurrence of this phenomenon in the coronary circuit in patients with angina pectoris: during angina, a myocardial region supplied by a narrowed coronary artery not only shows less of an increase, but actually has a decrease in perfusion when flow to neighboring regions increases.[159] Hypothetically, training might reduce proximal steal during exercise when total $M\dot{V}O_2$ is reduced.

However, the enthusiasm for such optimistic speculations on how training might improve myocardial oxygen supply should be tempered by the finding of Detry and Bruce[5] that the slope of the relation between RPP and the extent of ST-depression during exercise is unchanged after training, even up to the provocation of pain, so that the ST-depression at pain is even deeper after training. If the degree of ST-segment depression reflects the degree of myocardial ischemia, this finding would speak against improved myocardial oxygen supply after training.

In conclusion, it cannot be decided at present whether the increase in RPP in response to training results from altered left ventricular functional conditions or from increased oxygen supply to potential ischemic regions. The finding of both a higher RPP at the onset of pain and a deeper ST-depression[5] could be interpreted to indicate that the patients tolerated a greater degree of ischemia before they experienced pain.

The possibility that the patients ignored the pain to a greater extent after training in these controlled laboratory tests is not very likely. Most patients cooperate satisfactorily and are able to indicate the time of onset, the location, and the progression in severity of pain rather precisely. Moreover, the reproducibility of the individual RPP threshold value is not reduced after training.[97] In many patients, training definitely changes the anginal attacks as to severity and character, the pain being milder, with slower progression, and without transient postexertional accentuation. Although such nuances in the severity of angina have been used to support the effect of drugs in some studies, in our study[97] the time for onset of pain both before and after training was defined as the moment at which the patient experienced even the slightest sensation known to lead to an anginal attack.

COMPARISON OF DIFFERENT MODES OF TREATMENT IN ANGINA PECTORIS

In many patients with exertional angina pectoris, the main trouble is the limitations the anginal attacks cause to activities in daily life rather than the chest pain per se. Even a moderate increase in physical performance capacity may mean a marked difference in quality of life by allowing physical activities such as walking, climbing stairs, gardening, and light manual labor. The improvement that can be obtained by training is often sufficient to achieve this.

However, the question arises how this effect compares to that of other modes of treatment currently used: nitroglycerin and other organic nitrate esters, pharmacologic beta-receptor blockade, and direct surgical revascularization by aortocoronary bypass. As long as none of these treatments nor physical training have been proven to affect survival in CAD,[9,12,161,162] it seems reasonable to judge their value from the ability to increase exercise capacity. In this context, we will rely exclusively on results obtained during suitable exercise tests in the laboratory setting.

Direct comparisons of the effect on exercise capacity of different modes of treatment in angina pectoris are not frequent. Even though several authors who report on the effect of aortocoronary bypass operations claim that preoperatively, the patients had angina pectoris "refractory to medical treatment," there are no studies including objective measurement of the effect of nitroglycerin, of beta-receptor blockade, and of physical training on exercise capacity performed in the same patients before the surgical intervention. There are a few studies comparing the effectiveness of nitrates and beta-receptor blockers in preventing or alleviating angina on exertion,[163–165] and in one study, the effect of nitroglycerin has been compared with that of physical training.[97]

Nitroglycerin

Eleven patients with typical exertional angina pectoris were exercised on the same individually chosen work load before and after 0.25–0.50 mg of nitroglycerin was administered sublingually.[97] Nitroglycerin caused a decrease in RPP of 5.4% at the time of onset of pain in the control study due to a decrease in SBP of 13%—which decrease overrode a concomitant increase in HR. As mentioned previously, in 25 patients, training caused a decrease of RPP of 10% due to a corresponding decrease in HR.

Nine patients were restudied after a training period lasting from 3 to 5 mo. In these patients, the effect of training could be related to that of nitroglycerin in the pretraining study. Rate pressure product at the time of onset of pain in the control study was 195 after nitroglycerin and 190 after training. The increase in total amount of work (wattsec) performed until onset of pain was 108% after nitroglycerin and 77% after training. This difference was not significant.

Nitroglycerin did not augment the RPP threshold value in this study,[97] but other investigators have reported an increase of this value of about 9%–12%. [93,166,167] This increase corresponds to that which has been reported after training.[5,11,12,96] Detry and Bruce[5] saw an increase in $\dot{V}O_{2\,max}$ of 14.5% after nitroglycerin was administered to patients with angina. This is about one half of the increase which can be obtained after training.[5,6,11,12] The percentage of the total number of patients who became limited by fatigue rather than by pain was 30%–67% after nitroglycerin[93,166,167] as compared to 18%–30% after training.[5,6,97]

From these findings, it seems reasonable to conclude that the effect of training on exercise capacity is quite similar to that seen after nitroglycerin. The main difference is that it may take less than a minute to obtain the effects of nitroglycerin, but several weeks or months before training is efficient. On the other hand, the benefits from training are present all day, and if CAD is stable, they will last as long as the improved physical condition is maintained, whereas the effect of nitroglycerin disappears after about 30 min.[167]

Both training and nitroglycerin act by reducing RPP at submaximal work loads and by increasing the RPP pain threshold. While training predominantly reduces HR and, to a lesser extent and less consistently, SBF, nitroglycerin causes a marked decrease in SBP, but increases HR.[93,97,166-168] Due to this difference regarding changes in HR and blood pressures, the fall in RPP obtained by training and by nitroglycerin may have different implications for coronary blood flow. A decrease in HR augments the length of cardiac diastole and thus the time for coronary collateral flow, whereas a decrease in diastolic pressure can be anticipated to have a deleterious effect on coronary circulation. Nonetheless, nitroglycerin has at least the same potency in alleviating or preventing angina as training, even though the reduction in RPP is less pronounced. Obviously, nitroglycerin influences the functional conditions of the heart in a complex manner. The effect of nitroglycerin is assumed to be mediated by dilatation of systemic resistance and capacitance vessels.[101,166] Among the multiplicity of hemodynamic changes caused by this general vasodilation,[168] a decrease of SBP and in ventricular size can be expected to lower $M\dot{V}O_2$, while the concomitant reflex increase in HR and inotropic state will tend to increase $M\dot{V}O_2$. Apparently the net result is an improved relationship between oxygen requirements and supply in the coronary circuit.[95]

Beta-receptor Blocking Agents

In normal subjects and in patients with CAD, ingestion of beta-receptor blocking agents* causes a decrease in HR and $\dot{Q}$ during exercise, together with a reduction of SBP.[102,115,116,122,151,169-178] At the same time, there is an increase in left and right ventricular filling pressures and in heart volume during supine exercise in normal subjects. [169,170,172] Consequently, we are faced with signs of cardiac functional impairment that normally would call for medical intervention, and in normal subjects, exercise capacity expressed as $\dot{V}O_{2\,max}$ and/or endurance time at maximal work loads is reduced.[116,122,151]

Nonetheless, beta-receptor blocking agents increase exercise capacity in most patients with angina pectoris, and their elevated $LVED_p$ or PCW during supine exercise does not increase further.[173-177] Maximal oxygen uptake seems not to have been measured in patients with angina pectoris before and after beta-receptor blockade, but an increase in time to onset of pain or complete prevention of pain has been observed during exercise at a given work load, as well as at progressive multistage exercise tests.[163-165,174,176,179-181] The effectiveness of beta-blocking agents in improving exercise capacity in angina pectoris has been compared to that of nitrates in a few studies. One investigator found propranolol and isosorbide dinitrate to be equally potent in preventing and mitigating angina during exercise,[163] whereas in two other studies, the effect of beta-receptor blockade was not quite as effective as that of nitrates.[164,165] In one study, after beta-receptor blockade, 17%–24% of the patients were limited by fatigue instead of by angina during a progres-

---

*No distinction has been made between different types of beta-blocking agents, since their circulatory effects during exercise in equipotent doses seem to be almost the same.

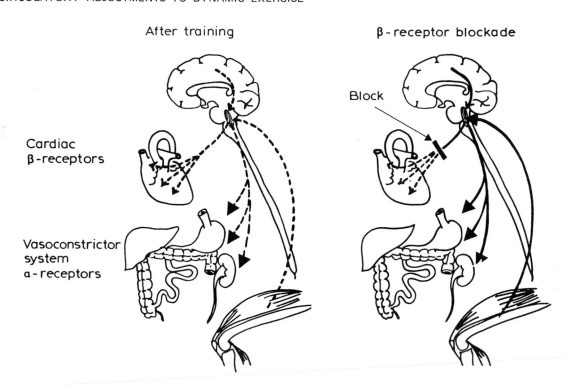

Fig. 14. Comparison of the mode of action of training and beta-receptor blockade on sympathetic stimulation of the heart and peripheral resistance vessels during exercise. Training reduces the sympathetic stimulation of the heart as well as the vasoconstriction. Beta-receptor blockade prevents the heart from responding to the sympathetic stimulation, but causes compensatory increased peripheral vasoconstriction mediated by alpha-receptors (from Trap-Jensen and Clausen,[194] with permission).

sive multistage exercise test;[179] i.e., a result comparable to that seen after training and nitroglycerin. The advantage of beta-receptor blockade as compared to nitroglycerin is that the protective action is of longer duration.

The beneficial effect of beta-blocking drugs can be explained by a substantial reduction in RPP during exercise due to fall in both HR and SBP. In connection with a decrease in myocardial contractility, this probably causes a net reduction in $M\dot{V}O_2$[62] despite concomitant augmentation in ventricular volume that tends to increase $M\dot{V}O_2$.[169,172]

In contrast to what is seen after training and after nitroglycerin, the pain threshold values for RPP and for HR are reduced respectively by 17%–30%[164,174,179] and by 15%–25%[164,165,174,179,181] after beta-receptor blockade. This could be the result of an enlarged $LVED_{vol}$ as seen during supine exercise.[169,172] However, if measurements of coronary flow and $M\dot{V}O_2$ are reliable in man, this is probably not the main reason. In healthy young subjects, the relation between $M\dot{V}O_2$ and

RPP was unchanged during upright exercise, but the relation between coronary blood flow and RPP was reduced.[62] If this finding applies to patients with angina pectoris, it means that pain could be expected to occur at a lower RPP and HR because the ability to increase myocardial flow is impaired after beta-receptor blockade.

The effects of beta-receptor blockade have often been compared to those of training because both cause a fall in HR and in SBP during exercise. However, as shown in Fig. 14, the reduction in HR and SBP is accomplished by a completely different mechanism after training as compared to beta-receptor blockade. While training reduces HR and SBP by a less pronounced sympathetic stimulation of the heart and a less pronounced peripheral sympathetic vasoconstriction at a given submaximal $\dot{V}O_2$, beta-receptor blockade prevents the heart from responding to the sympathetic stimulation, but elicits a compensatory increase in alpha-receptor-controlled peripheral vasoconstriction. Thus, while the perfusion of abdominal viscera is less reduced during exercise after training, it is,

sistance vessels in the contracting muscles, where it might act to oppose the local dilator mechanism.

In man, the activity of the sympathetic vasoconstrictor fibers to the forearm can be augmented by application of subatmospheric pressure to the lower part of the body.[68] Strandell and Shepherd[69] applied this method during exercise of forearm muscles. Muscle blood flow was measured by venous occlusion plethysmography and by radioactive xenon clearance. When exercise was mild, forearm muscle blood flow could be reduced by the increased adrenergic activity; this effect lessened as the exercise increased in severity so that with maximal muscle activity, no significant effect was observed. The decrease in flow during and after exercise caused by the increased sympathetic action was compensated for by greater oxygen extraction so that no debt occurred and the metabolic recovery was not prolonged. From these studies, it appears that the sympathetic nerves modulate the local dilator mechanism in active muscles to maintain the most economical ratio of blood flow to oxygen consumption.

This interaction has also been studied in unanesthetized dogs during graded exercise by comparing the blood flow in a normal limb with that of a sympathectomized one.[70] The magnitude of the limb blood flow during exercise and the decline of postexercise hyperemia were similar in both limbs. However, electric stimulation of the lumbar sympathetic chain by chronically implanted electrodes reduced limb blood flow at all levels of exercise, demonstrating that if sufficient activation of sympathetic nerves occurs, this can partly oppose the dilatation caused by the local metabolic changes.

In the gracilis muscle of the dog, a comparison of norepinephrine infusion and sympathetic stimulation showed that these sympathetic responses were reduced more during exercise than the responses to norepinephrine.[71] Thus, during exercise, there may be some inhibition of sympathetic neurotransmission. Local metabolites such as potassium, which is found in increased concentration in the blood from the active muscles,[72,73] may play a role in this inhibition, since this ion can inhibit the release of norepinephrine.[74]

RECEPTORS CONCERNED WITH THE REFLEX HEMODYNAMIC ADJUSTMENTS DURING MUSCULAR EXERCISE

The receptors concerned with the cardiovascular changes during muscular exercise are still a matter of discussion. Two main theories have been proposed: according to the "central" theory, the changes are caused by the cortical centers in the brain influencing the vasomotor center; the "peripheral" theories implicate the arterial baroreceptors or receptors in or around the muscles.

According to the central theory,[75] there is, during exercise, an "irradiation" from the motor cortex to the cardiovascular and respiratory centers. The fact that electric stimulation of hypothalamic or subthalamic structures elicits a cardiovascular response similar to that observed at the beginning of muscular exercise recommends this theory.[76] This response is reminiscent of the so-called "defense reaction."[42,77]

Of the peripheral theories, it was first postulated that the cardiovascular response to muscular exercise would be regulated mainly by the carotid sinus and aortic baroreceptors;[78-81] the vasodilatation in exercising muscles can cause a decrease of systemic arterial blood pressure, resulting in inhibition of baroreceptor activity and reflex increase in systemic blood pressure and vascular tone. However, in the absence of these receptors, the ability of the dog to exercise is not impaired.[82-84]

Alam and Smirk[85,86] postulated that the contracting muscles play an important role. They found that the increase of blood pressure and heart rate during exercise of the forearm muscles in man was augmented by temporary arrest of the forearm circulation. Also, the blood pressure remained elevated as long as the circulation was arrested after exercise was stopped. These changes were not observed in a patient with unilateral syringomyelia.[87,88] This suggested that metabolites in the contracting muscles might activate receptors within the muscles to cause the increase in blood pressure and heart rate.

Stimulation in the anesthetized cat of the central end of the cut hamstring nerve at low frequency and voltage decreased blood pressure and caused dilatation of renal, mesenteric, cutaneous and muscular vessels; at higher frequency and voltage, the blood pressure increased and the vascular beds were constricted.[89,90]

Tetanic contraction of the hind limb muscles elicited by stimulating the ventral roots L6–S1 caused an increase in arterial blood pressure, usually accompanied by small increases in heart rate and pulmonary ventilation; the pressor response increased with increasing strength of contraction and was abolished either by muscle paralysis or by section of the dorsal roots L6–S1.[91] Thus, the response was reflexly induced from the exercising limb.[91,92]

In anesthetized dogs with carotid sinuses isolated and vagi cut, rhythmic contraction of the muscles of the thigh caused reflex decreases in blood pressure, dilatation of the resistance vessels in muscle and skin, and constriction of the cutaneous veins; tetanic muscular contraction caused the blood pressure to increase and caused constriction of the resistance vessels along with dilatation of the cutaneous veins.[93,94] After muscle paralysis, the pressor response was abolished while the depressor response was maintained. The afferent pathway for this reflex was in the nerves innervating the stimulated limb, because section of the femoral, sciatic, and obturator nerves of that side abolished the response.[93] The efferent pathway utilizes the sympathetic nerves because sympathectomy abolishes the response[93] and because changes in sympathetic traffic can be demonstrated during muscular contraction.[95] In the dog, the receptors initiating these reflexes are localized in the muscles because skinning of the stimulated limb and separation of the muscles from their tendons did not influence the response; however, in the cat, the pressor responses to passive limb movement are slightly reduced by section of sensory fibers from the knee joint.[96]

Whether the receptors concerned are activated mechanically or as a consequence of metabolic changes in the contracting muscles, or both, is not known. It is unlikely that the muscle spindles are involved in the pressor response, because stimulation of their afferent nerve fibers does not cause an increase of blood pressure;[97] this was recently confirmed by electrophysiologic studies.[98,99] By use of anodal block of the dorsal roots receiving afferents from the exercising muscles, it appears[92] that the pressor responses are mediated by small medullated and nonmedullated fibers (groups III and IV). The size of the afferent fibers responsible for the depressor response is not known.

INTEGRATED REGULATION OF THE CIRCULATION DURING MUSCULAR EXERCISE

In order to provide the active muscles with their metabolic requirements, the heart and blood vessels have to be regulated appropriately. At the onset of muscular contraction, the capacitance vessels in the active parts become mechanically compressed, resulting in an increased return of

blood to the right heart; in addition to reducing the volume of blood contained in the legs, the pumping action of the muscles will reduce the venous pressure in the leg and foot veins and therefore increase the perfusion pressure to the lower limbs. The muscle pump, which is especially important during upright exercise, is aided by reflex venoconstriction mediated by sympathetic adrenergic nerves. Unlike the resistance vessels, the veins, which are well equipped to respond to humoral[100] as well as neurogenic influences,[101,102] react as a whole through a centrally integrated neurogenic mechanism rather than through the influence of local factors. However, as body temperature increases during exercise, the cutaneous venoconstriction lessens while the constriction of the splanchnic veins remains the same. The latter maintains the central blood volume that is necessary to provide an adequate filling pressure of the heart during muscular exercise.

In addition to causing venoconstriction, the increased sympathetic outflow constricts the resistance vessels of the nonexercising muscles, of the splanchnic bed, and of the kidney and may adjust the vasodilatation in the active muscles.

The increase in blood pressure and heart rate and the constriction of resistance vessels in nonexercising parts are tempered by the baroreceptors but not prevented by them.

The importance of these reflex actions can be best demonstrated in conditions in which the function of the sympathetic system is disturbed. After adrenergic blockade in normal subjects, systemic arterial blood pressure is decreased rather than increased during muscular exercise.[103] Patients with idiopathic orthostatic hypotension experience a pronounced decrease in systolic and diastolic blood pressure even during mild supine exercise, in spite of a normal increase in cardiac output.[104] Thus, the decrease in blood pressure is the result of a failure of compensatory constriction of blood vessels and not of cardiac output to increase.[104,105]

When the increase in cardiac output during exercise is prevented by severe mitral stenosis, blood pressure is maintained by a stronger constriction of the vessels outside the active muscles.[106–108] The same is true in normal subjects when the cardiac response to exercise is depressed by administration of propranolol.[109] By contrast, peripheral vasodilatation may occur during leg exercise in patients with aortic stenosis and a history of exertional syncope.[110] Inhibition or reversal of forearm vasoconstrictor responses in aortic stenosis was associated with significant increases in left ventricular pressure. This abnormal response may be caused by activation of mechanoreceptors in the left ventricle.

CONCLUSIONS

To prevent a decrease in systemic arterial blood pressure during muscular exercise, rapidly adapting mechanisms must compensate for the metabolic vasodilatation in the active muscles. The peripheral vessels play an important role in this adaptation. Reflex venoconstriction, along with mechanical compression of these vessels by the contracting muscles in the active parts, provides for an in-creased venous return to the heart. Reflex constriction of the resistance vessels in the nonactive parts results in a diversion of the cardiac output, mainly toward the exercising muscles. In the resistance vessels of the skin, there is a balance between this reflex constriction and dilatation to maintain a constant body temperature.

The receptors responsible for these reflexes are still a matter of discussion; recent work shows that besides central influences, receptors in the active muscles may play a role. The importance of these reflex changes in vascular tone is demonstrated in conditions where the controlling influence of the sympathetic nerves is disturbed.

REFERENCES

1. Gaskell WH: On the changes of the blood stream in muscles through stimulation of the nerves. J Anat 11: 360-402, 1877

2. Grant RT: Observations on the blood circulation in voluntary muscle in man. Clin Sci 3:157-173, 1938

3. Corcondilas A, Koroxenidis GT, Shepherd JT: Effect of a brief contraction of forearm muscles on forearm blood flow. J Appl Physiol 19:142-146, 1964

4. Guyton AC, Ross JM, Carrier O, et al: Evidence for tissue oxygen demand as the major factor causing auto-regulation. Circ Res 14-15 (Suppl I):60-69, 1964

5. Dawes GS: The vaso-dilator action of potassium. J Physiol (Lond) 99:224-238, 1941

6. Kjellmer I: The potassium ion as a vasodilator during muscular exercise. Acta Physiol Scand 63:460-468, 1965

7. Mellander S, Johansson B, Gray S, et al: The effects of hyperosmolarity on intact and isolated vascular smooth muscle. Possible role in exercise hyperemia. Angiologia 4:310-322, 1967

8. Mellander S, Johansson B: Control of resistance, exchange and capacitance functions in the peripheral circulation. Pharmacol Rev 20:117-196, 1968

9. Lundvall J: Tissue hyperosmolarity as a mediator of vasodilatation and transcapillary fluid flux in exercising skeletal muscle. Acta Physiol Scand (Suppl 379):1-142, 1972

10. Skinner NS, Powell WJ: Regulation of skeletal muscle blood flow during exercise. Circ Res 20-21 (Suppl I):59-69, 1967

11. Hilton SM, Vrbova G: Inorganic phosphate—a new candidate for mediator of functional vasodilatation in skeletal muscle. J Physiol (Lond) 206:29P-30P, 1970

12. Bojad IA, Forrester T: The release of adenosine triphosphate from frog skeletal muscle in vitro. J Physiol (Lond) 199:115-135, 1968

13. Folkow B: Range of control of the cardiovascular system by the central nervous system. Physiol Rev:40 (Suppl 4):93-101, 1960

14. Love AHG: The rate of blood flow and the oxygen saturation of the effluent blood following contraction of the muscles of the human forearm. Clin Sci 14:275-283, 1955

15. Ross JIr, Kaiser GA, Klocke PJ: Observations on the role of diminished oxygen tension in the functional hyperemia of skeletal muscle. Circ Res 15:473-484, 1964

16. Glover WE, Roddie IC, Shanks RC: The effect of intra-arterial potassium chloride infusions on vascular reactivity in the human forearm. J Physiol (Lond) 163:22P-23P, 1962

17. Barcroft H, Foley TH, McSwiney RR: Experiments on the liberation of phosphate from the muscles of the human forearm during vigorous exercise and on the action of sodium phosphate on forearm muscle blood vessels. J Physiol (Lond) 213:411-420, 1971

18. Duff F, Paterson G, Shepherd J: A quantitative study of the response to adenosine triphosphate of the blood vessels of the human hand and forearm. J Physiol (Lond) 125:581-589, 1954

19. Forrester T: An estimate of adenosine triphosphate release into the venous effluent from exercising human forearm muscle. J Physiol (Lond) 224:611-628, 1972

20. Barcroft H, Millen JLE: The blood flow through muscle during sustained contraction. J Physiol (Lond) 97:17-31, 1939

21. Humphreys PW, Lind AR: The blood flow through the forearm during hand-drip contractions at different tensions and muscle temperature. J Physiol (Lond) 161: 53P-54P, 1962

22. Humphreys PW, Lind AR: Blood flow through active muscles of the forearm during sustained hand-grip contractions. J Physiol (Lond) 163:18P, 1962

23. Humphreys PW, Lind AR: The blood flow through active and inactive muscles of the forearm during sustained hand-grip contractions. J Physiol (Lond) 166:120-135, 1963

24. Lind AR, Taylor SH, Humphreys PW, et al: The circulatory effects of sustained voluntary muscle contraction. Clin Sci 27:229-244, 1964

25. Maréchal R, Pirnay F, Petit JM: Débit circulatoire musculaire pendant la contraction isométrique. Arch Int Physiol Biochim 81:273-281, 1973

26. Barcroft H, Dornhorst AC: Blood flow through the human calf during rhythmic exercise. J Physiol (Lond) 109:402-411, 1949

27. Rother FD, Rochelle RH, Hyman C: Exercise blood

flow changes in the human forearm during physical training. J Appl Physiol 18:789–793, 1963

28. Folkow B, Gaskell P, Waaler BA: Blood flow through limb muscles during heavy rhythmic exercise. Acta Physiol Scand 80:61–72, 1970

29. Sjöstrand T: The regulation of blood distribution in man. Acta Physiol Scand 26:312–327, 1952

30. Wang Y, Marschall RJ, Taylor HL, et al: Cardiovascular response to exercise in sedentary man and athletes. Physiologist 3:173, 1960

31. Daly WJ, Krumholz RA, Ross JC: The venous pump in the legs as a determinant of pulmonary capillary filling. J Clin Invest 44:271–277, 1965

32. Blair DA, Glover WE, Roddie IC: Vasomotor responses in the human arm during leg exercise. Circ Res 9:264–274, 1961

33. Bevegård BS, Shepherd JT: Reaction in man of resistance and capacity vessels in forearm and hand to leg exercise. J Appl Physiol 21:123–132, 1966

34. Eklund B, Kaijser L, Knutsson E: Blood flow in resting (contralateral) arm and leg during isometric contraction. J Physiol (Lond) 240:111–124, 1974

35. Uvnäs B: Cholinergic vasodilator nerves. Fed Proc 25:1618–1622, 1966

36. Eliasson S, Folkow B, Lindgren P, et al: Activation of sympathetic vasodilator nerves to the skeletal muscles in the cat by hypothalamic stimulation. Acta Physiol Scand 23:333–351, 1951

37. Folkow B, Mellander S, Öberg B: The range of effect of the sympathetic vasodilator fibres with regard to consecutive sections of the muscle vessels. Acta Physiol Scand 53:7–22, 1961

38. Renkin EM, Rosell S: Effects of different types of vasodilator mechanisms on vascular tonus and on transcapillary exchange of diffusible material in skeletal muscle. Acta Physiol Scand 54:241–251, 1962

39. Abrahams VC, Hilton SM: Active muscle vasodilatation and its relation to the "flight and fight reactions" in the conscious animal. J Physiol (Lond) 140:16P–17P, 1958

40. Abrahams VC, Hilton SM, Zbrozyna A: Reflex activation of vasodilator nerve fibers to skeletal muscle in decerebrate and intact cats. J Physiol (Lond) 152:54P–55P, 1960

41. Abrahams VC, Hilton SM, Zbrozyna A: Active muscle vasodilatation produced by stimulation of the brain stem: its significance in the defense reaction. J Physiol (Lond) 154:491–513, 1960

42. Abrahams VC, Hilton SM, Zbrozyna AW: The role of active muscle vasodilatation in the alerting stage of the defense reaction. J Physiol (Lond) 171:189–202, 1964

43. Ellison G, Zanchetti A: Diffuse and specific activation of sympathetic cholinergic fibers of the cat. Am J Physiol 225:142–149, 1973

44. Blair DA, Glover WE, Roddie IC: Abolition of reactive and post-exercise hyperaemia in the forearm by temporary restriction of arterial inflow. J Physiol (Lond) 148:648–658, 1959

45. Barcroft H, Brod J, Hyl Z, et al: The mechanism of the vasodilatation in the forearm muscle during stress (mental arithmetic). Clin Sci 19:577–586, 1960

46. Greenfield ADM: Survey of the evidence for active neurogenic vasodilatation in man. Fed Proc 25:1607–1610, 1966

47. Mason GT, Braunwald E: Effects of guanethidine, reserpine and methyldopa on reflex venous and arterial constriction in man. J Clin Invest 43:1449–1463, 1964

48. Bevegård BS, Shepherd JT: Regulation of the circulation during exercise in man. Physiol Rev 47:178–213, 1967

49. Bradley SE: Variations in hepatic blood flow in man during health and disease. N Engl J Med 240:456–461, 1949

50. Wade OL, Combes B, Wheeler AW, et al: The effect of exercise on the splanchnic blood flow and the splanchnic blood volume in normal man. Clin Sci 15:457–463, 1956

51. Rowell LB, Blackmon JR, Bruce RA: Indocyanine green clearance and estimated hepatic blood flow during mild to maximal exercise in upright man. J Clin Invest 43:1677–1690, 1964

52. Bishop JM, Donald KW, Wade OL: Changes in the oxygen content of hepatic venous blood during exercise in patients with rheumatic heart disease. J Clin Invest 34:1114–1125, 1955

53. Bishop JM, Donald KW, Taylor SH, et al: Changes in arterial hepatic venous oxygen content difference during and after supine leg exercise. J Physiol (Lond) 137:309–317, 1957

54. Lacroix E, Leusen I: Splanchnic hemodynamics during induced muscular exercise in the anesthetized dog. Arch Int Physiol Biochim 74:235–250, 1966

55. Van Citters RL, Franklin DL: Cardiovascular performance of Alaska sled dogs during exercise. Circ Res 24:33–42, 1969

56. Vatner SF, Higgins CB, White S, et al: The peripheral vascular response to severe exercise in untethered dogs before and after complete heart block. J Clin Invest 50:1950–1960, 1971

57. Rowell LB: Human cardiovascular adjustments to exercise and thermal stress. Physiol Rev 54:75–159, 1974

58. Scher AM, Ohm WW, Bumgarner K, et al: Sympathetic and parasympathetic control of heart rate in the dog, baboon and man. Fed Proc 31:1219–1225, 1972

59. Higgins CB, Vatner SF, Franklin D, et al: Effect of experimentally produced heart failure on the peripheral vascular response to severe exercise in conscious dogs. Circ Res 31:186–194, 1972

60. Vatner SF, Higgins CB, Franklin D: Regional circulatory adjustments to moderate and severe chronic anaemia in conscious dogs at rest and during exercise. Circ Res 30:731–740, 1972

61. Vatner SG, Higgins CB, Millard RW, et al: Role of the spleen in the peripheral vascular response to severe exercise in untethered dogs. Cardiovasc Res 8:276–282, 1974

62. Millard RW, Higgins CB, Franklin D, et al: Regulation of the renal circulation during severe exercise in normal dogs and dogs with experimental heart failure. Circ Res 31:381–388, 1972

63. Chapman CB, Henschel A, Minsckler J, et al: Effect of exercise on renal plasma flow in normal male subjects. J Clin Invest 27:639, 1948

64. Grimby G: Renal clearances during prolonged su-

pine exercise at different loads. J Appl Physiol 20:1294–1298, 1965

65. Merritt FL, Weissler AM: Reflex venomotor alterations during exercise and hyperventilation. Am Heart J 58:382–387, 1959

66. Seaman RG, Wiley RL, Zechman FW, et al: Venous reactivity during static exercise (handgrip) in man. J Appl Physiol 35:358–360, 1973

67. Zitnik RZ, Ambrosioni E, Shepherd JT: Effect of temperature on cutaneous venomotor reflexes in man. J Appl Physiol 31:507–512, 1971

68. Brown E, Goei JS, Greenfield ADM, et al: Circulatory responses to stimulated gravitational shifts of blood in man induced by exposure of the body below the iliac crest to sub-atmospheric pressure. J Physiol (Lond) 183:607–627, 1966

69. Strandell T, Shepherd JT: The effects in humans of increased sympathetic activity on the blood flow to active muscles. Acta Med Scand [Suppl] 472:146–167, 1967

70. Donald DE, Derek JR, Ferguson DA: Similarity of blood flow in the normal and the sympathectomized dog hind limb during graded exercise. Circ Res 26:185–199, 1970

71. Burcher E, Garlick D: Antagonism of vasoconstrictor responses by exercise in the gracilis muscle of the dog. J Pharmacol Exp Ther 187:78–85, 1973

72. Donald KW, Lind AR, McNicol GW, et al: Cardiovascular responses to substained (static) contractions. Circ Res (Suppl I) 20–21:15–32, 1967

73. Wildenthal K, Mierzwiak DS, Skinner Jr NS, et al: Potassium-induced cardiovascular and ventilatory reflexes from the dog hindlimb. Am J Physiol 215:542–548, 1968

74. Lorenz R, Vanhoutte PM: Inhibition of adrenergic neurotransmission in isolated veins of the dog by potassium ions. J Physiol (Lond) (in press)

75. Krogh A, Lindhard J: The regulation of respiration and circulation during the initial stage of muscular work. J Physiol (Lond) 47:112–136, 1913

76. Rushmer RF, Smith Jr OA: Cardiac control. Physiol Rev 39:41–68, 1959

77. Hess WR: Das Zwischerhim. Schwabe, Basel, 1949

78. Jarisch A, Gaisböck F: Uber das Verhalten des Kreislaufes bei der postanämischen Hyperämie. Arch Exp Pathol Pharmacol 139:159–171, 1929

79. Sarnoff SJ, Gilmore JP, Brockman SK, et al: Regulation of ventricular contraction by the carotid sinus. Circ Res 8:1123–1136, 1960

80. Sarnoff SJ, Mitchell JH: The control of the heart, in: Handbook of Physiology, Section 2: Circulation, vol. I. Baltimore, Williams and Wilkins, 1962, pp 489–532

81. Remensnyder JP, Mitchell JH, Sarnoff SJ: Functional sympatholysis during muscular activity: observations on influence of carotid sinus on oxygen uptake. Circ Res 11:370–380, 1962

82. Leusen I, Demeester G, Bouckaert JJ: Pressorécepteurs artériels et débit cardiaque au cours de l'exercise musculaire. Arch Int Physiol Biochim 64:564–570, 1956

83. Leusen I, Demeester G, Bouckaert JJ: Chémo- et presso-récepteurs artériels et respiration au cours de l'exercise musculaire. Acta Physiol Pharmacol Neerlandica 6:43–52, 1957

84. Leusen I, Demeester G, Bouckaert JJ: Influence du travail musculaire sur la circulation et la respiration chez le chien. Acta Cardiol (Brux) 13:153–172, 1958

85. Alam M, Smirk FH: Observations in man upon a blood pressure raising reflex arising from the voluntary muscles. J Physiol (Lond) 89:372–383, 1937

86. Alam M, Smirk FH: Observations in man on a pulse-accelerating reflex from the voluntary muscles of the legs. J Physiol (Lond) 92:167–177, 1938

87. Alam M, Smirk FH: Unilateral loss of a blood pressure raising, pulse accelerating reflex from voluntary muscle due to a lesion of spinal cord. Clin Sci 3:247–258, 1938

88. Lind AR, McNicol GW, Bruce RA, et al: The cardiovascular responses to sustained contractions of a patient with unilateral syringomyelia. Clin Sci 35:45–53, 1968

89. Johansson B: Circulatory responses to stimulation of somatic afferents. Acta Physiol Scand [Suppl. 198] 57:1–91, 1962

90. Khayutin VM: Specific and non-specific responses of the vasomotor centre to impulses of spinal afferent fibres. Acta Physiol Acad Sci Hung 29:131–143, 1966

91. Coote JH, Hilton SM, Perez-Gonzales JF: The reflex nature of the pressor response to muscular exercise. J Physiol (Lond) 215:780–804, 1971

92. McCloskey DI, Mitchell JH: Reflex cardiovascular and respiratory responses originating in exercising muscle. J Physiol (Lond) 224:173–186, 1972

93. Clement DL, Pelletier LC, Shepherd JT: Role of muscular contraction in the reflex vascular responses to stimulation of muscle afferents in the dog. Circ Res 33:386–392, 1973

94. Clement DL, Shepherd JT: Influence of muscle afferents on the cutaneous and muscle vessels in the dog. Circ Res 35:177–183, 1974

95. Clement DL, Shepherd JT: Changes in renal nerve traffic with stimulation of muscle afferents. Circulation 48:28 (Suppl IV), 1973

96. Barron W, Coote JH: The contribution of articular receptors to cardiovascular reflexes elicited by passive limb movement. J Physiol (Lond) 235:423–436, 1973

97. Laporte Y, Bessou P, Bouisset S: Action réflexe des différents types de fibres afférentes d'origine musculaire sur la pression sanguine. Arch It Biol 98:206–221, 1960

98. Coote JH, Perez-Gonzales JF: Response of some sympathetic neurons to volleys in various different nerves. J Physiol (Lond) 208:261–278, 1970

99. Perez-Gonzales JF, Coote JH: Activity of muscle afferents and reflex circulatory responses to exercise. Am J Physiol 223:138–143, 1972

100. Clement D, Vanhoutte P, Leusen I: Capacitance reactions of isolated veins to mono-amines and acetylcholine. Arch Int Physiol Biochim 75:73–87, 1969

101. Vanhoutte P, Clement D, Leusen I: Response characteristics of isolated veins to electrical stimulation. Arch Int Pharmacodyn Ther 167:495–497, 1967

102. Vanhoutte P, Leusen I: The reactivity of isolated venous preparations to electrical stimulation. Pfluegers Arch 306:341–353, 1969

103. Taylor SH, Donald KW: Circulatory effects of bretylium Tosylate and guanethidine. Lancet 2:389–349, 1960

104. Marshall RJ, Schirger A, Shepherd JT: Blood pressure during supine exercise in idiopathic orthostatic hypotension. Circulation 24:76–81, 1961

105. Bevegård S, Jonsson B, Karlöf I: Circulatory response to recumbent exercise and head-up tilting in patients with disturbed sympathetic cardiovascular control (postural hypotension): Observations on the effect of norepinephrine infusion and antigravity suit inflation in the head-up tilted position. Acta Med Scand 172:623–636, 1962

106. Muth HAC, Wormald PN, Bishop JM, et al: Further studies of blood flow in the resting arm during supine leg exercise. Clin Sci 17:603–610, 1958

107. Zelis R, Mason DT, Braunwald E: Partition of blood flow to the cutaneous and muscular beds of the forearm at rest and during exercise in normal subjects and in patients with heart failure. Circ Res 24:799–806, 1969

108. Zelis R, Longhurst J, Capone RJ, et al: Peripheral circulatory control mechanisms in congestive heart failure. Am J Cardiol 32:481–490, 1973

109. Robinson BF, Wilson AG: Effect on forearm arteries and veins of attenuation of the cardiac response to leg exercise. Clin Sci 35:143–152, 1968

110. Mark AL, Kioschos JM, Abboud FP, et al: Abnormal vascular responses to exercise in patients with aortic stenosis, J Clin Invest 52:1138–1146, 1973

Quantification of Exercise Capability and Evaluation of Physical Capacity in Man

Per-Olof Åstrand

THE basal metabolic rate in humans is quite high; 5500–7000 kJ* during a 24-hr period being a realistic figure for an adult, which is equivalent to the extra energy demand of walking about 18 miles (30 km). The single factor which will significantly increase energy output above resting levels is muscular activity. Working skeletal muscles may increase the rate of the oxidative processes to more than 50 times their resting level.

Figure 1 presents examples of some activities and their energy demand expressed in kJ (and kcal) as well as the corresponding need for oxygen transport to the mitochondria. From an oxygen uptake ($\dot{V}O_2$) of 0.20–0.30 liters/min for a supine, resting individual, many daily activities, including walking, carrying, lifting etc., will increase the $\dot{V}O_2$ to about 1 liter/min, heavy manual labor to 1.5 or even 2 liters/min. In competitive sports we have measured oxygen uptakes exceeding 6 liters/min ("world record" so far is 7.4 liters/min!).[35]

A consequence of the unique ability of skeletal muscle to vary its metabolic rate, is that this activity can seriously interfere with the *milieu interne,* i.e., change the composition and property of the fluid within cells and of their surroundings. While the consumption of fuel and oxygen increases up to 50-fold, the rate of removal of heat, carbon dioxide, water, and waste products must be increased similarly. To maintain the chemical and physical equilibrium of the cells there must be a concomitant increase in the exchange of molecules and ions between intra- and extracellular fluid; "fresh" fluid must continuously flush the exercising cells. The maintenance of a relatively stable environment within the body during exercise represents a significant challenge to various "service functions," not the least respiration and circulation. The circulatory system is normally dimensioned to provide optimal service not only at resting conditions but also in connection with vigorous physical activity. It should also be emphasized that optimal function can only be achieved by regularly exposing the heart, circulation, muscles, skeleton, and nervous system to some loading, that is to say training.

Functional tests have gained wide application in medical practice, and have proved to be of great diagnostic value. The bases for all such functional tests is the assumption that an organic abnormality or functional inadequacy is more apt to become apparent when the organ or organ function is subjected to functional stress than is the case at rest when the demand is minimum.

ENERGY YIELD

At rest and during muscular activity of relatively moderate severity, the necessary energy is yielded by *aerobic processes,* i.e., an oxidation in the mitochondria of free fatty acids, carbohydrates, and protein. For each liter of oxygen consumed about 20 kJ are yielded (the exact figure depends upon the fuel, but the range is small, or from 19.7 to 21.2 kJ). The energy is of course utilized for the resynthesis of ATP from ADP and P. During the transition from rest to vigorous exercise the oxygen supply to the working muscles will eventually be delayed, and in very heavy exercise there will ensue a continuous oxygen deficit. Under those conditions part of the energy will be derived from *anaerobic processes:* ATP and creatine phosphate may yield 20–30 kJ, and a breakdown of glycogen to pyruvic acid and lactic acid may contribute an additional 100 kJ (at the most). This anaerobic reserve can cover the energy demand for only a few minutes of vigorous exercise. If we disregard competitive sport activities and some unusual situations (more of an emergency nature) the anaerobic processes play actually a minor role in our daily life, at least from a quantitative point of view. If we add that an exact measurement of the power of the anaerobic machinery is presently not possible (except for in a few well standardized conditions), there is a good excuse for excluding

---

*1 kJ (kilojoule) = 1000 J (joule); 1 kcal = 4.2 kJ.

Manuscript submitted for publication: March, 1975.

From the Department of Physiology, Gymnastik-och Idrottshögskolan, Stockholm, Sweden.

Reprint requests should be addressed to Dr. Per-Olof Åstrand, Department of Physiology, Gymnastik-och Idrottshögskolan, S-114 33 Stockholm, Sweden.

on the listed (and other) factors. It becomes very difficult or impossible to predict the performance in one activity from data obtained in studies from a different activity. However, there is one factor operative in all types of muscular movement; i.e., an increased energy demand, and (disregarding the anaerobic contribution) this is mirrored by an elevated oxygen uptake. Therefore, knowing the potential for an individual's oxygen transporting system one can actually predict his potential for vigorous muscular exercise. On the other hand, a high maximal aerobic power does not guarantee a good performance in a specific event, for technique, strength, and motivation, etc. may be poor. For a top performance in cross-country skiing in international competitions the participant's maximal oxygen uptake should be around 80 ml · kg^{-1} · min^{-1} or higher. There are quite a few athletes with such a high aerobic power but who exhibit a poor performance in skiing. They may lack the skill and specific training although they may be superb runners!

WHAT IS THE LIMITING FACTOR(S) FOR OXYGEN TRANSPORT DURING EXERCISE?

There are many studies showing that pulmonary function does not limit oxygen uptake in normal individuals.[6] During maximal exercise there is a hyperventilation due to an extra respiratory drive caused by a lowered blood pH. The alveolar oxygen tension will increase and the P_{CO_2} is reduced. There may be a slight reduction in the arterial P_{O_2}, but this is not necessarily caused by a limitation in the diffusion of oxygen across the alveolar and erythrocyte membranes. It should also be noted that one can voluntarily further increase pulmonary ventilation during maximal exercise, indicating that the respiratory muscles are not normally taxed to their maximal power.

When discussing the links between the capillaries in the lungs and those in the working muscles, it is wise to consider the Fick formula for O_2 transport:

$$\dot{V}O_2 = \underbrace{HR \times SV}_{\dot{Q}} \times (C_{a_{O_2}} - C_{\bar{v}_{O_2}})$$

(HR = heart rate; SV = stroke volume; $\dot{Q}$ = cardiac output; C = content). The increased oxygen demand during exercise is met by an elevated cardiac output as well as a gradually wider a-$\bar{v}$ O_2 difference.[6,34]

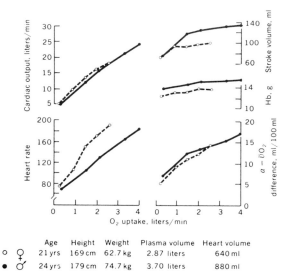

Fig. 4. The figure is based on average values from measurements on 11 women and 12 men, all of them relatively well trained and working on a bicycle ergometer in the sitting position. (Since the abscissa gives the oxygen uptake in absolute values, the calculated mean curves can be misleading. The less-fit subjects have both a low maximal oxygen uptake and low stroke volume. Those with a high capacity for oxygen uptake also have a larger stroke volume. A man with a maximal aerobic power of 5 liters/min eventually attains maximal stroke volume first at a work load giving an oxygen uptake of 2 liters/min. The one with a maximal oxygen uptake of 3.5 liters/min reaches his plateau for stroke volume when the oxygen uptake exceeds 1.3 liters/min.)[6]

Figure 4 presents mean curves for the mentioned functions on well-trained subjects exercising at submaximal and maximal rates of work on a bicycle ergometer. Cardiac output was measured with a dye dilution technique. The increase in cardiac output with the increase in oxygen uptake was slightly curvi-linear. Studies have indicated that cardiac output at a given oxygen uptake is essentially identical in trained and untrained subjects,[6,34] in arm and leg exercise, respectively,[6] in running and bicycling,[19] and during running and swimming.[22] There are individual variations in the absolute values, but we can conclude that *oxygen uptake gives an indirect evaluation of the cardiac output.* During maximal exercise there is a linear relation between maximal oxygen uptake and maximal cardiac output. Subjects with a maximal oxygen uptake of 3.0 liters/min will attain a cardiac output of about 20 liters/min; with a $\dot{V}O_2$ max of 6.0 liters/min, the $\dot{Q}$max will be about 40 liters/min!

During exercise plasma extravasates and the resulting hemoconcentration, causes a slight increase in the oxygen content of arterial blood. During maximal work the blood leaving the muscles has a very low oxygen content and in mixed venous blood the C_{O_2} will be around 20 ml/liter blood.

In upright exercise the stroke volume will increase some 50% above the "resting" value but a maximum is reached at an oxygen uptake corresponding to about 40% of the individual's maximal $\dot{V}O_2$. Therefore, the main factor behind the rise in cardiac output during exercise is an increase in heart rate. The increase in heart rate with oxygen uptake is essentially linear, at least for a wide range of submaximal exercise loads. However, in work with smaller muscle groups (i.e., arm exercise) and isometric (static) exercises the heart rate at a given oxygen uptake is significantly higher than in dynamic leg exercise.

There is a tendency towards a higher heart rate at a given oxygen uptake (and cardiac output) attained during running than in bicycling, but this difference has no practical consequence, for the individual variations in the heart rate response to the two types of exercises are rather marked.

Despite a reduced peripheral resistance in the vascular bed during dynamic exercise, there is an increased intra-arterial blood pressure during exercise in young, healthy subjects. The aortic systolic pressure will reach about 175 mm Hg, but the increase in diastolic pressure is usually less than 10 mm Hg.[6,34] In older normotensive individuals the systolic pressure may go up to about 225 mm Hg.[3] Arm exercise and static work will elevate the blood pressure more than dynamic exercise.

A working knowledge of the variables inherent to the Fick formula is requisite for an understanding of the concepts to be developed in this review. Therefore the following brief summary of some specific issues is provided.

Oxygen Content in Arterial Blood

Acute hypoxia (altitude 4000 m) will reduce the oxygen content of the arterial blood. During submaximal work there is a compensatory increase in the cardiac output (due to an elevated heart rate), but during maximal efforts the cardiac output is not different from control values. There is no mechanism which allows a more efficient utilization of oxygen in the blood, and therefore the maximal oxygen uptake and physical performance will be reduced.[6]

With part of the hemoglobin blocked by carbon monoxide (up to 20%) the oxygen transport at a given submaximal rate of work can be maintained. The heart rate is increased and the cardiac output is at control levels or somewhat higher. During maximal work the oxygen uptake is reduced more or less in proportion to the varied oxygen content of the arterial blood. However, with 15% HbCO the cardiac output averaged 5% lower than in the control experiments.[15]

An increased oxygen tension in the inspired air will increase the maximal oxygen uptake and improve the performance.[15,16] Recent studies by Ekblom et al.[15] on nine subjects breathing 50% oxygen in nitrogen at sea level showed an average 12% increase in maximal aerobic power. The cardiac output was only slightly elevated, but the a-v̄ oxygen difference became significantly wider.

With controlled blood loss and reinfusion of red cells the effect of acute variations in hematocrit can be studied. The effect of blood loss is a deterioration of physical performance, which is related to a reduced maximal oxygen uptake. A reinfusion of red cells (equivalent to 800 ml of blood) in subjects who have recovered after blood loss could dramatically ("over a night") improve the maximal oxygen uptake and the performance to supernormal values (in average an increase in $\dot{V}O_2$ max of 9%). In five subjects running at maximal speed which could be maintained for about 5 min the oxygen content of the arterial blood averaged 13% higher after reinfusion of red cells compared with the situation after blood loss. The difference in maximal oxygen uptake was actually about 13% (but the individual variations were rather large). The maximal heart rate and stroke volume respectively were more or less identical in the different experiments.[13]

Stroke Volume

The heart rate during submaximal and maximal exercise can be varied markedly by various drugs. Figure 5 presents data on subjects submitted to submaximal (on bicycle ergometer) and maximal (treadmill) exercise four times: (1) control; (2) after infusion of 10 mg propranolol; (3) after infusion of 2 mg atropine and (4) after double blockade (propranolol and atropine). At a given oxygen uptake the heart rate varied about 40 beats/min, taking the extremes, but the cardiac output was almost similar in the four situations, since stroke volume compensated for the changes in the heart rate. (In the propranolol experiments there was in average 1.5-2 liters/min reduction in cardiac out-

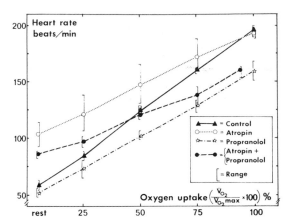

Fig. 5. Relationship between heart rate (means and ranges) and relative oxygen uptake $\dfrac{\dot{V}O_2}{\dot{V}O_{2\,max}} \times 100$ in five sets of experiments (four subjects) during normal conditions (control) and after blockade. Resting heart rate was recorded in the sitting position.[14]

put.) It should be noted that the subjects reached their normal maximal oxygen uptake despite a reduction in maximal heart rate from 195 to about 160 beats/min. The performance time was significantly shorter after β-blockade and the intra-arterial blood pressure was reduced.[14]

There are large individual differences in stroke volume during exercise. Values range between the extremes of 40 up to about 200 ml. There is an almost proportional variation in maximal cardiac output (8 up to 40 liters/min) and maximal oxygen uptake (from about 1 up to 6 liters/min). Genetic factors and the individual's habitual physical activity affect stroke volume. Longitudinal studies have shown that physical conditioning increases the stroke volume, and prolonged inactivity, e.g., bed rest, reduces it.[6,34,36] In one well controlled study[36] the $\dot{V}O_2$max decreased by 28% (mean value) in five subjects bed-ridden for 3 wk (three previously very sedentary subjects and two well-trained ones). This drop was entirely due to a decrease in stroke volume. During 2 mo of daily physical training the maximal oxygen uptake for three of the sedentary subjects increased 33% above the prebed rest control level and it was aportioned about equally between increased stroke volume and a-v̄ O_2 difference. (Their improvement in $\dot{V}O_2$max above the postbed rest control was about 100%!) A 15 to 20% increase in $\dot{V}O_2$max is a common report from training studies.

The lower the starting $\dot{V}O_2$max the greater the increase with physical conditioning. In many

studies the improved $\dot{V}O_2$max was entirely due to an increase in stroke volume, particularly in older subjects, in others up to 50% of the increase in $\dot{V}O_2$max with training was caused by an increment in the a-v̄ O_2 difference, thus supporting the increase in stroke volume.

The maximal heart rate is unchanged or slightly reduced (less than 10 beats/min) during a period of bed rest or physical conditioning, respectively. However, with advancing age a reduction in maximal heart rate occurs in most individuals.

Muscle Mass

Working at maximal rate with one leg on a bicycle ergometer brought in one study[11] the oxygen uptake to 2.4 liters/min. With both legs working the maximum became 3.5 liters/min only, i.e., a relatively small increment.

In swimming with arms only and the legs tied together a well-trained girl swimmer attained an oxygen uptake of 2.7 liters/min, and during swimming with leg kicks (with the arms placed on a cork plate) 3.4 liters/min. In the normal stroke she did not reach 2.7 + 3.4 but "only" 3.6 liters/min.[22] Working with arms and legs simultaneously on two bicycle ergometers increased the $\dot{V}O_2$max by less than 10% compared with maximal leg exercise (see the following).

The purpose of this brief summary is to illustrate that the maximal oxygen uptake (maximal aerobic power) in exercise engaging large muscle groups is apparently not limited by the capacity of the muscle mitochondria to consume oxygen. Slight variations in the volume of oxygen offered to the tissue ($\dot{Q} \times C_{aO_2}$) will produce almost proportional changes in the oxygen consumed. Exercise with the arms (in swimming) as well as with one leg does include some muscle groups which are also engaged in two-leg work. It is remarkable, however, that the combined exercise does not markedly increase the $\dot{V}O_2$max. This finding supports the hypothesis that the central circulation is the limiting factor.

It should be emphasized that a period of physical conditioning will increase the volume of mitochondria in trained muscles increasing the aerobic energy capacity.[21,23] Gollnick et al.[18] have, however, concluded from their studies of enzyme systems in skeletal muscles of untrained and trained men, that the metabolic capacity of both conditioned and unconditioned muscles normally exceed the actual oxygen uptake of the muscles. The increase in enzymes noticed with conditioning also far exceeds the improvement in $\dot{V}O_2$ max.

In prolonged heavy exercise (i.e., hours) the limiting factor may be a depletion of glycogen stores in working muscles and the liver. With training, the energy yield from free fatty acids will become proportionally greater, it will take a longer time to exhaust a given quantity of glycogen stores and performance will be improved. This shift in the metabolic pattern may be a consequence of the changes induced in the enzyme systems by physical training.[6,21]

The conclusion is that it is *the cardiovascular system that imposes the upper limit on oxygen uptake.* At present it is unknown whether cardiac output (central circulation) or the peripheral perfusion is the critical factor limiting $\dot{V}O_2$ max. (For further discussion see Rowell[34] including an analysis of the blood pressure regulation during exercise.)

There are, however, some intriguing findings which do not fit this general scheme. A champion swimmer attained over some years the same $\dot{V}O_2$ max when running on a treadmill, but his maximum when swimming varied in accordance with the intensity of his swim training, and so did his performance when swimming. Two identical twins reached similar $\dot{V}O_2$ max when running (3.6 liters/min), but the sibling who had been in training for swimming attained a 30% higher oxygen uptake (3.6 liters/min!) than her nonswim-trained sister (who some years earlier was a swimmer as successful as her sister).[22] Evidently there is a specificity in the effect of training.

EVALUATION OF PHYSICAL CAPACITY

The conclusions of the preceding review are as follows: (1) All muscle activity demands extra energy, and therefore exercise will impose an extra load on the oxygen transporting system in the body; (2) The oxygen uptake at a given *submaximal* rate of work on a bicycle ergometer or treadmill is very constant even if the work is performed under different conditions (e.g., subjects conditioned or unconditioned, exposed to hypoxia or hyperoxia, hot environment, dehydrated;[6,34] (3) The cardiac output is highly correlated to the oxygen uptake; (4) An individual's $\dot{V}O_2$ max is modified roughly in proportion to the oxygen volume offered to the tissue. Of particular importance is in this context the size of the stroke volume; (5) If due to a change in habitual physical activity there

is an *increase in the stroke volume,* there is *a concomitant decrease in heart rate at a submaximal rate of work;* a decrease in $\dot{V}O_2$ max is almost always accompanied by an increase in submaximal heart rate. Generally speaking, an individual with a high $\dot{V}O_2$ max is characterized by a large stroke volume, and a relatively low heart rate at a given submaximal oxygen uptake. (6) It should be added that prolonged exercise will gradually elevate the heart rate at a given $\dot{V}O_2$ (and cardiac output). The $\dot{V}O_2$ max may be at the control level, but the physical performance is often impaired. In this case the submaximal heart rate response gives a better prediction of the actual fitness than the $\dot{V}O_2$ max.

Conclusion

A measurement of the $\dot{V}O_2$ max gives a very good estimate of the potential of the cardiovascular system. Impaired function of the heart will more likely be evident under a stress test than at rest. The heart rate response to a given submaximal oxygen uptake will in a longitudinal study [limited to some years,[5]] reflect eventual fluctuations in the maximal aerobic power.

ARE THERE ANY NORMAL DATA ON MAXIMAL $\dot{V}O_2$?

Figure 6 presents data on maximal oxygen uptake and its relation to age of the subject. All subjects (most of them were Swedes) were *clinically healthy and relatively well conditioned.* A peak is

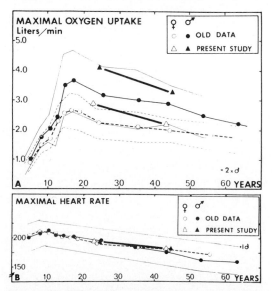

Fig. 6. Maximal oxygen uptake (A) and maximal heart rate (B) from cross-sectional studies on 350 moderately well-trained subjects of 4–70 yr of age. Filled dots males, unfilled dots females. Included are data from a longitudinal study on 66 well-trained subjects ("present study[5]").

attained at age 20 yr and from then on $\dot{V}O_2$ max declines. Part of this gradual reduction in $\dot{V}O_2$ max is due to a decrease in the maximal heart rate, but the stroke volume also decreases with age. It should be noted that individual variations in $\dot{V}O_2$ max are large; the 95% confidence range is about ±40% in this relatively homogenous group of subjects. If we include sedentary subjects and also endurance athletes in such an illustration the scatter will be still more pronounced. From this four important facts emerge.

(1) In our opinion maximal data from a *single* test on $\dot{V}O_2$, cardiac output, stroke volume, and performance (e.g., when running at a given speed or for a given time) do not reveal whether the subject was untrained (physically unconditioned), habitually moderately active, or well trained (excluding the extremes). Consequently it is also rare that one can from these *physiologic* measurements evaluate with certainty whether a relatively poor test result be due to "inferior" endowment, poor physical condition or a disease in the cardiovascular system. The response is similar regardless of etiology. Therefore it is of doubtful value to compare an individual's test score with "normal" data. The question is: What is actually normal for that particular person? The effects on the oxygen transport system of bed rest, physical conditioning, hypoxia, dehydration and disease must include repeated studies with each subject serving as his own control.

(2) When an exercise test is performed for clinical reasons (diagnosis, prognosis) one must at least include measurements of ECG, blood pressure, and register symptoms and signs. It is still better if invasive methods can be included for measurements of intravascular pressures and gas contents and pressures.

(3) The maximal oxygen uptake gives an excellent estimate of the subject's aerobic fitness, i.e., her or his ability to perform a task with the aerobic demands well defined (but a *guarantee* for a good performance cannot be based on only the $\dot{V}O_2$max). Also a submaximal exercise test can yield sufficient information: There is a rule of thumb that a worker involved in manual labor, who is more or less free to set his own pace, normally accepts working with an energy output which is approximately 40% of his maximal aerobic power. During shorter periods of time one can without fatigue work at about 50% of $\dot{V}O_2$ max.[6] Therefore, if an individual can work for at least 5 min with a rate of work demanding an oxygen uptake of 2.5 liters/min (it may be a submaximal load) he can most likely work under steady-state conditions for hours with an oxygen uptake of 1.0 liter/min. Another approach is to let him exercise on a treadmill or bicycle ergometer with an oxygen uptake of 1.0 liter/min (or somewhat higher if this demand is predicted and not measured). If he is free from clinical symptoms and signs, does not feel any fatigue, there is no increase in blood lactate concentration, and the heart rate is low (<120 beats/min), he can probably fulfil a hobby or job which demands an oxygen uptake of 1.0 liter/min. (Work with small muscle groups and static work are, as mentioned, extra demanding.)

(4) As emphasized the oxygen uptake gives important and exact information on the aerobic energy yield and, with less precision, it mirrors the cardiac output. The maximal oxygen uptake, in *liters/min* has therefore a specific meaning.

The individuals potential to move and lift his body is better evaluated when we correct the maximal oxygen uptake for his body size. With a $\dot{V}O_2$ max 2.8 liters/min for a 70-kg man the corrected value will be 40 ml $\times$ kg^{-1} $\times$ min^{-1}. However, we need both figures in our evaluation of the circulatory *and* aerobic fitness. In our opinion there is in the literature too much emphasis on aerobic power corrected for body size. Assuming that our subject will gain 30 kg (fatty tissue) in weight, than his corrected $\dot{V}O_{2max}$ will decrease to 28 ml $\times$ kg^{-1} $\times$ min^{-1}. Definitely his power to lift his body (and therefore to walk or run on a treadmill at an uphill grade) will be impaired. However, his $\dot{V}O_2$ max may still be 2.8 liters/min, and therefore his cardiac output and stroke volume i.e., heart function may not be different compared with the 70-kg situation.

During a period of a year a patient may achieve a 15% gain in $\dot{V}O_2$ max (i.e., from 2.0 to 2.3 liters/min). An increase in body weight from 55 to 64 kg would completely mask this improved circulatory fitness if the maximal aerobic power is expressed in relation to the body weight. Exercise testing is often applied for an evaluation of a surgical or pharmacological treatment of heart disease. Six to 12 mo may elapse between two tests, and the body weight may change more or less markedly.

During adolecense well-trained girl swimmers did improve their $\dot{V}O_2$ max (cardiac output and stroke volume) but a calculation of $\dot{V}O_2$ max per kilogram body weight indicates a reduced fitness, for the increase in body fat is proportionally larger than the improvement in $\dot{V}O_2$ max.

We must differentiate between evaluation of general fitness and cardiac fitness. For a rower and swimmer, not facing any uphill transport, the performance is better predicted from $\dot{V}O_2$ max in liters, but for the runner we need the ml/kg value. Fatty tissue has a very low metabolic rate and blood supply, and there is no reason for including the amount of fatty tissue (which is often a considerable part of the body weight) when we evaluate the cardiac performance. The abscissa should then be the $\dot{V}O_2$ in liters/min, not in ml/kg and per min.

Another way to express the oxygen uptake during exercise is to relate it to the energy expenditure at rest (1 = MET), equivalent to approximately 3.5 ml $O_2 \times kg^{-1} \times min^{-1}$. This new, and quite popular unit has, however, no particular advantage in an evaluation of the cardiac performance (for it includes the correction for body weight). It does *not* directly reflect the total load on the oxygen transporting system and it is therefore *not* well correlated to the myocardial metabolic demand.

It is certainly of interest, both from a physiologic and clinical viewpoint, to relate the maximal oxygen uptake (and cardiac output and stroke volume) to various dimensions (for a discussion see Åstrand and Rodahl[6] chap. 10). We can choose fat-free body weight (lean body mass), heart size (evaluated from roentgenograms), blood volume, total amount of hemoglobin, and other parameters. Such functions, as well as performance tests may be highly correlated to $\dot{V}O_2$ max. The deviation from the regression line is, however, much more critical when it comes to an evaluation of the individual case, than is the correlation coefficient. In fact the prediction of $\dot{V}O_2$ max from the values of the mentioned parameters is loaded with large errors.

In conclusion, there is no single figure or measurement which answers all questions as to state of fitness.

EXERCISE TESTING

In our studies in work physiology, mostly on clinically healthy subjects of both sexes and various ages, we find it as important to measure $\dot{V}O_2$ max as taking record of age, body weight, and height. It is very useful to analyze responses to a submaximal $\dot{V}O_2$ expressed in absolute terms as well as in relation to the subject's $\dot{V}O_2$ max. The question as to which exercise test should be used must be considered.

In the last years there has appeared several publications with discussions on exercise testing in health and disease.[6,9,26,28,32,38-40] The following presents a condensed discussion of basic principles and methodology. (Our personal experience comes from applications of step tests, bicycle ergometer, and treadmill tests.)

Type of Exercise

In laboratory experiments three methods of producing standard rates of work have been applied: Walking or running on a motor-driven treadmill, working on a bicycle ergometer, and using a step test (with or without a hand support). Ideally any test of the oxygen transport system should meet the following minimal requirements: (1) the work in question must involve large muscle groups; (2) the rate of work must be measurable and reproducible; (3) the test conditions must be such that the results are comparable and repeatable; (4) the test must be tolerated by most individuals; (5) the mechanical efficiency (skill) required to perform the task should be as uniform as possible in the population to be tested.

Table 1 summarizes some studies on relatively well-trained healthy subjects submitted to various exercises.

These data are average figures. It should be emphasized that the individual variations are very pronounced. Trained bicyclists usually attain a higher $\dot{V}O_2$ max bicycling than when running. Rowers and canoests may reach a higher $\dot{V}O_2$ in

Table 1. Mean Values for Maximal Oxygen Uptake Attained in Various Types of Exercises.*

Type of Work	$\dot{V}O_2$ max	Reference
Running uphill ($\geqslant 3°$)	100%	6, 19, 20, 25
Running horizontal	95%-98%	20
Bicycling, upright†	93%-96%	6, 19, 20, 25
Bicycle supine	82%-85%	6
One leg, upright	65%-70%	11
Arms (cranking)	65%-70%	6
Arm + legs‡	100%	
Swimming	85%	22
Step test	97%	24, 37

*100% = $\dot{V}O_2$ max during uphill running.

†60 rpm is for most subjects optimum.

‡10%-20% of the total load on the arms; with higher relative load on the arms the $\dot{V}O_2$ max will be lower. Bergh et al: Maximal oxygen uptake during exercise with various combinations of arm and leg work. J Appl Physiol 1976 (in press)

arm exercise than in leg work. It is frequently reported that Americans have difficulties working hard on the bicycle ergometer due to leg fatigue.[32] It is emphasized that they are less experienced cyclists than Europeans. We can, however, conclude that *there is a surprisingly small difference in $\dot{V}O_2$ max in a step test or a test on the bicycle ergometer and treadmill.* Therefore, one can actually choose anyone of them. When studying subjects with physical handicaps the one-leg or arm exercise can be an alternative.

The *treadmill* has an advantage when (1) one wants to establish the highest $\dot{V}O_2$ that a subject can reach in a laboratory test (2) one needs a supplementary information of the work time on a maximal rate of work, (3) one studies children.

During maximal efforts the *bicycle ergometer* imposes more of a leg stress. When testing on an ergometer with a "constant load" (i.e., the power is within certain limits independent of the pedal frequency) the subject must usually stop the exercise when fatigued—he cannot continue to work with reduced pace for the force per push will become too high. Those ergometers which provide a power proportional to the pedal frequency (usually with a mechanical brake) have the advantage that a measurement can be accomplished whilst the subject is working, even if the power as reduced. However, some subjects have difficulties in keeping a preset rhythm and for them the constant-load ergometer is preferable.

Experiments with indwelling catheters and recordings of ECG and blood pressure are more "fool-proof" with a subject on a bicycle ergometer than on a treadmill or stepping up and down.

The *step test* is rather difficult to drive to a maximum. The pace of stepping must be high, and it is always a risk that the subject stumbles when he approaches a maximal rate of work. Secondly, the aftermath is, in the unaccustomed subject, sore muscles. The difficulties in various recordings are, if anything, exaggerated compared with the treadmill experiments.

The motor-driven treadmill is the most expensive equipment; a universally adaptable machine should cover a speed range from 1.5 to 16 km/hr (1–10 mph), and a slope from horizontal to about 20% ($12°;1° = 1.75\%$).

The bicycle ergometer can be electrical (more expensive, must be recalibrated at periodic inter-

vals), or mechanical (rather inexpensive; the rate of work is proportional to the pedal frequency). The subject should in fitness tests exercise in an upright position, and the seat should be almost vertically above the center of the cranks.

The step test can be performed on simple benches and the cost for the equipment is therefore very modest.

When oxygen uptake is not measured it can be predicted from the rate of work on the bicycle ergometer ($\dot{V}O_2$ in liters/min), speed and slope on the treadmill ($\dot{V}O_2$ in $ml \times kg^{-1} \times min^{-1}$), bench height and step frequency on the step test ($\dot{V}O_2$ in $ml \times kg^{-1} \times min^{-1}$). The bicycle ergometer has some advantage in prediction of the $\dot{V}O_2$ due to its slightly lower coefficient of variation.[6,9 (p. 269)] (Of course the $\dot{V}O_2$ can be expressed in any way with the total volume of $\dot{V}O_2$ and body weight are known.) During very severe exercise the predicted oxygen uptake may be too high since anaerobic processes can assist in the total energy yield.

Procedure

An exercise test should be standardized. When all variables are considered we regard the bicycle ergometer and treadmill test superior compared to the step test, and will limit our discussion to these modalities of testing.

A maximal test should always be preceded by submaximal exercise. There is a general agreement that a multi-stage exercise test (the work load is increased at regular intervals until the endpoint is reached) has definite advantages compared with the single-stage procedure (one submaximal and constant rate of work). Figure 7 presents schemat-

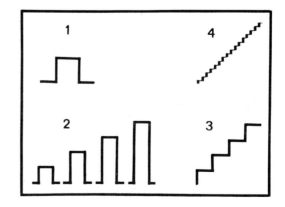

Fig. 7. Various principles for exercise test ("abscissa" = time; "ordinata" = rate of work).

ically the various methods applied in exercise testing.

The Master Two-Step Test[30] is an example of a single-stage, submaximal test, now-a-days considered old-fashioned.

In the *multi-stage tests* the load may be increased step wise with several submaximal, eventually also maximal and "supermaximal" loads; the work time is a minimum of 3 min on each step with (Fig. 7:2) or without (7:3) intervening resting periods. Alternatively, the rate of work may be increased step wise every or every second minute (Fig. 7:4). With the prolonged work time there is a better chance for a steady state, i.e., the oxygen uptake equals the oxygen demand of the tissues. (Examples: in *Bruce's multi-stage treadmill test*[10] there are up to VI stages, each of 4-min duration without resting periods. I: 1.7 mph, 10% grade; II: 2.5 mph, 12%; III: 3 mph, 14%; IV: 4.2 mph, 16%; V: 5.0 mph, 18%; VI: 5.5 mph, 20% grade.) The end point is the individually determined limits of maximal possible or tolerated exertions, or pathological ECG changes of specific significance, or symptoms or signs indicating disease.

In the protocol by Taylor et al.[38] the speed is maintained constant (7 mph), but the slope of the treadmill is increased in steps (0%, 2.5%, 5%, etc.). Work time is about 3 min on each step, and the subject rests inbetween (various length of time— 5 min up to 24 hr or more—depending on project.) This test is rather demanding for the aim is to map out the subject's $\dot{V}O_2$ max.

Balke's test[7] belongs to group 4 in Fig. 7. The speed is maintained constant (usually 3.4 mph) and the grade is increased by 1% per min or in a modified protocol by 2% every second minute.

Nagle et al.[31] have recommended that patients with assumed low maximal aerobic power be started at 2 mph on a zero percentage grade. Speed is then held constant and the grade increased 3.5% every 3 min.

When examining patients the *Scandinavian Committee in ECG Classification*[4] recommended the bicycle ergometer and a step wise increment in rate of work every 6 min. The initial load and the increase in resistance are adopted to the subject's physical fitness.)

At present there are many protocols utilized for exercise testing. Exercise testing was introduced quite recently into clinical physiology and it is therefore natural that "pioneers" have developed their own protocols. It will be difficult to get *one* internationally accepted standard method, and we do not think that this is desirable. The questions behind an exercise test vary; the subject may be a cardiac patient, someone who wants advice before joining a training program, an athlete evaluating his physical condition etc. If the aim of a test is to establish a diagnosis it can be enough with a submaximal stress; if one wants a direct measure of the subject's functional limit it must be brought to a maximum. In research it may be a study of how environmental factors affect various functions, and the measurements involved must be adapted to the specific problems. These factors must inevitably influence the choice of protocol, including exercise time, demand for steady-state conditions etc.

Something may go wrong during an experiment due to technical difficulties, the response from the subject—patient may call for extra attention and therefore, it is a disadvantage to be strictly tied to a rigid protocol. An exercise test is inevitably a compromise with regard to equipment, time available as compared to desirable stress and inconvenience for the subject.

Test Endpoints

For measurements of $\dot{V}O_2$ max the different protocols (Fig. 7), when carefully conducted, are regarded to give the same maximum.[6,8] Froelicher et al.[17] however have recently reported a greater mean $\dot{V}O_2$ max (+7- +10%) with the Taylor protocol compared with the Bruce and Balke protocols. It is an absolute demand in this context that an *objective criteria* is used for an evaluation that the individual's $\dot{V}O_2$ max has really been established (no further increase in $\dot{V}O_2$ despite an increment in rate of work; high concentration of muscle or blood lactates). In well motivated and fit subjects the $\dot{V}O_2$ max is actually attained at a submaximal rate of work—it is not necessary to "exhaust" the anaerobic power also, (Fig. 2). When one leaves the decision to the subject as to endpoints, or stops the work for other reasons (e.g., marked S-T depression) the measured oxygen uptake at that stage should *not* be named "$\dot{V}O_2$ max."

It should be pointed out that subjects with a high maximal aerobic power submitted to the same protocol as unconditioned subjects or cardiac patients will endure the multi-stage test for long periods of time. With a room temperature above 20°C and poor conditions for air movement (no fan) the heat load and heat tolerance and not the $\dot{V}O_2$ max will eventually limit the performance.

Bruce advocates the use of maximal testing even for cardiac patients (with some exceptions), while others believe it is safer to limit the testing to submaximal rates of work. Blomqvist and others (Blackburn[9] p. 281) have reported that the degree of S-T depression, if present in the ECG will increase with higher oxygen uptake (and cardiac output) up to maximum. In testing patients for diagnostic and prognostic purposes it is in our opinion still an open question as to what gain is obtained with a maximal test as compared to the disadvantages of such a test. There may actually appear more so called false-positive cases in the maximal test; the submaximal one may end up with some false-negative cases. But what are the respective numbers?

The Scandinavian Committee on ECG Classification[4] recommended that submaximal exercise testing be terminated at a certain predetermined heart rate: in the age group 20-29 yr at 170 beats/min; 30-39 yr at 160; 40-49 yr at 150; 50-59 yr at 140; 60-69 yr at 130 beats/min. The background for this target heart rate is as follows. The maximal heart rate declines with age (Fig. 6). Mean values are of the order 220 minus the subjects' age in years.[6,9,32] The standard deviation (SD) is about 10 beats/min. Taking 195 minus the age in years as the endpoint means that only one subject out of 200 is taxed to his maximal heart rate (2.5 × 1 SD = 25 beats/min). In average the subjects are working up to about 85% of their maximal heart rate which corresponds to 75%-85% of their $\dot{V}O_2$ max. It is during the interval between 80% and $\dot{V}O_2$ max that lactate concentration rises rapidly thereby producing hyperventilation and fatigue.

It must be remembered that this endpoint is based on mean values and that inter-individual variability is marked. Therefore, in a group of 200 45-yr-old subjects exercised to the target heart rate 150 beats/min (195-45) one of them may be working at maximum, but another one is stopping 50 beats/min from his ceiling (220-45 + 2.5 × 10 = 200 beats/min!)

Considering the wide scatter in maximal heart rates reported in the literature[9 p.285] it is quite meaningless to be very sophisticated in the choice of a target heart rate. Moving it up or down 5-10 beats/min will not help significantly when evaluating the result of an individual test. Again, the SD was ±10 beats/min and therefore the extreme range for the 1% level of significance is 50 beats/min!

The Scandinavian norms are quite simple to remember, and they have passed the test of time. At present there is not any better alternative available for the choice of a submaximal endpoint. (An analysis of the blood lactate concentration after the end of the exercise will give a hint whether the subject was working close to his maximum or not, i.e., whether or not the anaerobic energy yield was significant.)

Another approach is just to simulate on a treadmill or bicycle ergometer the energy demand of the individual's job and/or activity during leisure time (Fig. 1), and note heart rate, ECG, and symptoms. When prescribing a specific training program, its predicted circulatory effects can first be studied in a standardized exercise test simplifying the recordings of ECG and blood pressure. One should in such tests include a reasonable safety margin with regard to the metabolic rate.

Note. Particularly in the testing of patients with cardiovascular disease the termination of the test may be due to discomfort or symptoms like angina, inappropriate dyspnea, severe leg pain, faintness or dizziness, abnormal ECG changes such as successive ventricular beats or ischemic ST-changes, or a systolic pressure that fails to rise or even falls as the rate of work increases.

Measurements

It is advantageous to measure *oxygen uptake* during the test. When using electronic gas analysers care must be taken to correct for water pressure in the expired gas in relation to the gas used for calibration. Otherwise the error may be as large as 25% in the calculated $\dot{V}O_2$!) It takes a minimum of 3 min before a steady state is attained. During *maximal* exercise it is an advantage to do at least two successive measurements. If the second value for $\dot{V}O_2$ does not exceed the first one (difference less than 0.1 liter/min) the maximum was probably reached. With well calibrated bicycle ergometers and treadmills the oxygen uptake can, as mentioned, be predicted from the rate of work. However, during very strenuous work part of the energy demand may be supplied by anaerobic processes. Expressing the work capacity in watts or work time can therefore include both an aerobic fraction loading the circulation *and* an anaerobic fraction with no relation to the heart work.

The energy cost of running (jogging) at a low speed is much higher than when walking (Fig. 3) and therefore it can be a disadvantage to change the speed in the treadmill test. There will be a speed at which some subjects prefer to walk (long legs!) but others will run. The oxygen uptake will be quite different, and it cannot be predicted from the speed alone.

The *heart rate* should be measured at least every minute. In a test for medical reasons the ECG should be monitored (and the paper speed frequently calibrated!).[9,26] In patients with arrythmias (established or suspected) a continuous ECG recording is mandatory.

The *blood pressure* can be measured indirectly with a cuff. The diastolic pressure (at the point where the Korotkow sounds change in character— 4th phase) may be difficult to note. Figure 8 presents data on middle-age people with normal blood pressures at rest.

According to Kitamura et al.[27] there is in young healthy male subjects a high correlation ($r = 0.88$– 0.90) between coronary blood flow and myo- cardial oxygen consumption and the product of the heart rate and systolic blood pressure mea-

sured in the aorta. It should be emphasized that in healthy subjects the systolic pressure measured in a peripheral artery is higher than in the aorta.[29] (This is at least partly due to a distortion in the transmission because of summation of the centri- fugal wave and reflected waves from the periphery. However, in older patients with arterial degenera- tive disease the pressure wave is apparently trans- mitted virtually unchanged.) Secondly, with the blood pressure cuff one is only measuring the pressure energy (side pressure) and not the kinetic energy of the blood, which increases markedly with increased cardiac output. For these reasons it is presently difficult to interpret the significance of the product of heart rate and systolic blood pressure measured indirectly, and its relation to the heart work. The more blood and oxygen the heart can offer the exercising muscles at a given coronary blood flow and myocardial metabolic rate the better the cardiac fitness. Again, the oxygen uptake should be calculated for this evalua- tion in liters/min and not be corrected for the subject's body weight. It should be noted that with physical training the heart rate, and in many cases also the systolic blood pressure decrease at a given total oxygen uptake. This tends to reduce the heart rate—blood pressure product which in turn indicates improved cardiac function.

Blood lactate concentration is a good indirect measure as to how close a subject is working to his maximal aerobic power. A drop of blood taken from the finger tip is enough for the analysis (for method see ref. 2, pp. 14–16). Another sign of a partly anaerobic energy yield is relative hyper- ventilation, i.e. the expired volume of CO_2 exceeds the produced one. Inevitably the *respiratory quo- tient* (the ratio of the volumes CO_2/O_2 in the expired air) will increase, and it may be above 1.0.

At the end of each exercise stage it has proven quite useful to ask the subject about the *subjective rating of perceived exertion*. Borg[28,p.141] has sug- gested a scale consisting of 15 grades from 6 to 20 (7 = "very, very light;" 9 = "very light;" 11 = "fairly light;" 13 = "somewhat heavy;" 15 = "heavy;" 17 = "very heavy;" 19 = "very, very heavy"). In most situations the heart rate mirrors the physical strain experienced subjectively.[12] The questionnaire can be diverted to a rating of general fatigue, leg fatigue, dyspnea etc.

These simple measurements provide good infor- mation about the subject's aerobic power and

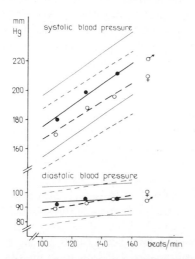

Fig. 8. Systolic and diastolic blood pressure measured indirectly (cuff and mercury manometer) in relation to heart rate during exercise on a bicycle ergometer. Subjects were 103 women (filled lines) and 80 men dashed lines) with normal blood pressures at rest, mean age 55 yr (range 48–63). The thin lines denotes ±1 SD. The average systolic end diastolic blood pressures respectively for dif- ferent heart rate groups are also given (○ = women, ● = men).[3]

heart function. Specific questions demand application of additional more or less complicated methods to be analyzed and answered, but it is beyond the scope of this review to cover that topic.

GENERAL COMMENTS ON THE PROCEDURES

Variability in Test Results

The first time someone is submitted to an exercise test the heart rate may be as much as 10 to 15 beats/min higher than in a second test conducted the next day. The oxygen uptake may also be higher (>0.1 liter/min) at a given rate of work during the first test compared with the second one.[1,9 p.271] The reason for these discrepancies is at least partly emotional involvement with the test procedure and its outcome, and to a smaller extent a function of learning to walk or run on the treadmill or ride the bicycle. In a research project it is therefore important to repeat the initial test and eventually the first test results should be disregarded. Otherwise, when the measurements are obtained under properly standardized conditions the day-to-day variability is very small in $\dot{V}O_2$ max, maximal heart rate, submaximal $\dot{V}O_2$ and heart rate ($\dot{V}O_2$ 2%-4%, heart rate 2-4 beats/min).[6,34]

As previously discussed a change in submaximal heart rate at a standard oxygen uptake is in most situations a consequence of a proportional but reciprocal change in stroke volume. Again it should be emphasized that the oxygen uptake calculated per kilogram body weight in exercise on a treadmill is not directly mirroring the total oxygen uptake, cardiac output, and myocardial function. In longitudinal studies the bicycle ergometer has therefore an advantage compared to treadmill and step tests, for one can from time to time easily expose the same stress to the oxygen transport system (eventually limiting the test protocol to one rate of work). A change in body weight will on a standard treadmill or step test cause a proportional variation in oxygen uptake, and therefore in cardiac output and heart rate (and myocardial metabolism) but the cardiac function in itself may be unaffected.

It has been mentioned that at a given speed on the treadmill running gives a different energy cost than walking. Varying the stride frequency may also change the $\dot{V}O_2$. If the subject supports himself by gripping the hand rail the energy output

will drop. On a bicycle ergometer a change in the pedal frequency may modify the efficiency. If the oxygen uptake is not measured but predicted from the external rate of work it is essential to standardize all these factors in order to keep the variability at a minimum.

Work Time

When measurements are important during submaximal exercise it is advantageous to perform studies during steady state (oxygen uptake = oxygen demand) or near steady-state conditions (Fig. 7: 2 and 3). In a continuous procedure (Fig. 7: 3) 3 min per stage may be sufficient. With traditional methods for determination of the oxygen uptake the collection of expired air takes at least 1 min during mild exercise and a total of 3 min will eventually not be sufficient. These protocols also give better flexibility in the procedure, and one can compare test results even if the work time is varied to allow for more or less time consuming measurements. In the multi-stage, steady-state test one can by interpolation calculate heart rate and other parameters at any oxygen uptake within the range studied. The drawback of increased time with a protocol designed to obtain steady state conditions can be compensated for by reducing the number of stages necessary to load the subject to the target endpoint. If the main purpose of a test is to determine the subject's work tolerance the quicker procedure illustrated in Fig. 7: 4 has advantages.

Work Increment

The clinical examination of the resting subject and the medical history should be the base of information upon which the decision as to type of exercise procedure is made. The initial rate of work and the increase in work intensity should for practical reasons not be similar for severely limited cardiac patients, healthy "normal" individuals, and athletes. The initial load on the bicycle ergometer can be anything from pedaling with no extra friction up to 150 W (900 kpm/min), and the steps from about 25 up to 100 W with the "steady-state" protocol. When increasing the rate of work every minute the steps can be 10 to 20 W (eventually with larger steps at the beginning and smaller steps when it becomes critical). On the treadmill there is some advantages to keep the speed constant and the first stage can be with the belt running horizontally or at a slope. The grade increment may be 1.0%, 2.5%, or 5% per step.

Miscellaneous

In our research on the human being as a "working machine" we often choose a bicycle ergometer to study the response to submaximal exercise but apply a treadmill test when maximal work capacity is a concern. A comprehensive evaluation of a patient should in many cases follow two protocols, i.e. according to the steady-state procedure (Fig. 7: 2 or 3) *and* the quicker, nonsteady-state staircase (Fig. 7: 4).

It should be pointed out that many physical activities in jobs and leisure time are of an intermittent nature. Actually quite heavy work can be performed with moderate stress on the oxygen transport system and little fatigue if the work periods are limited to less than 30 sec with frequent short intervening periods of rest or light activity.[6] During exercise, oxygen stored with the myoglobin can be utilized, and during the interspaced resting periods the oxygen stores can be refilled. Therefore individuals with a relatively low maximal aerobic power can carry out relatively demanding physical tasks if they can adapt it to an intermittent schedule. It is not realistic to simulate an intermittent type of standardized work in a laboratory test. As the demand on the oxygen transport system is less in intermittent work as compared with a continuous exercise at the same rate of work, one is on the safe side when evaluating the individual's potential in the traditional exercise tests.

Precautions

In clinical programs it is a recommended and accepted practice that the exercise test should be supervised by a physician. The risk for serious episodes in connection with the test is very small. Bruce reports[32 p.46] that in over 10,000 multi-stage treadmill tests ventricular fibrillation occurred only twice, once in a normal subject after a hot shower, and once in a patient with angina pectoris immediately after exertion. The mortality rate so far was zero. Myocardial infarction was reported in less than one in 2500 properly selected patients. Others have reported deaths but the statistics are uncertain.

In Sweden several 100,000 submaximal exercise tests have been conducted by nonmedical assistants in unselected, presumably healthy subjects, not submitted to a clinical examination prior to the test, without any reported hazards or accidents. These tests are part of a physical education program under the motto "sport for all!"

Since risks cannot be excluded, a clinical examination should be done prior to testing in all patients. There should be professional monitoring of the ECG during testing, and criteria should be formulated for stopping the exercise. Patients should be discouraged from taking a hot shower or bath within 30 min after the test. During the recovery period it is in some cases better to have the patient sitting on a chair than in the supine position (e.g., in patients with pulmonary hypertension). An emergency plan should be worked out. There should be a ready access to emergency equipment (e.g., for oxygen supply, defibrillator) and appropriate drugs for medical care.[26 p.22]

PREDICTION OF PHYSICAL FITNESS FROM SUBMAXIMAL EXERCISE TESTS

Several methods have been developed to predict maximal oxygen uptake from data attained during submaximal tests. As discussed above there are no measures on the resting individual with a sufficiently high correlation with $\dot{V}O_2$ max for application in such a prediction. Most of these indirect methods are based on the more or less linear relation between the exercise heart rate and oxygen uptake: an extrapolation is made up to the measured or from the subject's age predicted maximal heart rate, and the corresponding oxygen uptake is read on the abscissa. The Åstrands' nomogram[2] has been used quite extensively. It is in fact not based on any sophisticated theories on such relationships but merely on empirical findings. When young men were working at 50% of their $\dot{V}O_2$ max their heart rates were in average 128 beats/min; for women the heart rates were 138. From similar data a nomogram was constructed. A correction factor for older individuals was derived from the quotient between the actually measured $\dot{V}O_2$ max and the predicted one. The maximal heart rates were not considered.

Any prediction of $\dot{V}O_2$ max from submaximal tests has a standard error of estimate of 10%–15%. One source of error is the wide variation in maximal heart rate, and another one the lack of linearity in the heart rate–$\dot{V}O_2$ relationship in many subjects at high rates of work.

As screening tests rough predictions can be made. We usually apply the mentioned nomogram and submit the subject to a work load which demands the predicted $\dot{V}O_2$ max + ca 10% of that value. As the work proceeds there is eventually an adjustment of the rate of work due to the subject's symptoms, degree of exhaustion and breathing rhythm. The aim is to get a work time of 3–5 min. With one submaximal and one maximal load this protocol takes a minimum of time. For patients with more or less continuous arrhythmia no predictions can be made from the heart rate measurements.

SUMMARY

(1) Every type of exercise is in a sense a unique situation. However, all forms of muscular work do increase the metabolic rate and therefore it is of particular interest to analyse the involvement of the oxygen transport system. The oxygen uptake gives an accurate measure of the aerobic power, and it is highly related to the cardiac output. The $\dot{V}O_2$ max is under standardized conditions a highly reproducible characteristic of the individual's aerobic fitness. It is, however, subject to variations under certain conditions (i.e., after prolonged inactivity, after training, as a consequence of cardiac diseases). The main factor behind such variations in $\dot{V}O_2$ max is proportional changes in the stroke volume. Therefore a recording of the heart rate during exercise at a given oxygen uptake will reflect these variations in longitudinal studies. Generally speaking, a high heart rate is usually associated with a low stroke volume. However, from this information it is not possible to tell whether this (poor) exercise response was caused by genetic factors, lack of training, impaired heart function, or other factors.

(2) Data have been presented suggesting that the maximal transport of oxygen (cardiac output × oxygen content of arterial blood) is limited by the central circulation rather than by the tissues' ability to utilize the oxygen.

(3) A multi-stage exercise test on a treadmill or bicycle ergometer will provide a measurement of the rate of work an individual is able to tolerate

without symptoms or electro-cardiographic abnormalities.

(4) For a prediction of the subject's ability to move his body the maximal oxygen uptake per kilogram body weight should be calculated. However, an evaluation of the cardiac performance should be based on the total oxygen transport (liter $\dot{V}O_2$/min), for that is correlated to the cardiac output, the myocardial oxygen consumption and blood flow. Variation in the body-fat content is not followed by similar changes in the dimensions of muscles, heart, blood volume etc., and demands for local blood flow. In other words, in a heterogenous group of individuals the $\dot{V}O_2 \times kg^{-1} \times min^{-1}$ value is *unrelated* to the actual load on their hearts. One good measure of the cardiac performance is the ratio of oxygen uptake/heart rate.

(5) There is not one test protocol ideal for all situations. It is recommended that one adapts the initial rate of work and the increment in work intensity to the assumed maximal power of the tested person. The work time on each stage should if possible be at least 3 min; the larger the increments in rate of work, the longer the work time on each stage. If the main purpose of the exercise test is to establish the $\dot{V}O_2$ max or symptom-limited work tolerance one can apply a nonsteady-state protocol with 1–2 min on each stage.

(6) For the investigator who is willing to accept the small but definite risk involved, a multi-stage test carried to symptom-limited or maximal power will provide the clearest results, particularly for a differentiation between normals and coronary heart disease patients.

(7) It is an alternative to terminate the multi-stage exercise test at a heart rate close to 195 minus the age (years) of the subject. For most individuals that means a submaximal test. The third alternative is to simulate on a bicycle ergometer or treadmill the metabolic rate of the subject's job and recreational activities.

Repeated single-stage or multi-stage tests give excellent measures of variations in physical conditioning (changes in body weight must be considered in a treadmill test).

REFERENCES

1. Åstrand I: The physical work capacity of workers 50–64 years old. Acta Physiol Scand 42:73, 1958
2. Åstrand I: Aerobic work capacity in men and women

with special reference to age. Acta Physiol Scand 49 (Suppl 169), 1960, p 92
3. Åstrand I: Blood pressure during physical work in a

group of 221 women and men 48–63 years old. Acta Med. Scand 178:41, 1965

4. Åstrand I: The "minnesota code" for ECG classification. Adaptation to CR leads and modification of the code for ECG's recording during and after exercise. Acta Med Scand (Suppl 481), 1967

5. Åstrand I, Astrand P-O, Hallbäck I, et al: Reduction in maximal oxygen uptake with age. J Appl Physiol 35: 649, 1973

6. Åstrand P-O, Rodahl K: Textbook of Work Physiology. New York, McGraw-Hill, 1970, p 669

7. Balke B, Ware RW: An experimental study of physical fitness of air force personnel. US Armed Forces Med J 10:675, 1959

8. Binkhorst RA, Leuwen P. van: A rapid method for the determination of aerobic capacity. Intern Z Angew Physiol 19:459, 1963

9. Blackburn H: Measurement in Exercise Electrocardiography. Springfield, Ill. Charles C. Thomas, 1969

10. Bruce RA: Exercise testing of patients with coronary heart disease. An Clin Res 3:323, 1971

11. Davies CTM, Sargeant AJ: Physiological response to one- and two-leg exercise breathing air and 45% oxygen. J Appl Physiol 36:142, 1974

12. Ekblom B, Goldbarg AN: The influence of physical training and other factors on the subjective rating of perceived exertion. Acta Physiol Scand 83:399, 1971

13. Ekblom B, Goldbarg AN, Gullbring B: Response to exercise after blood loss and reinfusion. J Appl Physiol 33:175, 1972

14. Ekblom B, Goldbarg AN, Kilbom Å, et al: Effects of atropine and propranolol on the oxygen transport system during exercise in man. Scand J Clin Lab Invest 30:35, 1972

15. Ekblom B, Huot R, Stein EM, et al: Effect of changes in arterial oxygen content on circulation and physical performance. J Appl Physiol 39:71, 1975

16. Fagraeus L: Cardiorespiratory and metabolic functions during exercise in hyberbaric environment. Acta Physiol Scand (Suppl 407), 1974

17. Froelicher VF Jr, Brammell H, Davis G, et al: A comparison of three maximal treadmill exercise protocols. J Appl Physiol 36:720, 1974

18. Gollnick PD, Armstrong RB, Saubert CW IV, et al: Enzyme activity and fiber composition in skeletal muscle of untrained and trained men. J Appl Physiol 33:312, 1972

19. Hermansen L, Ekblom B, Saltin B: Cardiac output during submaximal and maximal treadmill and bicycle exercise. J Appl Physiol 29:82, 1970

20. Hermansen L, Saltin B: Oxygen uptake during maximal treadmill and bicycle exercise. J Appl Physiol 26:31, 1969

21. Holloszy JO: Biochemical adaptations to exercise: Aerobic metabolism, in Wilmore JH (ed): Exercise and Sport Sciences Reviews, vol I. New York, Academic Press, 1973, p 46

22. Holmér I: Physiology of swimming man. Acta Physiol Scand (Suppl 407), 1974

23. Hoppeler H, Lüth P, Claessen H, et al: The ultrastructure of the normal human skeletal muscle. Pflügers Arch Ges Physiol 344:217, 1973

24. Kasch FW, Phillips WH, Ross WD, et al: A comparison of maximal oxygen uptake treadmill and step-test procedures. J Appl Physiol 21:1387, 1966

25. Kamon E, Pandolf KB: Maximal aerobic power during laddermill climbing, uphill running and cycling. J Appl Physiol 32:467, 1972

26. Kattus AA: Exercise Testing and Training of Apparantly Healthy Individuals. New York, American Heart Association, 1972

27. Kitamura K, Jorgensen CR, Gobel FL, et al: Hemodynamic correlates of myocardial oxygen consumption during upright exercise. J Appl Physiol 32:516, 1972

28. Larson LA: Fitness, Health, and Work Capacity: International Standards for Assessment. New York, Macmillan, 1974

29. Marx HJ, Rowell LB, Conn RD, et al: Maintenance of aortic pressure and total peripheral resistance during exercise in heat. J Appl Physiol 22:519, 1967

30. Master AM, Rosenfeld I: The two-step test: Current status after twenty-five years. Mod Conc Cardiovasc Dis 36:19, 1967

31. Nagle FS, Balke B, Baphista G, et al: Compatibility of progressive treadmill bicycle and step tests based on oxygen uptake responses. Med Sci Sports 3:149, 1971

32. Naughton JP, Hellerstein HK, Mohler IC: Exercise Testing and Exercise Training in Coronary Heart Disease. New York, Academic Press, 1973

33. Pugh LGCE: Air resistance in sport with a note on the effect of altitude, in International Symposium on Exercise and Sports Physiology. Patiala, India, Oct. 1974, p 38

34. Rowell LB: Human cardiovascular adjustments to exercise and thermal stress. Physiol Rev 54:75, 1974

35. Saltin B, Åstrand P-O: Maximal oxygen uptake in athletes. J Appl Physiol 23:353, 1967

36. Saltin B, Blomqvist G, Mitchell JH, et al: Response to submaximal and maximal exercise after bed rest and training. Circulation 38 (Suppl 7), 1968

37. Shephard RJ, Allen C, Benade AJS, et al: Standardization of submaximal exercise tests. Bull WHO 38: 765, 1968

38. Taylor HL, Buskirk E, Henschel A: Maximal oxygen uptake as an objective measurement of cardio-respiratory performance. J Appl Physiol 8:73, 1955

39. World Health Organization Report Series: Exercise Tests in Relation to Cardiovascular Function: Report of a WHO Meeting. No. 388, 1968

40. Zohman LR, Phillips RE: Medical Aspects of Exercise Testing and Training. Intercontinental Medical Book Corporation, New York, 1973

Age Changes in Myocardial Function and Exercise Response

Gary Gerstenblith, Edward G. Lakatta, and Myron L. Weisfeldt

AS the average life span and the number and proportion of our population older than 65 years of age increases, knowledge of the normal physiology of aged individuals becomes more important. There were 21 million Americans 65 years of age or older in 1972 and the number is expected to increase to 24 million, or more than ten per cent of the population by 1980.[1,2] Of this number, approximately one in four is hospitalized each year.[3] Cardiovascular disease is the most frequent reason for these hospitalizations, and cardiac disease alone accounts for more than 40% of the deaths in this age group.[3]

It is important to establish norms for cardiovascular function of the aged before conclusions can be drawn with regard to effects of pathologic conditions, but studies of aging present several obstacles. One is the lack of an easily obtainable, appropriate animal model. Most common mammals, with the exception of the rat, have life spans of at least 8-10 yr.[4] Thus, aged animals are scarce and expensive. It must be certain that one is studying aging, i.e., changes which occur after reaching adulthood, rather than changes due to growth and development. Therefore, fully grown, adult individuals must be compared with senile individuals. Cross-sectional and longitudinal studies are used to examine aging. Both types of studies have certain disadvantages. In a cross-sectional study, groups of individuals of different ages are studied at one time, and any differences among the groups are attributed to the aging process. In such a study it is difficult to eliminate genetic or environmental differences between groups. Also, as a result of lack of survival of some of the individuals to senility, the older groups studied may represent a select, long-lived subset of the younger population. A longitudinal study examines the same individuals as they age. Obviously a prolonged time is required for human studies, and in animal studies the subject cannot be sacrificed. In addition, there may be time-related drifts in methodology that cannot be differentiated from age changes. In any study of aging, the participants should be as nearly free of disease as possible. This requirement can present great difficulties in studies of the cardiovascular system in man because of the prevalence of atherosclerosis. For example, more than a quarter of all coronary artery disease in some age groups may remain undetected by routine history and physical examination.[5,6]

Stress is a common tool employed in studies of cardiovascular aging because it allows quantification of the limits of an individual's physiologic function. However, those parameters dependent upon cardiovascular function may not be easily separable from those dependent on other systems. An aged population may not be able to exercise as long or as hard as a younger one because of limitations of the respiratory or neuromuscular, rather than the cardiovascular system. Finally, the functional importance of the phenomenon recorded must be considered. If a given parameter changes with age, it is necessary to examine whether this change is physiologically significant enough to influence the individual's performance capacity. As an example, the activity of a specific enzyme

From The Department of Medicine, The Johns Hopkins University School of Medicine and Hospital, Baltimore, Md. and The Gerontology Research Center, National Institute of Aging, NIH, Baltimore, Md.

Supported in part by USPHS Grant HL 15565.

Reprint requests should be addressed to Myron L. Weisfeldt, M.D., 508 Blalock Building, The Johns Hopkins Hospital, 601 N. Broadway, Baltimore, Md. 21205.

may decrease with age, but if this enzyme is not the rate-limiting step, this finding may have no functional significance.

In this presentation, the available information describing age changes in the cardiovascular system of man at rest and during exercise will first be summarized. Emphasis will be placed on information that may indicate the presence or absence of physiologically important changes in the function of the heart and of the peripheral circulation. Secondly, studies of cardiac muscle structure and function in aged animals will be discussed in the light of possible mechanisms for age-associated alterations in the response of the heart to exercise. Thirdly, age changes in the peripheral circulation will be examined. Interrelationships between age changes in the peripheral vessels and cardiac function will be emphasized. Although it is not possible to reach final conclusions, some perspective of the problem areas can be gained.

CARDIOVASCULAR AGING IN MAN

Resting State

Although age changes are more pronounced with stress, several parameters of cardiovascular function measured at rest do show aging changes.

Noninvasive studies have indicated a prolongation of mechanical systole and isovolumic diastole in the aged. Strandell[7] compared the interval between the first and second heart sounds in a group of men 61–83 yr of age with that in a group 21–25 yr of age. The average value for the older group, 345 msec, was 11 msec longer than that of the younger group, but this difference was not statistically significant. In another study, left ventricular ejection time, measured from carotid pulse recordings and corrected for heart rate and blood pressure, was estimated to increase 2 msec/decade.[8] However, other studies have shown no change in ejection time with age but have described an increase in the preejection period and therefore, in the $Q-S_1$ and $Q-S_2$ intervals.[9–13] The major change observed in a 10–14-yr, longitudinal ballistocardiographic study of 65 clinically healthy subjects was a decrease in the I and J waves, indicating a diminished acceleration of ejection. Starr and Hildreth concluded that "as the heart grows older, it lifts its load more slowly."[14] Harrison and associates[13] found that the isovolumic relaxation time, measured from the carotid incisura to the onset of outward precordial movement and corrected for heart rate, increased by

40% between the third and ninth decade. This was ascribed to a slower rate of ventricular relaxation.

Although these studies indicate prolonged contraction and relaxation times in aged, unstressed individuals, it is unclear whether these findings reflect intrinsic differences in myocardial function or alterations in work load, impedance, or properties of other tissues. Alterations in the relative stiffness and degree of fibrosis of the aortic and mitral valves with age[15] could alter the timing of valve motion and, therefore, the phonocardiographic assessment of mechanical systole. The carotid pulse is dependent upon a pressure-induced, lateral displacement of the arterial wall, which itself stiffens with age. The rate of transmission of the pulse to the carotid would be more rapid in the older individual with stiffer central arteries. Since the apexcardiogram records low frequency chest wall movements, it would be affected by the properties of the cartilage, bone, muscle, and skin layers between the sensor and the moving ventricle. The ballistocardiogram would also be altered by any age changes in the compliance of vessel walls and body tissues. Therefore, although these techniques provide useful information in an individual patient with cardiac pathology, they are not likely to provide an adequate assessment of age changes in cardiac muscle function and contractility in large groups of participants.

Resting heart rate does not vary with age in man.[16] The electrocardiograms of healthy male subjects otherwise show[17–21] small but significant increases in the P-R, QRS, and Q-T intervals, a decrease in the amplitude of the QRS complex, and a leftward shift in the QRS axis with increased age.

Invasive studies have shown that resting cardiac output determined by Fick or dye dilution techniques and stroke volume decline with age.[22–25] In a group of 67 male subjects between the ages of 19 and 86 yr, cardiac output was estimated to fall an average of 1% a year from a mean of 6.49 l/min in the third decade to 3.87 l/min in the ninth.[22] Stroke volume fell from 85.6 ml to 60.1 ml over the same time period. In a different study, cardiac output averaged 7.89 l/min in ten young, healthy male subjects, and in another, 5.85 l/min in 17 healthy male subjects 60–83 yr of age.[23] Unfortunately, the two age groups were studied at different times. These results have been interpreted as indicating a decline in resting cardiac function with age. However, this may not be the correct explanation. Since the mean pulmonary artery pressure was less in the older group,[23] a difference in preload resulting from differences in peripheral factors—rather than an intrinsic alteration in cardiac performance—probably accounts for this age difference. In addition, there was no age difference in resting cardiac output or stroke volume in this same study[23] when the subjects were in the sitting position. Furthermore, the validity of using measurements obtained with pulmonary or brachial artery catheters in place to describe "resting state" function is subject to question. In a less stressful situation, Proper and Wall[26] measured cardiac output and stroke volume by precordial counters following intravenous injection of labeled material. They reported no age-associated changes in either parameter in a group of 500 men 20–70 yr of age.

In summary, measurements of pump function of the heart obtained at rest do not show any striking changes with age. There are some minor changes in the electrocardiogram. Noninvasive techniques have indicated prolonged isovolumic diastolic and systolic time periods and possibly delayed relaxation. Invasive studies have shown a small decline in stroke volume that accounts for the decline in cardiac output, since heart rate remains constant. This decline in cardiac output at rest does not appear to reflect a limitation in cardiac contractile function.

Exercise

Although age differences in cardiovascular parameters measured at rest are often difficult to interpret, it is generally agreed that the ability of the cardiovascular system to respond to stress clearly and significantly decreases with advancing age. Dock[27] has compared this phenomenon to the aging of visual accommodation. Presbyopia is characterized by functional changes that become apparent under the stress of near vision. Similarly, the predisposition to the development of cardiac arrhythmias and failure when the aged heart is stressed has been called "the essence of myocardial aging" and has been termed "presbycardia."[28]

One of the earliest reports of a reproducible, objective measurement of the cardiovascular response to exercise with aging was reported by Master and Oppenheimer[29] in their original description of the two-step test. The maximum number of steps that could be climbed in a $1\frac{1}{2}$-min period, and the pulse, and systolic blood pres-

sure return to preexercise levels within 2 min were determined. It was found that men reached a maximum of 3795 foot-pounds of work at 27 yr of age, which declined to 2250 foot-pounds at 74 yr of age. The values for female subjects were 2950 foot-pounds at 24 yr of age and an estimated 1700 foot-pounds at 74 yr of age.

Information as to the limits of an individual's performance capacity requires prolonged exercise to the maximum attainable. The cardiovascular system supports this performance by taking up and distributing oxygen to the working muscles. A standardized, accurate measure of this ability is the maximal oxygen consumption ($\dot{V}O_{2\,max}$). This value for any individual is not altered by increasing the percentage of inspired oxygen or by adding other muscular work when more than 50%–60% of the muscle mass is being exercised.[30] Therefore, maximal oxygen consumption is not thought to be influenced by respiratory factors or to be limited by the ability of muscle to extract oxygen. These observations were made in younger individuals. Final conclusions with regard to the mechanism of age-associated decreases in $\dot{V}O_{2\,max}$ will depend upon documentation that ventilation is not limiting in aged individuals. Such information is not presently available.

Robinson's studies of age changes in oxygen consumption during exercise revealed that after a 2–5 min, exhausting treadmill run, $\dot{V}O_2$ declined from a mean of 3.53 1/min for men at a mean age of 24.5 yr to 1.71 1/min at a mean age of 75 yr.[31] Although the experimental procedure has been criticized,[32,33] subsequent studies have confirmed age-related decreases in maximal oxygen uptake for both physically active and inactive men and women (Fig. 1).[25,34–47] In a longitudinal study, Astrand and associates[36] compared maximal oxygen uptake in physically active men and women whose age range was 20–33 yr at the time of entrance into the study. After a 21-yr interval, $\dot{V}O_{2\,max}$ fell by approximately 20%. The extent of the age-associated decline in $\dot{V}O_{2\,max}$ is influenced by physical conditioning, smoking, and obesity. Robinson and associates,[42] in a longitudinal study, found a 25% decline in $\dot{V}O_{2\,max}$ in men from the ages of 18–22 to 40–44 yr. However, long-term physical conditioning coupled with elimination or reduction of cigarette smoking and a reduction in body weight enabled a subset of this group to increase their $\dot{V}O_{2\,max}$ an average of 11% during an ensuing 5-yr period. Thus, although

duration of active state[75] and since aged myocardium has been reported to have a decreased catecholamine content,[76,77] it might be hypothesized that depleted catecholamine stores in aged myocardium account for the prolonged contraction duration. To examine this possibility, trabeculae carneae were studied under control conditions and after the addition of 1×10^{-6} M d-1-propranolol to the bathing fluid. This concentration of propranolol was sufficient to result in a 50% reduction in the response to 1×10^{-6} M norepinephrine. The results of these studies are shown in Fig. 9. A statistically significant prolongation of contraction duration was again present under control conditions and after blockade with propranolol. In addition, the muscles were studied after depletion of tissue catecholamines with 6-hydroxydopamine using the technique of Roberts.[78] With this regimen, catecholamines were depleted by 95% in control animals and by 97% in the aged group. Following catecholamine depletion, there was again no age difference in either active tension or dT/dt at L_{max}, and the prolongation of contraction duration persisted (Fig. 10). Thus, it appears that the mechanism responsible for active state prolongation in aged myocardium is not related to catecholamine content.

Prolonged active state may indicate a prolonged presence of calcium at the troponin site. This could result from either a higher affinity of the

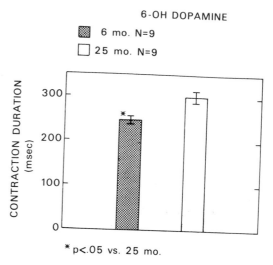

6-OH DOPAMINE

*p<.05 vs. 25 mo.

Fig. 10. Contraction duration in muscles from 6- and 25-mo-old rats that have been previously depleted of myocardial catecholamines with 6-hydroxydopamine. The prolongation of duration in the muscles from the 25-mo-old group persisted after depletion.

troponin for calcium or from delayed calcium removal from the contractile proteins because of decreased function of the relaxing system. If prolongation of contraction also occurs in the intact working heart and specifically occurs with age in intact man, this could account at least in part for the age-associated increase in pulmonary capillary wedge pressure noted during exercise in aged subjects in the reclining position. Prolonged contraction duration or a prolonged duration of systole, particularly at rapid heart rates, may compromise the diastolic filling period and thus lead to an elevation of left atrial pressure. Should this prolonged contraction duration be great enough to result in incomplete relaxation between beats at rapid rates,[51,79] left ventricular end-diastolic pressure might also be elevated and end-diastolic fiber length might be shorter on the basis of prolonged contraction duration in the older human subjects. It should be emphasized that even from the point of view of studies of isolated rat heart, this is only one of a number of mechanisms that may explain the elevation in filling pressure with exercise. Other explanations will be presented subsequently.

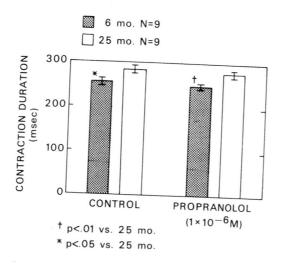

† p<.01 vs. 25 mo.
* p<.05 vs. 25 mo.

Fig. 9. Contraction duration in muscles from 6- and 25-mo-old rats before and after addition of 1×10^{-6} M d-1-propranolol to the bathing fluid. Prolonged contraction duration in the muscles from the older rats persisted after addition of propranolol.

Response to Stress

It has been previously mentioned that the cardiac response to stress is markedly diminished with advanced age. The mechanisms which enable the myocardium to increase its performance when confronted with stress are mediated via an increase in heart rate, the Frank–Starling mechanism, and an increase in contractility. Maximal heart rate is clearly decreased with age, but it is unclear whether the pathologic changes present in the cardiac impulse formation system (see previous discussion) are etiologically related to this phenomenon. Although Cavoto and associates[80] did record significant slowing of the rate of rise and the time to 95% repolarization of the action potential of rat atrium before 6 mo of age, no change was found in rats between 6 and 12 mo of age. The fact that there is no age difference in the active length tension curves of the left ventricular trabeculae up to L_{max}[68] suggests that there is no age difference in the ability to utilize the Frank–Starling mechanism to increase performance. The sympathetic nervous system plays an important role in the exercise-associated increase in contractility and heart rate. The fact that some age differences in cardiovascular performance are obliterated by the administration of propranolol[24] suggests the possibility that an age difference in either the elaboration or effectiveness of the sympathetic response to stress may account for the diminished performance of the stressed aged myocardium.

To examine the effect of age on the intrinsic reactivity of cardiac muscle to catecholamines, the inotropic response of isolated rat trabeculae carneae from 6-, 12-, and 25-mo-old rats was examined by Lakatta and associates.[81] As discussed previously, baseline dT/dt and active tension are not age-related. However, the increase in dT/dt (Fig. 11) under isometric conditions was significantly less in the 25-mo-old group than it was in the 6-mo-old group at the same concentration of norepinephrine or isoproterenol. Although the base-line contraction duration was longer in the muscles from the older group, the extent of shortening of contraction duration with catecholamines was similar in muscles from senile and adult animals. The combination of the decreased inotropic response (as indexed by dT/dt) and the similar extent of relative shortening of contraction duration resulted in striking differences in the extent of increase in active tension with catecholamine stimulation. Under conditions of 1.0 mM calcium and a pacing rate of 24 beats/min there was, in fact, no increase in active tension in muscles from the 25-mo-old group at norepi-

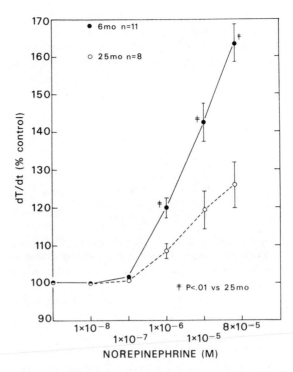

Fig. 11. The effect of age on the response of maximal rate of tension development (dT/dt) to increasing concentrations of norepinephrine. Redrawn from Lakatta et al.[81]

nephrine concentrations up to $1 \times 10^{-5}\ M$; whereas the muscles from 6-month-old rats showed an increase in active tension of $21 \pm 4\%$ and $22 \pm 4.1\%$, respectively (Fig. 12). Some insight into the mechanism responsible for this age change can be gained by examining the two means by which catecholamines are thought to alter active state properties. First, they are believed to shorten the duration of active state by stimulating the cardiac relaxing system.[82] Since contraction duration is shortened equally in the young and aged muscles, it appears that the sequence of events responsible for this effect is intact in aged cardiac muscle. Catecholamines are also believed to increase the intensity of active state[82] by increasing the amount of calcium delivered to the contractile element. As judged by the response of dT/dt, it appears that this effect is diminished in aged muscles. This could be due to either a smaller amount of calcium being delivered to the contractile element in the aged muscle, or to an equal amount of calcium being delivered, but with an impaired contractile element response to the calcium. In order to explore the latter possibility, the effect of age on the inotropic response to increasing concentrations of calcium from 0.5

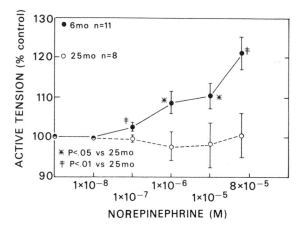

Fig. 12. Effect of age on the response of active tension to increasing concentrations of norepinephrine. Redrawn from Lakatta et al.[81]

mM to 2.5 mM, the concentration at which the maximal response occurs, was also determined. There was no age difference in the increase in developed tension or maximal rate of tension development. These findings indicate that the ability of the contractile element to respond to increased calcium is intact and that the diminished inotropic response to catecholamines in aged myocardium probably results from an impairment in the ability of the catecholamines to increase the amount of calcium delivered to the contractile element.

Oxygen Delivery

Rakusan and Poupa[83] initially suggested that aging is characterized by a progressive obliteration of capillaries within the heart of the rat. These investigators found a decrease in the capillary-fiber ratio in senile rats. The diffusion distance for oxygen was increased to a somewhat greater extent by virtue of myocardial cell hypertrophy in the absence of proliferation of capillaries. Tomanek[84] later repeated similar investigations, but studied both exercised and nonexercised rat. In non-exercised rats, the results of Tomanek[84] are consistent with those of Rakusan and Poupa.[83] There was a lower capillary-fiber ratio and a decreased capillary density in senile rats. After exercise, rats from both age groups had a higher capillary-fiber ratio. Furthermore, following exercise, the capillary-fiber ratio of the senile rats increased to a level equal to the level of the non-exercised adult rats. This increase in capillary-fiber ratio was associated with an increased capillary

density. Thus, these studies suggest that the hearts of animals in the oldest group are not limited with regard to their ability to increase capillarity with increasing demands. However, the increase in capillary-fiber ratio with training in the oldest group can also be attributed to a dropout of myocardial fibers associated with exercise. This possibility is suggested by the studies of Bloor, Pasyk, and Leon,[85] who showed that heart weight decreased with severe exercise in aged rats.

Hypoxia, either on the basis of decreased myocardial capillarity or on the basis of altered diffusion characteristics for oxygen,[86] has been suggested as an important mechanism of age changes in myocardial function. To examine this hypothesis from a functional point of view, the capacity of the coronary vascular bed to deliver oxygen was examined in isolated non-blood-perfused rat heart preparations from 12- and 24–27-mo-old rat hearts.[60] Hearts were perfused in retrograde fashion through the aorta with modified Krebs–Ringer biocarbonate solution at 36°C and at a constant perfusion pressure of 70 mm Hg. The hearts were paced at 220 beats/min. The hearts performed no external work, since a short poly-ethylene tube was placed through the apex of the left ventricle. The drip-off from the heart was taken as the coronary flow. The hearts were subjected to progressive hypoxia, and oxygen extraction and coronary flow were measured. Coronary flows for the adult and senile rat under conditions of maximal hypoxic stimulation to coronary vasodilation are shown in Fig. 13. As shown in the left panel of this figure, the total maximal coronary flow per heart did not differ significantly between animals of these two age groups. When, as shown on the right, coronary flow was normalized for dry heart weight, there was a small but statistically significant difference in coronary flow. The hearts from the oldest age group had a maximal coronary flow per gram dry heart weight that was 8.5% less than hearts from the adult group. The total weight of hearts from the older group was 7.3% higher than the adult group. Thus, these data suggest that there is some hypertrophy of the myocardium associated with age and that this hypertrophy is not accompanied by a concomitant increase in the size of the coronary vascular bed. This study suggests that there may be a relative but not an absolute decrease in the functional size of the coronary vascular bed of the entire heart with age. Oxygen extraction was

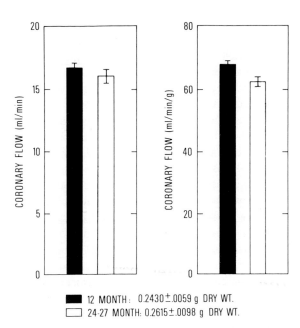

■ 12 MONTH: 0.2430±.0059 g DRY WT.
□ 24-27 MONTH: 0.2615±.0098 g DRY WT.

Fig. 13. Coronary flow at constant coronary perfusion pressure in rat hearts subjected to maximal hypoxic stimulus to coronary vasodilatation. Twelve and 24–27-mo-old rats were compared. The maximum coronary flow per heart shown in the left panel is not significantly different between hearts in the two age groups. When coronary flow is expressed per gram dry heart weight (right panel), the coronary flow of the hearts from the older group is 8.5% lower than that of the younger age group. Redrawn from Weisfeldt et al.[60]

measured in the same hearts under the conditions of progressive hypoxia. The hearts from 12-month-old rats were able to extract $86.3 \pm 1.8\%$ of the oxygen presented, and the hearts from the 24 to 27-month-old group were able to extract $86.6 \pm 0.9\%$ (not significant) of the oxygen presented. Thus, these observations do not support the notion that there is a major age change in the delivery of oxygen or essential nutrients to the myocardial cell in association with aging.

At present, there is conflicting evidence with regard to alterations in myocardial oxidative phosphorylation with age. In one study by Gold, Gee, and Strehler,[87] no significant difference was noted in terms of efficiency and respiratory control, or in phosphorylation rates in mitochondria isolated from hearts of senile rats. In the hamster, Inamdar and associates[88] again found no significant difference between young and old animals. In contrast, Chen, Warshaw, and Sanadi[89] found that state-(ADP-stimulated) respiration of myocardial mitochondria declined in rats after the age of 20 mo, and Frolkis and Bogatskaya[90] found higher P/O ratios and less mitochondrial content.

Future studies examining functional and other metabolic correlates of alterations in mitochondrial respiratory function will be important in assessing the physiologic significance of this observation. At present, it is difficult to conclude that alterations in the coronary vasculature, oxygen extraction ability, or oxidative phosphorylation account for major functional changes in the heart with age.

Myocardial Compliance

In addition to changes in the active contractile properties of aging cardiac muscle, there is considerable evidence to suggest that there are alterations in the passive compliance, or stiffness properties of the ventricle. The stiffness of rat left ventricular trabeculae carneae has been evaluated in terms of the resting length–tension curve and the time course and magnitude of stress relaxation (fall in resting tension at constant length). Resting force was normalized for cross-sectional area, and resting length-tension curves were compared.[68] The mean cross-sectional area from the adult and senile muscles did not differ significantly. Resting tension was measured during stepwise increases in muscle length. Initially, the length of the muscle at zero resting tension (L_0) was determined. Then the length of the muscle was increased by 5% at 4-min intervals, and the resting tension determined at the end of a 4-min period allowed for stress relaxation. It was found that resting tension of muscles from the senile rats was significantly greater at lengths equal to or greater than 115% of L_0. The length of the muscles at L_{max} (length at maximal active tension) expressed in terms of per cent of L_0 did not differ between young and old rats. There was significantly greater resting tension in the muscles from older rats at L_{max}.

Using a similar preparation, the magnitude of stress relaxation in resting cardiac muscle was determined. Many tissues show a decrease in tension after a sudden change in length, which decrease is linearly proportional to exponential time. It was found that the magnitude of stress relaxation and the rate of decrease of tension with time were greater in muscles from adult rats than in muscles from senile rats. Thus, the muscles from the older animals exhibited less stress relaxation or change in stiffness with time. It is likely that the alterations in the resting length–tension curve were at least in part due to age-associated differences in the magnitude and the extent of stress relaxation. One recent preliminary report suggests

fluence of hypoxia on isolated papillary muscle stiffness and its elastic and viscous components. Circulation (Suppl IV) 48:67 (abs), 1973

75. Rolett EL: Adrenergic mechanisms in mammalian myocardium, in Langer GA, Brady J (eds): The Mammalian Myocardium. J Wiley and Sons, New York, 1974, pp 219–250

76. Gey KF, Burkard WP, Pletscher A: Variation of the norepinephrine metabolism of the rat heart with age. Gerontologia 11:1–11, 1965

77. Frolkis VV, Bezrukov VV, Bogatskaya LN, et al: Catecholamines in the metabolism and functions regulation in aging. Gerontologia 16:129–140, 1970

78. Roberts J: Effect of age on cardiac pacemakers and their reactivity to drugs. Fed Proc 33:459 (abs), 1974

79. Mitchell JH, Linden RJ, Sarnoff SJ: Influence of cardiac sympathetic and vagal nerve stimulation on the relation between left ventricular diastolic pressure and myocardial segment length. Circ Res 8:1100, 1960

80. Cavoto FV, Kelliher GJ, Roberts J: Electrophysiological changes in the rat atrium with age. Am J Physiol 226:1293–1297, 1974

81. Lakatta EG, Gerstenblith G, Angell CS, et al: Diminished inotropic response of aged myocardium to catecholamines. Circ Res 36:262–269, 1975

82. Buccino RA, Sonnenblick EH, Spann JF, et al: Interactions between change in the intensity and duration of the active state in the characterization of inotropic stimuli on heart muscle. Circ Res 21:857–867, 1967

83. Rakusan K, Poupa O: Capillaries and muscle fibers in the heart of the old rats. Gerontologia 9:107–112, 1964

84. Tomanek RJ: Effects of age and exercise on the extent of the myocardial capillary bed. Anat Rec 167:55–62, 1969

85. Bloor CM, Pasyk S, Leon AS: Interaction of age and exercise on organ and cellular development. Am J Pathol 58:185–199, 1970

86. Sobel H, Masserman R, Parsa K: Effect of age on the transvascular passage of I^{131} labelled albumin in hearts of dogs. J Gerontol 19:501–504, 1964

87. Gold PH, Gee MV, Strehler BL: Effect of age on oxidative phosphorylation in the rat. J Gerontol 23:509–512, 1968

88. Inamdar AR, Person R, Kohnen P, et al: Effect of age on oxidative phosphorylation in tissues of hamsters. J Gerontol 29:638–642, 1974

89. Chen JC, Warshaw JB, Sanadi DR: Regulation of mitochondrial respiration in senescence. J Cell Physiol 80:141–148, 1972

90. Frolkis VV, Bogatskaya LN: The energy metabolism of myocardium and its regulation in animals of various age. Exper Gerontol 3:199–210, 1968

91. Templeton GH, Platt MR, Willerson JT, et al: Influence of aging on left ventricular stiffness. Clin Res 23:210A, 1975

92. Tomanek RJ, Taunton CA, Liskop KS: Relationship between age, chronic exercise, and connective tissue of the heart. J Gerontol 27:33–38, 1972

93. Montford R, Perez-Tamayo R: The muscle–collagen ratio in normal and hypertrophic human hearts. Lab Invest 11:463–471, 1962

94. Verzar F: The stages and consequences of ageing of collagen. Gerontologia 15:233–239, 1969

95. Tsuchiya M, Kawasaki S, Masuya K, et al: The effect of age on hemodynamics. Jap J Geriatr 9:364–369, 1962

96. Learoyd BM, Taylor MG: Alterations with age in the viscoelastic properties of human arterial walls. Circ Res 18:278–292, 1966

97. Braunwald E: Regulation of the circulation. II. N Engl J Med 290:1420–1425, 1974

98. Fleisch JH, Maling HM, Brodie BB: Beta-receptor activity in aorta. Variations with age and species. Circ Res 26:151–162, 1970

99. Fleisch JH: Further studies on the effect of aging on Beta-adrenoceptor activity of rat aorta. Br J Pharmacol 42:311–313, 1971

100. Ericsson EE: Age dependent variations in Beta-receptor activity and cyclic AMP in vascular smooth muscle. Acta Pharmacol (Suppl 1) 31:45, 1972

101. Heymans C, Neil E: Reflexogenic Areas of the Cardiovascular System. Boston, Little Brown and Co, 1958, pp 72–82

102. Gribbin B, Pickering TG, Sleight P, et al: Effect of age and high blood pressure on baroreflex sensitivity in man. Circ Res 29:424–431, 1971

103. Parizkova J, Eiselt E, Sprynarova S, et al: Body composition, aerobic capacity, and density of muscle capillaries in young and old men. J Appl Physiol 31:323–325, 1971

104. Cournand A, Riley RL, Breed ES, et al: Measurement of cardiac output in man using the technique of catheterization of the right auricle or ventricle. J Clin Invest 24:106–116, 1945

105. Amery A, Bosseart H, Verstraete M: Muscle blood flow in normal and hypertensive subjects. Am Heart J 78:211–216, 1969

106. Lindbjerg IF: Diagnostic application of the ^{133}Xenon method in peripheral arterial disease. Scand J Clin Lab Invest 17:589–599, 1965

107. Hartley LH, Grimby G, Kilbom ASA, et al: Physical training in sedentary middle-aged and older men. III: Cardiac output and gas exchange at submaximal and maximal exercise. Scand J Clin Lab Invest 24:335–344, 1969

108. Roy CS: The elastic properties of the arterial wall. J Physiol (London) 3:125–159, 1880–1882

109. Aschoff L: Lectures in Pathology. New York, Paul Hoeber, Inc, 1924, p 131

110. Roach MR, Burton AC: The effect of age on the elasticity of human iliac arteries. Can J Biochem 37:557–570, 1959

111. Bader H: Dependence of wall stress in the human thoracic aorta on age and pressure. Circ Res 20:354–361, 1967

112. Gonzna ER, Marble AE, Shaw A, et al: Age-related changes in the mechanics of the aorta and pulmonary artery of man. J Appl Physiol 36:407–411, 1974

113. Yakovlev VM: Some data on the functional state of the arterial system in aged persons. Kardiologiia 11:99–103, 1971

114. Hallock P, Benson IC: Studies on the elastic properties of human isolated aorta. J Clin Invest 16:595–602, 1937

115. Bramwell JC, Hill AV: The velocity of the pulse wave in man. Proc Roy Soc (Series B) 93:298–306, 1922

116. Conway J, Smith KS: A clinical method of studying the elasticity of large arteries. Br Heart J 18:467–474, 1956

117. Abboud FM, Huston JH: The effects of aging and degenerative vascular disease on the measurement of arterial rigidity in man. J Clin Invest 40:933–939, 1961

118. Freis ED, Heath WC, Luchsinger PC, et al: Changes in the carotid pulse which occur with age and hypertension. Am Heart J 71:757–765, 1966

119. Dontas AS, Taylor HC, Keys A: Carotid pressure plethysmograms: Effects of age, diastolic pressure, relative body weight, and physical activity. Archiv Kreislaufforsch 36:49–58, 1961

120. Haynes FW, Ellis LB, Weiss S: Pulse wave velocity and arterial elasticity in arterial hypertension, arteriosclerosis and related conditions. Am Heart J 11:385–401, 1936

121. Wolinsky H: Long-term effects of hypertension on the rat aortic wall and their relation to concurrent aging changes. Morphological and chemical studies. Circ Res 30:301–309, 1972

122. Lansing AI: The Arterial Wall: Aging, Structure, and Chemistry. Baltimore, Williams and Wilkins, 1959, pp 136–160

123. King AL: Pressure-volume relation for cylindrical tubes with elastomeric walls: the human aorta. J Appl Physics 17:501:505, 1946

124. Morozov KA, Koryakin NN: The reactivity of the circulatory system in aged and senile persons. Kardiologiia 12:76–82, 1972

125. Carter SA: In vivo estimation of elastic characteristics of the arteries in the lower extremities of man. Can J Physiol Pharmacol 42:309–413, 1964

126. Busby DE, Burton AC: The effect of age on the elasticity of the major brain arteries. Can J Physiol Pharmacol 43:185–202, 1965

127. Landowne M: The relation between intra-arterial pressure and impact pulse wave velocity with regard to age and arteriosclerosis. J Gerontol 13:153–161, 1958

128. Remington JW: The physiology of the aorta and major arteries, in Hamilton WF, Dow P (eds): Handbook of Physiology. Circulation II. Washington, DC, American Physiological Society, 1963, p 808

129. Peterson LH, Roderick EJ, Parnell J: Mechanical properties of arteries in vivo. Circ Res 8:622–639, 1960

130. Tuttle RS: Age-related changes in the sensitivity of rat aortic strips to norepinephrine and associated chemical and structural abnormalities. J Gerontol 21:510–516, 1966

131. Urschel CW, Covell JW, Sonnenblick EH, et al: Effects of decreased aortic compliance on performance of the left ventricle. Am J Physiol 214:298–304, 1968

132. Salisbury PF, Cross CE, Rieben PA: Ventricular performance modified by elastic properties of outflow system. Circ Res 11:319–328, 1962

133. Walker WE (doctoral thesis): The influence of changes of aortic input impedance on the dynamics of left ventricular performance. Johns Hopkins University, 1975

134. Strandell T: Heart volume and its relation to anthropometric data in old men compared with young men. Acta Med Scand 176:205–232, 1964

135. Sjogren AL: Left ventricular wall thickness determined by ultrasound. In 100 subjects without heart disease. Chest 60:341–346, 1971

136. Maurea, Nqlin G, Sollberger A: Normal heart volume. Acta Cardiol 10:336–361, 1955

137. Meerson FZ: Senile changes in the compensatory cardiac hyperfunction and their experimental prevention. Zh Obshch Biol 23(2):114–118, 1962

138. Alpert NR, Hamrell BB, Halpern W: Mechanical and biochemical correlates of cardiac hypertrophy. Circ Res 34–35 (Suppl II): 71–82, 1974

139. Bing OHL, Matsushita S, Fanburg BL, et al: Mechanical properties of rat cardiac muscle during experimental hypertrophy. Circ Res 28:234–245, 1971

140. Meerson FZ, Kapelko VI: The contractile function of the myocardium in two types of cardiac adaptation to a chronic load. Cardiology 57:183–199, 1972

141. Gunning JF, Coleman HN III: Myocardial oxygen consumption during experimental hypertrophy and congestive heart failure. J Molec Cell Cardiol 5:25–38, 1973

142. Spann JF, Buccino RA, Sonnenblick EH, et al: Contractile state of cardiac muscle obtained from cats with experimentally produced ventricular hypertrophy and heart failure. Circ Res 21:341–354, 1967

143. Kaufmann RL, Homburger H, Wirth H: Disorder in excitation-contraction coupling of cardiac muscle from cats with experimentally produced right ventricular hypertrophy. Circ Res 28:346–357, 1971

144. Pickering GW: High blood pressure. London, JA Churchill, 1955, pp 154–183

Cardiovascular Adjustments to Exercise: Hemodynamics and Mechanisms

Stephen F. Vatner and Massimo Pagani

THE manner in which the intact organism responds to the stress of exercise has intrigued cardiovascular physiologists for the past century. The circulatory adjustments, necessary to meet the extraordinary demands of the working musculature and which begin even before the onset of exercise, remain areas of intense investigation and speculation. These adjustments must take place in almost every organ system of the body and involve all aspects of cardiac and peripheral vascular control, including regulation by the central and autonomic nervous systems. The goal of this review is to discuss many of the compensatory mechanisms that permit the capability for severe exercise, with emphasis on directly measured experimental data radiotelemetered from intact, conscious animals spontaneously running in the field.

NEURAL MECHANISMS

The mediation of the cardiovascular response to exercise, i.e., "exercise stimulus," has been variously attributed to carotid and aortic baroreceptor and chemoreceptor activation, to effects of increased venous return on reflexes originating from the right heart, to metabolic products in muscle producing local and/or spinal reflex changes, and to central neural mechanisms.[1] Neural mechanisms appear to be of great importance in mediating the initial response to exercise, which involves very rapid changes in heart rate and blood pressure. For instance, the time to reach peak tachycardia is prolonged in dogs with cardiac denervation.[2,3] In addition, in men instructed to begin isometric effort at the onset of an auditory stimulus, tachycardia was observed within 0.5 sec.[4,5] This was not considered to be related to changes in respiration or metabolic factors but appeared to be due to a central mechanism resulting in an abrupt inhibition of vagal tone.[4,5]

Reflex adjustments initiated by the stimulation of afferent nerve fibers from the exercising muscles are also likely to play a role in the cardiovascular response to exercise. There is evidence that reflex cardiovascular adjustments originating in the contracting muscles are not mediated by muscle spindle afferents[6] but rather by small myelinated and unmyelinated afferent fibers.[7] In anesthetized animals significant pressor effects (up to 60 mm Hg) occurred in proportion to the tension developed in muscle after stimulating its efferent innervation, which were abolished by administration of curare and augmented by rendering the muscle ischemic.[8] Similar pressor responses with tachycardia were elicited in man during sustained static contraction of the forearm muscles.[9] These studies,[9,10] as well as recent work by Liang and Hood,[11] suggest that afferent neural pathways are stimulated by metabolites in the contracting muscle. Liang and Hood further demonstrated an important role for neural transmission in mediating the increase in cardiac output in the response to tissue hypermetabolism.[11]

Since exercise is accompanied by major cardiovascular alterations, including marked tachycardia, increases in cardiac output and in arterial and

From the Department of Medicine, Harvard Medical School and Peter Bent Brigham Hospital, the Department of Cardiology Children's Hospital Medical Center, Boston, Mass., and the New England Regional Primate Research Center, Southboro, Mass.

Supported in part by USPHS Grants HL 15416, HL 17459, and American Heart Association Grants 73833, 76907, and NASA Grant NSG-2136. S. F. Vatner is an Established Investigator, American Heart Association; M. Pagani is an USPHS International Fellow.

Reprint requests should be addressed to Stephen F. Vatner, M.D., New England Regional Primate Center, 1 Pine Hill Drive, Southboro, Mass. 01772.

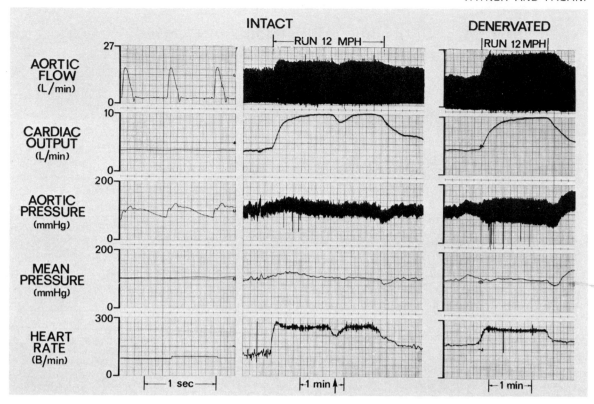

Fig. 1. Responses of aortic flow, cardiac output, phasic and mean aortic pressure, and heart rate to moderate exercise in an intact dog (left panel) and same dog after total arterial baroreceptor denervation (right panel). Note similarity of responses. (Reproduced by permission of *American Journal of Physiology.*[14])

atrial pressures, and a reduction in total peripheral resistance, it could be surmised that a cardio-vascular regulating mechanism as important as the arterial baroreceptor reflex would play a significant role in mediating and modifying the exercise response. Investigations into the role of the arterial baroreceptor reflex in the control of the cardiovascular system during exercise have yielded conflicting conclusions as to their importance. At first it was suggested that the baroreceptor reflex is just as active during exercise as at rest. On the other hand, if the baroreceptor reflex was important during exercise, the occurrence of tachycardia associated with an elevated pressure is opposite to the predicted response, since the baroreceptors should act to restrain heart rate in the face of an elevated pressure. There is now a large body of evidence suggesting the lack of importance of the baroreceptors during exercise. Studies conducted in dogs with and without baroreceptor isolation by Van Houtte et al.[12] revealed little difference in the cardio-

vascular response to exercise in the two groups of dogs, although measurements of cardiac output were made not during but immediately after the cessation of exercise. Krasney et al.[13] also found that the responses of normal and baroreceptor denervated dogs to the stress of moderate exercise were qualitatively similar. More recently, a study was conducted in our laboratory on the effects of more severe exercise in dogs before and after recovery from denervation of both sets of carotid sinus and aortic baroreceptor nerves.[14] In dogs with baroreceptor denervation, although there were minor differences in the preexercise levels of heart rate, arterial pressure, and stroke volume, all these variables rose to levels that were essentially identical to those observed in the dogs with intact baroreceptors during moderately severe exercise (Fig. 1).[14]

Further support for the position that the baroreceptors are of little importance during exercise can be derived from studies by Bristow et al.[15] and Cunningham et al.[16] who observed in man

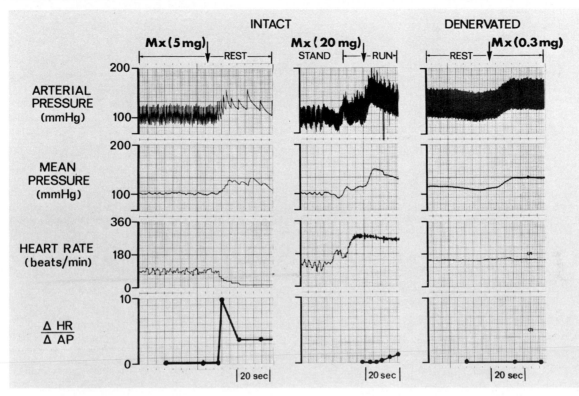

Fig. 2. Responses of arterial pressure, mean pressure, heart rate, and calculated Δ heart rate (HR)/Δ arterial pressure (AP) in an intact dog at rest in response to a bolus of 5 mg i.v. methoxamine (left panel) and to 20 mg i.v. methoxamine in same dog during moderately severe exercise (middle panel) and in a dog with total arterial baroreceptor denervation at rest to 0.3 mg methoxamine (right panel). Note similarity of ΔHR/ΔAP responses in intact dog during exercise and that of denervated dog at rest. (Reproduced by permission of *American Journal of Physiology*.[14])

that baroreflex sensitivity was reduced during exercise. They assessed baroreflex sensitivity by examining the slope of the regression line of systolic arterial pressure on heart rate. Arterial pressure was increased by intravenous injection of a pharmacologic agent, which constricts peripheral vessels and exerts little effect on the heart. Since the slope of the regression line was depressed during exercise, they concluded that the reflex was either reset or turned off during exercise and the magnitude was in proportion to the severity of exercise and resultant tachycardia.[15,16] Similar results were obtained during maximal exercise in dogs, where the vasoconstricting agent was injected remotely by activating a radio-controlled interrogator system connected to an intravenous line in the exercising dogs.[14] Heart rate did not slow appropriately with the sudden elevation of arterial pressure induced by intravenous injection of methoxamine during exercise (Fig. 2), supporting the hypothesis that the arterial baroreceptor reflex

is inhibited during this stress. The mechanism by which arterial baroreflex sensitivity is depressed during exercise is not known. However, it has been shown that this reflex can be profoundly affected by stimulation of a variety of afferent pathways as well as areas within the central nervous system.[17-20]

Another physiologic situation akin to exercise, where the arterial baroreceptor sensitivity is depressed allowing heart rate to rise in the face of elevated arterial pressure, is volume loading.[21] The original observation that tachycardia is induced by volume loading dates back to the work of Bainbridge[22] and has been demonstrated in the intact conscious animal only recently.[21,23] The rapid and large increases in venous return that occur with exercise[24] point further to an important role for the Bainbridge reflex. The mechanism of the tachycardia appears to involve vagal[21,23] and spinal sympathetic reflex circuits.[25-27] The latter mechanism is important to mention, since stimula-

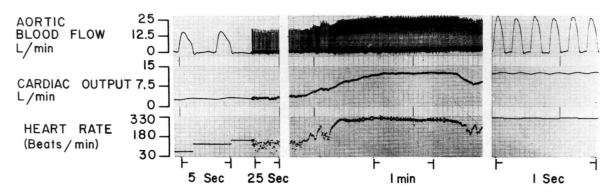

AORTIC
BLOOD FLOW
L/min

CARDIAC OUTPUT
L/min

HEART RATE
(Beats/min)

5 Sec   25 Sec   1 min   1 Sec

Fig. 3. A typical response of aortic blood flow measured and telemetered during severe exercise. The phasic waveforms representing instantaneous stroke volume during exercise at the right played back at fast paper speed can be contrasted to the ones at the left before exercise. (Reproduced by permission of *Journal of Clinical Investigation.*[33])

tion of cardiovascular sympathetic afferent fibers[28] produce cardiovascular reflexes that operate through a positive feedback mechanism,[25] and thus may be partially responsible for the increased sympatho-adrenal activity of exercise. This is opposed to reflex responses initiated by baroreceptors or vagally innervated cardiopulmonary receptors[29,30] that operate through negative feedback mechanisms.

CARDIAC OUTPUT

The major mechanism by which the elevated metabolic requirements of the exercising musculature are satisfied during exercise is through an increase in venous return and in cardiac output. Cardiac output can rise up to fourfold in man[31,32] and fivefold in the dog (Fig. 3).[33] Since the incremental blood flow is proportioned mainly to the exercising muscles, this additional blood flow provides the major capability for performing exercise.

That cardiac output rises during exercise has been documented extensively.[31,32] However, the manner in which the increase in cardiac output is achieved, i.e., either through an increase in heart rate or stroke volume, remains controversial. Moreover, the changes in stroke volume, whether due to enhanced inotropic stimulation or to the influence of the Frank–Starling mechanism, remains a subject under intense investigation. Recent data on these topics will be considered next.

HEART RATE

Heart rate is the predominant mechanism by which cardiac output rises during severe exercise under physiologic circumstances. Of course, in situations where the cardiac rate response is

limited, e.g., heart block, stroke volume plays a much more important role. Heart rate can rise to approximately 200 beats/min during maximal exercise in normal man[32,34,35] and will rise to slightly over 300 beats/min in the dog.[33] Considering the base-line heart rate of human athletes and healthy conscious dogs to be approximately 60 beats/min, it is clear that the major mechanism by which an increase in cardiac output can be achieved is through an elevation of cardiac frequency. Naturally, if base-line heart rate is elevated prior to exercise due to excitement or anxiety, the relative importance of changes in stroke volume becomes apparently greater. This point must be kept in mind in the evaluation of any study in which the relative roles of heart rate and stroke volume are compared.

Heart rate is generally regulated predominantly by the autonomic nervous system. The two major efferent mechanisms by which tachycardia occurs are either through a decrease in parasympathetic restraint or through an increase in sympathetic stimulation. The latter can occur either by neural stimulation or by an elevation in circulating catecholamines. In order to determine the extent to which these mechanisms operate under normal circumstances, exercise has been studied in healthy dogs before and after beta adrenergic blockade with propranolol and parasympathetic blockade with atropine. As mentioned above, heart rate rises to 300 beats/min in the normal dog during maximal exercise. The administration of atropine to these animals increases base-line cardiac rate to approximately 160 beats/min. The difference between that level and the one attained during maximal exercise is on the order of approximately 140 beats/min, which can be attributed to the sympathetic nervous system. Conversely, when propranolol is administered to these animals, resting heart rate is not altered. However, during maximal exercise in the presence of beta adrenergic blockade, heart rate rises to only 160-190 beats/min, which occurs through release of vagal tone confirming that the 110-140 beats/min difference is due to beta adrenergic stimulation. Thus both the sympathetic and parasympathetic arms of the autonomic nervous system play an important role in the regulation of cardiac rate during exercise.

A recent study by Schwartz and Stone provides an interesting concept regarding differential contribution of the right and left sympathetic cardiac innervations in mediating the adrenergic component of tachycardia during exercise.[36] In that study conscious dogs were studied during treadmill exercise after recovery from an operation where either the right or left stellate ganglion was removed. Ablation of the left stellate ganglion did little to the exercise tachycardia, but removal of the right significantly diminished the level of heart rate achieved during exercise, suggesting a more important role in mediating the response.

STROKE VOLUME

Since the classic work of Starling and co-workers[37,38] stroke volume has been assigned a preeminent role in mediating increases in cardiac output under a variety of circumstances, including exercise. It is now clear that Starling was forced to these conclusions from the experimental model that was employed, i.e., the heart–lung preparation. In that experimental model heart rate is already elevated substantially and rarely increases further. Accordingly, increases in cardiac output must occur through elevations in stroke volume.

Rushmer and colleagues challenged these classic views approximately two decades ago.[39] They developed techniques to study circulatory changes in intact conscious animals and found, in contrast to classical concepts, stroke volume was relatively constant even during exercise.[39] Studies conducted later in our laboratory[33] and also by Horwitz et al.[40] revealed that under more severe stress, during near maximal exercise, stroke volume does play a role in the increase in cardiac output, albeit not as great as the one attributed to tachycardia. In dogs running spontaneously in the field at speeds exceeding 20 mph, stroke volume rose

approximately 50% from the preexercise control level in the standing position.[33] However, it is well known that heart rate rises and stroke volume falls upon assuming the upright posture. Thus, when the peak response during exercise is compared to the control response in the supine position, the maximal rise in stroke volume with exercise in the dog is only approximately 25%.[41] In man the contribution of stroke volume appears to be more important.[42-47]

The effects of posture on the response of stroke volume are also important in man.[42] Increases in stroke volume play a greater role during erect exercise as opposed to supine exercise in man.[42-47] However, studies in which a large increase in stroke volume is demonstrated with exercise must be examined carefully to determine if the preexercise control heart rate was elevated due to anxiety or stress, since that would reduce the preexercise control stroke volume. Accordingly, when stroke volume then rose with exercise, its role would be apparently greater and falsely overemphasized.

The role of stroke volume during exercise in man becomes more important with training. It has been shown that cardiac output and arteriovenous oxygen difference during maximal work increase to a slightly greater level after training.[32] While the cardiac output response was greater, the maximal heart rate remains constant and only stroke volume increases by a greater amount.[32] In subjects previously active these changes are less marked than in those that were previously sedentary.[32]

Stroke volume can increase either through a reduction in afterload, an increase in preload, or an increase in the myocardial contractile state. Since the first mechanism (decrease in afterload) does not operate during exercise, stroke volume can increase due to either an increase in preload (Frank-Starling mechanism) or an increase in myocardial contractility. The former would result in an increase in ventricular end-diastolic dimensions, whereas the latter would act to reduce end-systolic dimensions. The importance of each of these mechanisms is discussed next under the ventricular response.

LEFT VENTRICLE

The manner in which the ventricles adapt to the augmented peripheral demands imposed by the

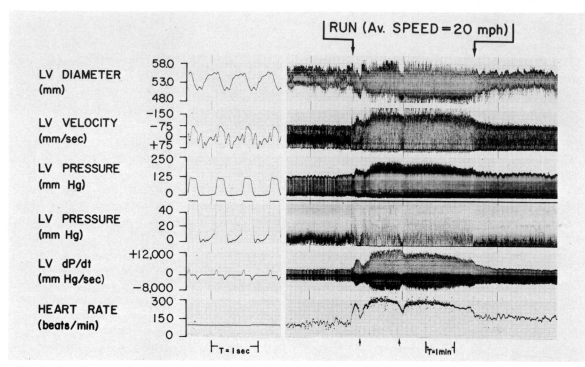

Fig. 4. A typical response to severe exercise for phasic left ventricular diameter (epicardial), velocity, pressure, diastolic pressure, dP/dt, and heart rate. Phasic waveforms at rapid paper speed in the control period (left) can be contrasted with those during severe exercise (right). The arrows denote the time when the dog paused to urinate. Note that end-diastolic diameter fell and then rapidly increased when severe exertion was resumed. (Reproduced by permission of *Journal of Clinical Investigation.*[33])

stress of severe exercise has been controversial and the subject of intense investigation for half a century. In particular, the role played by the Frank-Starling mechanism, i.e., an increase in end-diastolic myocardial fiber length, in mediating the increased contractile response of the heart has been of great interest. This mechanism was at one time considered to be of paramount importance.[37,38,48-50] Then, studies in animals during treadmill exercise[30,51,52] and in man[53-58] demonstrated that end-diastolic dimensions did not increase with moderately severe exercise. However, the level of exercise in earlier studies was not maximal, and it remained to be demonstrated whether increases in end-diastolic size could be elicited with more severe exertion. The development of the capability for telemetry of measurements of left ventricular pressure and dimensions[59] permitted an assessment of the left ventricular response to spontaneous severe exercise without the restraining or excitatory influences of the laboratory environment, leashes, tethers, or treadmills.

A recent study in our laboratory using these techniques indicated that the left ventricular response to severe exercise in healthy dogs running at speeds over 20 mph involved very profound increases in heart rate often exceeding 300 beats/min and increases in contractility, peak dP/dt increasing to fivefold.[33] With this level of exercise a reduction in end-systolic diameter and increases in end-diastolic diameter and pressure were noted (Fig. 4); relative changes were even more prominent when endocardial rather than epicardial dimensions were measured.[33,40] Thus, the Frank-Starling mechanism remains a mechanism by which the heart can augment its performance during severe exertion, although the extent of its application is limited since left ventricular end-diastolic dimensions attained during severe exercise do not exceed those at rest in the reclining position.

The major restraining influence on the increase in diastolic cardiac size during exercise is the concomitant tachycardia, which acts to shorten diastolic filling time. To dissect out the contribution of tachycardia to the exercise response, experiments were repeated after atrial rate had

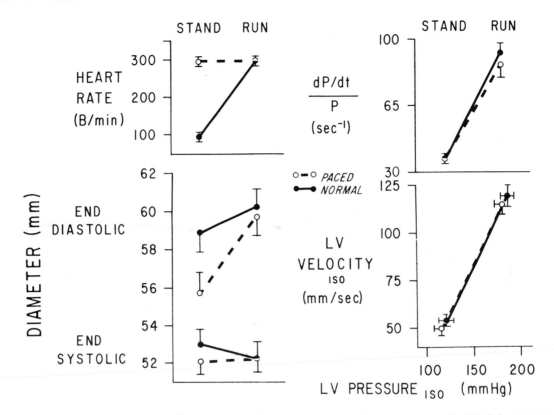

Fig. 5. The average ±SE values standing at rest and during severe exercise for seven dogs studied both in spontaneous rhythm and after heart rate had been elevated at rest to exercise levels with electrical stimulation of the atria. None of the values attained during steady-state severe exercise were significantly different in these two states. (Reproduced by permission of *Journal of Clinical Investigation.*[33])

been elevated in resting dogs and held constant at levels previously achieved during exercise.[33] Under these circumstances, similar increases in pressure and contractility occurred during exercise, as were observed in unpaced dogs, but the increases in end-diastolic dimensions were far greater (Fig. 5).[33] Thus, the major difference in the response to normal exercise, in comparison to exercise when heart rate is held constant at high levels, is the effect on left ventricular dimensions (Fig. 5); far greater increases in end-diastolic size are observed during exercise when heart rate is constant, indicating that the tachycardia which occurs during exercise counteracts the increase in dimensions which would otherwise occur and might be considered to mask the contribution of the Frank–Starling mechanism.

The role of the beta adrenergic system in mediating the ventricular response to exertion has been evaluated by examining the effects of exercise in dogs before and after beta adrenergic blockade

with propranolol (Fig. 6).[33,60] As mentioned above, this maneuver resulted in a significant reduction in the tachycardia that could be achieved. A more striking effect was observed in the inotropic response, where the increases in contractility, as reflected by the force–velocity relationship and by dP/dt, were largely prevented (Fig. 6).[33] Responses of stroke shortening and of stroke volume were also attenuated.[33,60] Thus, these factors that were influenced by beta adrenergic receptor blockade with propranolol imposed significant limitation on performance during exercise, which was most evident during maximal stress.

ABNORMAL VENTRICULAR RESPONSES TO EXERCISE

Heart Failure

The earliest manifestations of heart failure generally occur upon exertion. In the presence of

Table 1. Characteristics of Exercise Devices

Exercise Device	Tests Using Device	Intrinsic or Extrinsic Power Regulation*	Patient Acceptance Factors	Ease of ECG Recording	Considerations of Cost	Calibration for Work Rate Determination
"Two step" stair	Master two step	Intrinsic	Familiar, easy to use for mild exercise	Moderate exercise artifact	Low price, small size	Body weight × trips/minute × height of steps
Single step	Balke (Harvard step test)	Intrinsic	Familiar. Simplest and least costly mode of near maximal and maximal exercise	Moderate exercise artifact	Low price, small size	Body weight × trips/minute × height of step
Escalator	General purpose device	Extrinsic	Familiar and highly acceptable (not commercially available)	Moderate exercise artifact	If available would be relatively expensive and bulky	Body weight × vertical travel/minute (simple to measure)
Bicycle ergometer (conventional)	General purpose device	Intrinsic	Variable familiarity for USA patients. May cause knee pain before cardiovascular endpoint.	Least exercise artifact	Relatively low cost, requires little space	Pedaling rate × preset resistance (simple) plus a small error of estimating the chain and sprocket losses
Bicycle ergometer (regulated)	General purpose device	Extrinsic	Same as above; also regulator action may be disconcerting	Least exercise artifact	Expensive. Moderate space requirement	Moderately difficult to calibrate
Treadmill	General purpose device	Extrinsic	Most familiar form of exercise. Well tolerated.	Moderate exercise artifact	Moderately expensive. Somewhat noisy. Most models require considerable space.	Speed and elevation are simple to calibrate. External work = belt speed × grade × body weight

*See text for details.

diagnostic experiments reserved for only those requiring them.

Exercise Requirements for Stress Testing

The exercise ECG test is a classical example of the tolerance test approach: a particular system normally operates within a very wide range of performance capacity; at low or moderate performance levels a given measure of performance is normal, and abnormal performance is unmasked only when a near maximal or maximal demand is made of the system. Examples of this approach include the assessment of renal tubular secretion capacity,[3] blood glucose regulation capacity,[4] and myocardial perfusion capacity.[5]

Fortunately for man's heart but unfortunately for the sensitivity of the test, obstructive atherosclerotic arterial disease must be well advanced before evidence of reduction in maximal perfusion capacity is detectable; consensus is that obstruction must be $\geqslant 50\%$, and more likely $\geqslant 75\%$, before it will cause symptomatic or electrocardiographic evidence of myocardial hypoxia.[6,7] Because of this enormous reserve in coronary arterial cross sectional area, earliest possible detection of obstructive disease must require that myocardial O_2 consumption be very much increased, so that a disparity between supply and demand for myocardial perfusion will be induced and made detectable. A requirement for near maximal myocardial O_2 consumption, and therefore near maximal cardiac work implies the requirement of a very high cardiac output at increased ejection pressure. Only working muscle can make this magnitude of circulatory demand; brain, skin, gut, and glands' requirements drop from about 79% to around 12% of the total cardiac output during near-maximal exercise.[8]

Effective modes of exercise for test purposes must utilize the largest muscle groups, the antigravity muscles of our locomotion, and should employ as much of the total muscle mass as possible. The impossibility of raising the heart rate as high by cranking with the arms as by pedaling with the legs is due to the lower muscle mass of the arms and shoulders with respect to the legs and back.[9] This consideration is also the most likely explanation for the slightly higher total body O_2 consumption rates attainable on the treadmill in comparison with the bicycle ergometer, which exercises fewer muscle groups.[10]

Since it has been found possible to provoke angina pectoris in some patients by performing a forceful handgrip, the possibility of an improved stress test using isometric, rather than isotonic* exercise has been entertained.[11] However, it was found that isometric stress has its greatest effect on the blood pressure, and causes only modest acceleration of the pulse.[12] The resultant increase in heart rate-systolic blood pressure product, an index of cardiac work stress, is thus much less than the increase possible with isotonic exercise such as running, which markedly raises both heart rate and systolic pressure. This helps to explain the much lower sensitivity of isometric stress tests in detecting ischemic heart disease, as compared with treadmill or bicycle tests.[10,13]

Simulated self transportation has been found the exercise mode of choice for stress testing (Table 1). Only practicability, convenience, and the relative requirement of precision in work regulation limit the mode of this dramatized travel. Perhaps the main differentiating characteristic among the various modes is extrinsic control of work level as opposed to patient control. Climbing steps or pedaling an ordinary ergometer is done at a rate determined ultimately by the subject. If a prescribed level of work is generated, it is due to the effective cooperation of the subject with the laboratory staff. Many subjects do not cooperate well in maintaining a set work rate even when they wish to; poorly motivated subjects of course do worse. The treadmill avoids this dependence of work rate precision on the test subject's skill in cooperating: the subject either maintains his position on the treadmill unaided or he doesn't, and as long as he does so in the same gait his external work performance remains constant. The only two other exercise modes which ensure constant work rate are the stress test escalator, developed at Johns Hopkins University[14] and not in commercial production, and the electronically regulated bicycle ergometer. In the latter, pedaling velocity is constantly monitored, and the resistance to turning is continuously adjusted so that the product of speed and resistance is held constant at the selected level. This ingenious development has short-

---

*No common human exercise is truly isotonic according to the isolated-muscle physiologist's concept of it; however the need for an obvious antonym of isometric exercise justifies using the term *isotonic*.

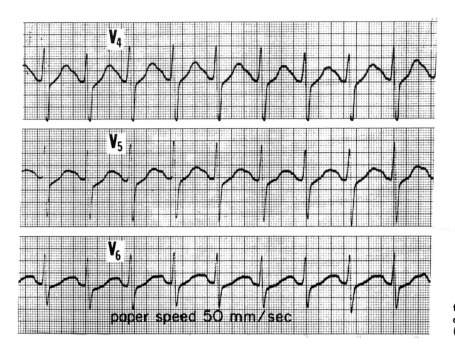

Fig. 3. Stable baseline and freedom from muscle artifact during strenuous exercise (heart rate 170/min).

paste electrolyte (Fig. 5). Platinum-platinum black electrodes are also very stable in this respect, but silver-silver chloride electrodes are much less expensive. It is not universally agreed however that drift-free electrodes should be used for exercise electrocardiography. Such electrodes should be used with electrocardiographic equipment which has "all DC coupling" and whose low frequency response therefore extends all the way to zero oscillations per second. But most investigators in exercise electrocardiography hold that perfect low

frequency response is undesirable in their work because a slight self-centering tendency in the equipment makes it possible to obtain highly legible records with much less difficulty. In other words, the preferred low frequency response happens also to be insensitive to electrode polarization drift. Thus it is reasoned: if the drift caused by stainless steel electrodes is not detected and registered on the graph, why use the more costly and delicate silver electrodes? But the low frequency response must not deviate much from DC, or the ECG wave

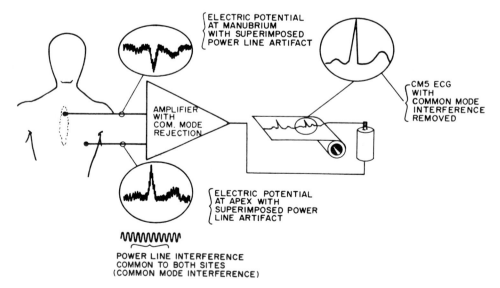

Fig. 4. Illustration of common mode rejection in electrocardiographic recorder.

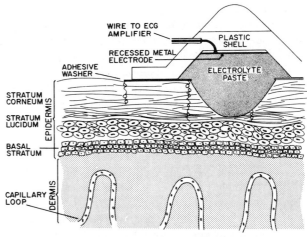

THE ELECTRODE – SKIN INTERFACE

Fig. 5. Illustrating the three principal considerations for obtaining high quality ECG signals: (1) The metal electrode does not make mechanical contact with the skin; (2) The electrode is held in place with adhesive rather than a strap or belt; and (3) The upper horny layer of the epidermis has been removed by abrasion to permit the electrolyte paste to contact the better conducting lower layers of skin.

forms, especially S waves and ST segments, will be measurably distorted as has been shown by Berson and Pipberger[36] (Fig. 6). This pitfall has been taken into account by the AHA Committee on ECG Equipment Standards.[37] Their recommendation requiring at least half-amplitude response at 0.05 Hz is a commendable one.

Additional improvements in exercise ECG quality have come with the use of very light, flexible cables connecting the electrodes of the patient to the ECG equipment. Manufacturers have been slow to satisfy this need, and it is ironic that while they are building computers into their recorders for improving noisy signals, the least noisy patient cables are still the hand made ones described by Grais, Campbell, and Adolph.[38]

ECG Leads

Conventional leads. A wealth of experience has accumulated in the use of the 12-lead "standard" ECG. The first exercise tests used some of these leads, and they have been in use ever since. Mason and Likar[19] made an important change in the limb leads in transferring the limb electrodes to appropriate locations on the torso. This torso modification causes a variable reduction in lead I ampli-

tude, and causes little or no alteration in leads II, III, and AVF. This is a fortunate situation, since lead I is redundant with respect to V_6, and therefore not required in exercise electrocardiography. Because the duration of ischemic ECG changes is known to be very brief in some subjects,[39,6] it is essential to record those leads of greatest diagnostic importance without delay at the end of exercise. If only a single channel electrocardiograph is available, as was usually the case in the past, it is necessary to record the leads with the greatest sensitivity to ischemia first, before the changes disappear. Thus the study of Blackburn and colleagues[40] of relative lead sensitivity to ischemia was of great practical utility as well as theoretic interest. Their now well known findings, that 89% of ischemic responses included abnormal ST depression in lead V_5, indicate that this lead should be among the first to be recorded after exercise. They found that 94% of positive responses were detectable using leads V_{3-6}, and 100% of the positives were detected by the further addition of leads II and AVF. Although this is the best information available on this issue, it unfortunately leaves some questions in doubt. Only ST segment *depression* was examined; ischemia is

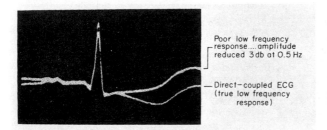

Poor low frequency response....amplitude reduced 3 db at 0.5 Hz

Direct–coupled ECG (true low frequency response)

Fig. 6. Conversion of downsloping ST segment to upsloping by inadequate ECG equipment. Reproduced by permission of *American Heart Journal*.[36]

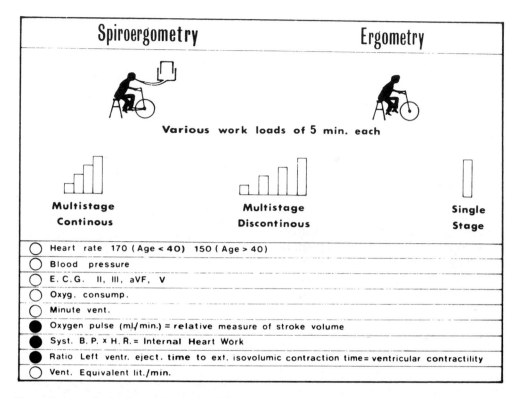

Fig. 1. Shows three methods of exercise testing: The multistage procedure with rest periods between the different work loads; the multistage procedure without rest periods (continuous); and finally the single stage test, based on a former performed multistage procedure. The highest work load reached at a multistage test is applied after a 1-hr test as a sudden, single load. The latter test is used mainly for diagnostic needs in patients with suspected, undiagnosed coronary disease.

oxygen uptake, since we believe such procedures may cause fatal arrhythmia or acute coronary episodes.

PHYSICAL WORKING CAPACITY OF HEALTHY INDIVIDUALS AND PATIENTS WITH CORONARY HEART DISEASE[9,18,76]

The mean normal PWC of healthy adult males is based on a mean body surface of 1.75 sq m and a mean body weight of 70 kg. The values obtained in our laboratories based on at least 100 patients in each category are: 150 ± 10.3 W for men, 18–39 yr old; 125 ± 10.7 W for men, 40–50 yr old; 112.5 ± 10.7 W for men, 51–60 yr old.

For women the normal near maximal physical working capacity is 30% less than in men (Fig. 1).

Less than 0.5% of examinees cannot perform the bicycle test as a result of their technical incapability to ride a bicycle ergometer. Therefore, only occasionally do we use steps and a treadmill. We initially attempted to determine whether or not there is an objective need for interrupting the continuity of the test by introducing breaks between the work loads but found that there were no significant changes at the highest work load reached at a given heart rate (PWC_{150}). The only difference found was a somewhat higher level of lactic acid concentration in arterialized capillary blood during the continuous procedure. In some of the individuals examined during both procedures (continuous and discontinuous), lactic acid levels of over 70 mg/100 ml were obtained in the continuous test.

The parameters recorded during the spiroergometric test are: pulse rate, blood pressure, oxygen consumption, minute ventilation, and electrocardiogram. From these parameters the following are calculated:

(1) oxygen pulse $= \dfrac{\text{oxygen consumption ml/min}}{\text{heart rate/min}}$

(2) ventilation equivalent

$$= \dfrac{\text{minute ventilation} \times 100}{\text{oxygen consumption/min}}$$

(3) systolic blood pressure $\times$ heart rate/min

These data are collected at rest, at various workloads, and after exercise (recovery time). The workloads are measured in W/min or kg/min. The test is started generally with a load of 25 W/min (150 kg/min) at a speed of 50 revolutions/min and raised gradually by 25 W/min. In healthy adults, we start with 50 W/min increments. Each phase of work is of 5-min duration, after which a 5-min rest period follows.

The spiroergometric test is interrupted, if any of the following occurs: (1) in patients with sinus rhythm, the heart rate exceeds: (a) 170 ± 5 beats/min (PWC_{150}) up to the age of 39; (b) 150 ± 5 beats/min (PWC_{150}) age 40 and above. (2) in patients with atrial fibrillation, the heart rate exceeds 180 ± 10 beats/min; (3) further pathologic changes appear in the electrocardiogram (ST segment depression, arrhythmias, etc.); (4) anginal pain; (5) systolic blood pressure decreases; (6) dyspnea and sweating; (7) heart rate and blood pressure does not increase from work load to work load.

Contraindications.[5,19,77] Exercise, stress testing, and an active supervised or advised rehabilitation program based on increased physical training are contraindicated in the following circumstances:

Absolute contraindications. (1) Congestive heart failure; (2) recent myocardial infarction; (3) decubital angina pectoris; (4) ventricular or dissecting aneurysm; (5) ventricular tachycardia (a) multifocal ventricular ectopic beats; (b) repetitive ventricular ectopic activity; (c) untreated high rate, supraventricular arrhythmia; (6) recent thromboembolic events (pulmonary or other); (7) significant respiratory impairment; (8) acute infections or other acute diseases.

Relative contraindications. (1) Aortic stenosis; (2) marked cardiomegaly; (3) pulmonary hypertension; (4) severe systemic hypertension; (5) significant conduction disturbances: (a) complete A-V block; (b) fixed rate pace makers.

Special precautions should be taken in patients with renal or hepatic insufficiency, severe anemia, uncontrolled metabolic diseases such as diabetes or thyrotoxicosis. In patients with moderate and severe musculoskeletal and arthritic diseases, the use of an exercise test procedure and/or the implementation of a physical training program is not possible.

Functional Assessment of PWC in Healthy Individuals as Compared to Coronary Patients

One of the most interesting conclusions obtained from our data on 2500 exercise test procedures, was that similar physiologic responses to exercise were found in both the control population and the coronary patients if the individuals near maximal working capacity were identical. This similarity is seen only so long as the exercise level is such that lactic acid concentrations in arterialized capillary blood remain below 65 mg/100 ml.

PWC, Heart Rate, Oxygen Consumption, and the Estimated Maximal Oxygen Uptake in Healthy Individuals and Coronary Patients

Figure 2 shows the results of exercise testing in 121 untrained healthy individuals and 195 patients with coronary heart disease. In the age group 40–49, 60 healthy subjects were examined, and the age group 50–59, 61 subjects. The main PWC_{150} for the first group was 125 W or 750 kg/min with a near maximal oxygen consumption of 1660 ml/min and a heart rate of 148 ± 7.9. The second group had a PWC of 112.5 W/min with an oxygen consumption of 1580 ml/min and a heart rate of 141 ± 17.7 min or 30 ml/kg body weight, and 25 ml/kg body weight (corrected for age) which represents a good average of the maximal oxygen intake for these age groups. The PWC of these two groups, expressed in W/min served as the normal capacity for the specific age groups. The second group represents patients after myocardial infarction who underwent the tests to find out whether or not they should return to their previous type of work after an acute attack, and whether they should be restricted from physical activity or be involved with a conditioning program. Thirty-five patients were of the age group 40–49 and 60 patients, 50–59. The mean near maximal PWC in the younger group was 102 W/min, 81% of the norm, and of the second age group 88 W/min, 78% of the norm. The mean near maximal oxygen consumption was 1507 ml/min for the younger and 1250 ml/min for the elder group.

The heart rates reached at near maximal levels were 151 ± 3.8 and 145 ± 5.6; maximal oxygen uptake/kg body weight was 25 ml and 21 ml, (corrected for age). The latter figures are lower than the corresponding values noted in age matched control patients. The third group mentioned here

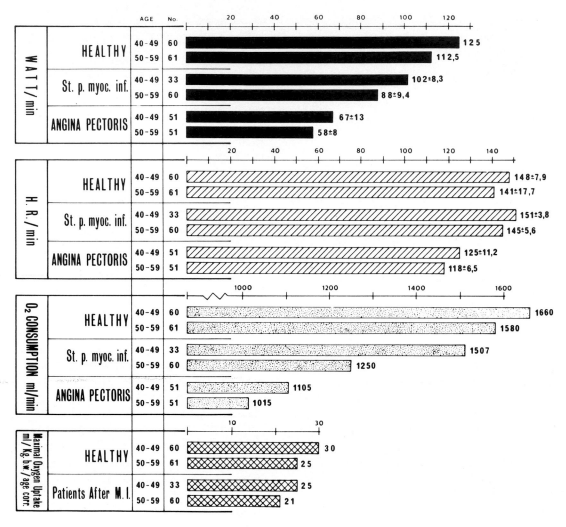

Fig. 2. Physical working capacity, heart rate, oxygen consumption, and estimated maximal oxygen uptake in healthy individuals and coronary patients.

are patients with angina pectoris who were sent mainly for diagnostic exercise tests to evaluate the findings of precordial pain with a normal EKG at rest. There were 51 patients in each age group with this problem. The younger group reached 67 W/min or 54% of the norm, and the elder group 56 W/min or 52% of the norm. The submaximal oxygen consumption was found to be 1105 ml/min and 1015 ml/min.

The mean heart rate obtained at endpoint levels (appearance of anginal pain) was 125 ± 11.2 and 118 ± 6.5. These findings indicate that patients after myocardial infarction, without a physical conditioning program, can reach a fairly high working capacity, and patients suffering from angina pectoris are disabled to a greater degree. We would like to add that the mean values of the lac-

tic acid concentration from the capillary blood were 45–50 mg/100 ml at near maximal levels in healthy individuals as well as patients after myocardial infarction, whereas in the angina pectoris patients, the mean lactic acid value was 25 mg/100 ml.

Metabolic Parameter of Testing Procedure

The lactic acid concentration of arterialized capillary blood was measured before and after ergometric tests. Figure 3 shows the results in 21 healthy individuals and 67 patients with coronary heart disease. As can be seen the postexercise lactic acid values were 45.7 mg/100 ml ± 11.3 in the healthy, and 42.5 mg/100 ml ± 6.9 in the patients with angina pectoris with coronary insufficiency. Here again, a similarity was seen between

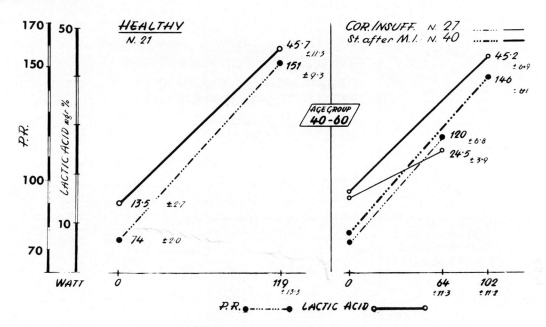

Fig. 3. Mean lactic acid values in submaximal ergometry.

the healthy group and the post myocardial infarction patients. In the angina pectoris group, the lactate levels noted after exercise are much lower due to the low PWC of these patients.

Figure 4 shows the heart rate, oxygen consumption, and the oxygen pulse at rest and after exercise, in healthy individuals and patients after myocardial infarction up to workloads of 100 W/min. It can be seen that quite similar results were obtained in both groups (heart rate for the healthy at rest 77, for the diseased, 80). At 100 W, the heart rate for the healthy patients was 139, for diseased patients, 136. Oxygen consumption was 344 ml/min at rest for the healthy and 317 ml/min in the diseased—for 100 W, 1.507 ml/min for the healthy, 1.433 ml/min for the diseased. The oxygen pulse/min was 1.0 ml/min in the healthy, 4.0 ml/min in the diseased and in 100 W/min 10.8 ml/min for the healthy 10.5 ml/min for the diseased. A further proof of similar findings in different physiologic parameters can be seen in the heart rate × systolic blood pressure product. This index is an indirect measure of myocardial oxygen consumption, (Sarnoff and others)[22] and was calculated before and after the exercise tests, in order to find out whether or not approximately the same near maximal work level (defined mainly by heart rate and endpoint) was obtained.

As shown in Fig. 5, identical results were obtained for the systolic blood pressure/heart rate product in 121 healthy individuals and 195 coronary heart disease patients, indicating that in both the healthy individuals and the postmyocardial patient, without angina, the same results were obtained at the end of the exercise, at heart rate 150, despite the fact that there were different work loads involved. In the angina pectoris group, however, much lower figures were obtained, and this for the reason that the test had to be interrupted at low heart rates (125,118, respectively) because of pain and EKG changes.[21]

In the beginning only light calisthenics, relaxation and breathing exercises involving 2–5 cal/min are introduced. Later uncompetitive ball games and jogging are used, reaching peak levels of 9 cal/min.

Our rehabilitation program (Table 1) starts at least 3 mo after the acute episode, and our experience in the last 12 yr is based mainly on the so-called maintenance phase–rehabilitation program. Initially, we started with small groups of patients. They were mostly welfare cases, who had not returned to work for a period between 1 and 7 yr after the acute coronary illness. Patients were accepted to a dormitory near the hospital, for a term of 4 mo. All had a low physical capacity. Training work started with daily sessions of 10 min in the morning and in the afternoons, in a special garden. By the end of 4-mo period, they attained 4–5 hr work/day in the garden, in addition to occupa-

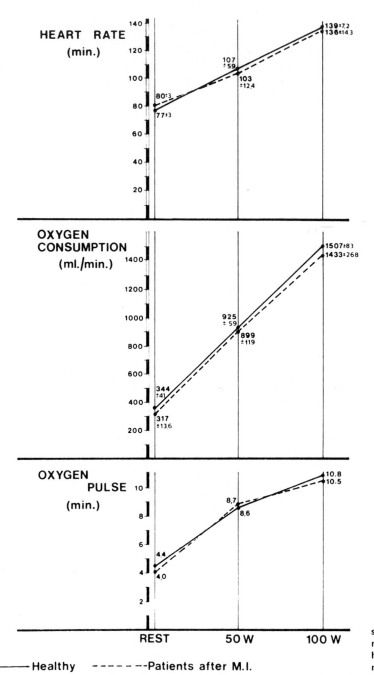

Fig. 4. Heart rate/min, oxygen consumption ml/min, and oxygen pulse/min at rest and after exercise in healthy individuals and patients after myocardial infarction.

——————Healthy   – – – – – –Patients after M.I.

tional therapy and a gymnastics course given three times weekly. While the calorie expenditure at gardening and occupational therapy was between 2-5 cal/min, the exercise program required 2-6 cal/min. All patients were advised to reduce or stop smoking. A low calorie diet was prescribed for obese patients.

Later in the study, we introduced a gradual physical exercise program for ambulatory patients.

These patients had sustained a myocardial infarction and suffered from angina pectoris. They had returned to work on their own initiative, mostly on a part-time basis. The great majority worked at sedentary occupations. They came to the hospital three times weekly during the morning. The exercise program for these groups was based on calisthenics and uncompetitive sport activities. The caloric expenditure was between 2 and 9 cal/min.

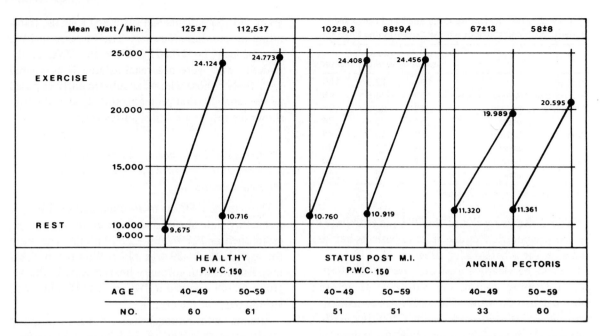

Mean Watt / Min.	125±7	112,5±7	102±8,3	88±9,4	67±13	58±8
	HEALTHY P.W.C.150		STATUS POST M.I. P.W.C.150		ANGINA PECTORIS	
AGE	40–49	50–59	40–49	50–59	40–49	50–59
NO.	60	61	51	51	33	60

Fig. 5. Systolic blood pressure—heart rate product in healthy individuals and coronary patients at rest and after exercise.

Each session at the hospital lasted for 50 min. These groups also participated in a 4-mo training course. At that time we had not decided whether further activity should be supervised, or whether the advice to continue the training would be sufficient to maintain the physiologic and psychologi-

cal achievements or even improve them. Soon we found that, because of the patients' lack of motivation and discipline, they did not continue the various physical activities as recommended; after the 4-mo supervised term 4 months later, a decrease in physical ability was documented. We, therefore, suggested that these programs should be supervised and continuously followed for the rest of the patient's life, if, of course, the patient's clinical and functional condition permits it.[24]

RESULTS

As described earlier, our program started with small groups of patients in a dormitory (welfare cases) and a few outpatients, who came to the hospital three times a week. It is obvious that most of the welfare patients, who did not return to work for many years after the acute coronary episode, had a very low physical working capacity. After a 4-mo training program, which included work in the garden (from 20 min/day to 5 hr/day), in addition to a gymnastic course three times per week and occupational therapy, 85% of these patients returned to work.

The ambulatory patients, who also participated in a 4-mo program, but only in the gymnastic course, (three sessions a week of about 50 min) returned to work on their own initiative, on a part-time basis.

Table 1. Rehabilitation Program

General measures
  Weight control
  No cigarette smoking

Physical measures: Physical training program

Frequency of training: 2–3 times/wk

Duration of each session: maximal 60 min

Method: Interval training

Intensity: Adapted to individual physical capacity peak levels at heart rate 70% of maximal

Caloric expenditure: 2 cal/min–9 cal/min

Clinical measure
  (a) Drug therapy if indicated: (1) Antiarrhythmic (2) Beta blocker (3) Nitrites (4) Antihyperlipemic
  (b) Systematic follow-up examinations clinical and functional reassessment, (3–4 times per year)

Psychological measures
  Group therapy if indicated
  Family counseling

Vocational counselor
  Occasionally

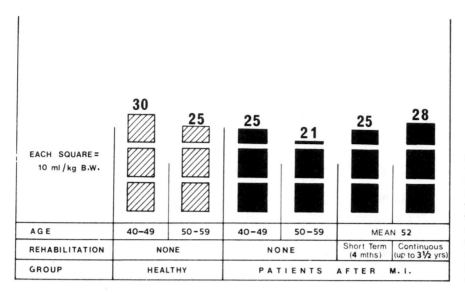

Fig. 8. Shows the maximal estimated oxygen uptake/kg body weight corrected for age in healthy male individuals and patients after myocardial infarction with and without rehabilitation. In patients with angina pectoris no significant elevation in maximal O_2 uptake could be obtained.

Fig. 9. Shows the oxygen consumption/heart beat/min in five patients who underwent a conditioning programme. It can be seen, that for a given work task, there is an increase of the oxygen pulse after training. Example: in case A the oxygen pulse before the conditioning was 7 ml/min and after training of 4 mo, 11 ml/min for the same work load. (Only increases of more than 0.9 ml/min were found to be significant in our series.) The oxygen pulse can be considered as a relative measure of the stroke volume (see Astrand and Rodahl[93]). Therefore the increase in oxygen pulse may indicate an increase in stroke volume for given submaximal work loads.

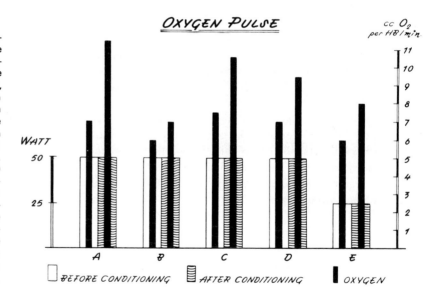

Table 3. Distribution of the Study Group by Sex, Age, and Status of Work

Status of work	Males					Females				
	Age group			Total		Age group			Total	
	<40	41–50	51–64	N°	%	<40	41–50	51–64	N°	%
Returned to the same work	12	63	129	204	77.3	—	6	22	28	80.0
Changed the type of work	7	6	18	31	11.7	—	1	2	3	8.6
Did not return to work	11	2	18	21	8.0	—	1	3	4	11.4
Did not work before	—	4	4	8	3.0	—	—	—	—	—
Total	30	75	169	264	100.0	—	8	27	35	100.0

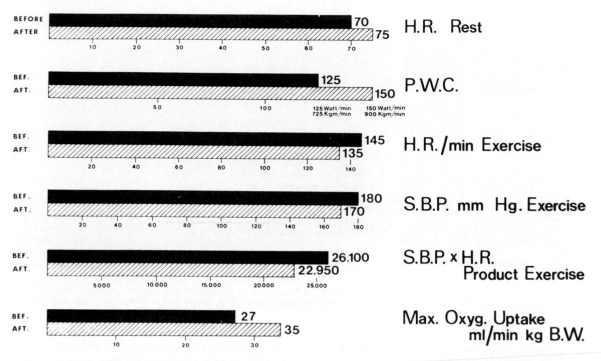

Fig. 10. Shows heart rate physical work capacity (PWC), the systolic blood pressure, the systolic blood pressure heart rate product and the estimated maximal oxygen uptake before and after a 4-yr physical training program in a 48-yr old patient after diaphragmatic myocardial infarction without angina pectoris. It can be seen that the main improvement is in the increase of the estimated maximal oxygen uptake from 27 ml/min to 35 ml/min (age adjusted) and the decrease of the systolic blood pressure times heart rate from 26.100 to 22.950 despite the increase in PWC from 125 W/min, 150 W/min.

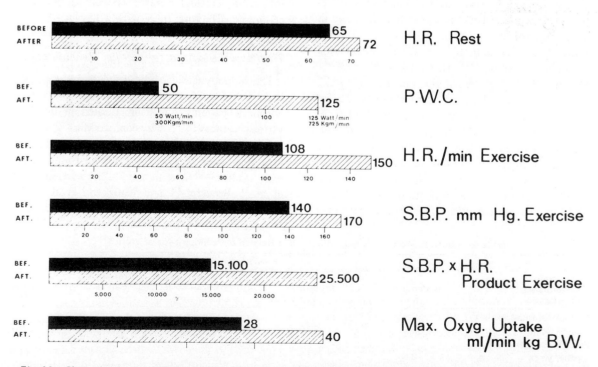

Fig. 11. Shows heart rate (PWC) physical work capacity, the systolic blood pressure, the systolic blood pressure heart rate product, and the estimated maximal oxygen uptake before and after a 4-yr physical training program in a 33-yr old patient with sever angina pectoris. It can be seen that the PWC is increased from 50 W to 125 W/min. The heart rate reached at exercise before the program was 108/min, when the exercise had to be stopped because of significant depression of the ST segment in the EKG. After the program work loads of 125 W at a heart rate of 150/min were tolerated without angina. The improvement in other parameters can be clearly seen from the figure.

that stroke volume is augmented due to more forceful contraction, with end-diastolic fiber length unchanged. Some findings obtained by noninvasive evaluation techniques, indicate that during physical exertion, the sedentary coronary patients may not experience the normally observed decrease of end-systolic and end-diastolic volumes and, therefore, the net result was that the rate of myocardial fiber shortening was decreased during the ventricular contraction. There is not enough evidence that physical training improves the mean systolic ejection rate in the patient with coronary heart disease who suffers from angina pectoris.

These theoretical considerations, notwithstanding the demonstrated physiologic effects of training in coronary patients are:[9-11,21,23-25,35,36,39,40,56] exercise tolerance improves after training; the systolic blood pressure decreases; the heart rate decreases; myocardial oxygen demand is decreased especially by reducing the internal heart work; stroke volume is increased; blood lactate concentration is decreased; muscular blood flow is decreased;

Psychological Results

The psychological evaluations of our patients during the different stages of our studies were done by Wintner[9] with the aid of a battery of tests, such as: Bender Gestalt, Rorschach, Cattels 16 P.F., Draw a Person Test and the Tennesse Self Concept Scale (Fitts tests). These tests showed that there is a marked increase in the emotional stability of the rehabilitated patient. There is a general increase in the total positive statements of the patient. There are highly significant rises in positive statements as regards the physical and family self and the behavioral dimensions. This means that the patients physical self-esteem is elevated. His perception of himself, as a good family member, becomes more positive and he perceives his way of functioning as more active and self-confident. Patients after rehabilitation were found to be more definite and certain in self-esteem and self-respect. They are significantly less confused, contradictive and they have less conflict with self-perception. Others have found that the psychological benefits of a physical training program includes a decrease of anxiety, frustration and depression, when compared with psychological evaluation done prior to these programs. Still we do not know to what extent the physical rehabilitation improves the psychological and/or the physiologic

state of the patient. It seems that there is not always a correlation in the improvements of both aspects. On the other hand, we believe, that the difficulty in the objective evaluation of psychological and/or physiologic improvements per se is the bias. It is rather hazardous to compare groups of patients, who are under constant medical care and are receiving much medical and paramedical attention, to others, who are not under any medical or paramedical regime. It seems impossible to eliminate this bias. It is interesting that the physiologist, Lange Anderson, believes that the most important effect of exercise is psychological rather than physiological.[94] On the other hand, physiologic improvements can be clearly stated. The increase of physical capabilities combined with a subjective feeling of well-being, can affect the patients life at work and at home, by increasing his self-confidence, decreasing his drug-dependency and his absence from work, and thus prove to him, that he is capable (in most of the cases) of leading an active productive life.

THE ROLE OF A COMPREHENSIVE REHABILITATION PROGRAM IN SECONDARY PREVENTION

There is still a lack of evidence that cardiac rehabilitation based on physical conditioning programs have any effect on the prevention of reinfarction and death and therefore can change the destiny of a patient who suffers from coronary heart disease.

To date there are insufficient numbers of studies available capable of answering this crucial question. Before reporting the results of our study in this field, one should take into consideration that, when talking about prevention of a multifactorial disease, it is hardly to be expected that the prognosis of the disease can be changed by involving the factor of physical activity only.

On the other hand supervised rehabilitation programs involve many other risk factors, mainly weight control, treatment of hyperlipemia, strong advice to change smoking habits and a close clinical follow-up.

Well designed studies involving large active and control groups are needed to determine whether or not morbidity and mortality can be reduced by comprehensive rehabilitation programs. It can not be expected that the "pure" effect of exercise can be isolated from all the other factors involved and there will always be a bias, which will interfere with a clear scientific statement, as to the negative or positive influence of prolonged physical training, on the prognosis of coronary heart disease.[52,53]

Our own study (Table 5) involves 194 male patients ranging from 35 to 64 yr, all of whom entered the study following a simple transmural myocardial infarction. The patients did not suffer from hypertension, diabetes, or significant arrhythmia. The number of patients having an anginal syndrome did not differ significantly in the study group and the control group. The patients were divided into three groups: As to the results, Groups I and II could be combined, because they did not continue any form of physical training or supervised and advised rehabilitation program of any kind.

Group I consisted of 92 patients who did not undergo an active rehabilitation program. According to the criteria used for the selection of patients for our rehabilitation program, all of them would have qualified for admission. Eight years later, we reexamined 53 of these patients and collected detailed information on the deaths among all 92 patients.

Group II consisted of 58 patients who underwent a 4-mo rehabilitation program. At the end of these 4 mo we instructed the patients to continue with exercises and walking at home. In the follow-up examinations it was found that these patients did not do any physical training because of lack of motivation, and, therefore, the increase in their physical capabilities achieved during the 4-mo training was lost and their physical working capacity decreased again to the level prior to enrolling in the program.

Group III consisted of 44 patients after myocardial infarction who underwent a training program for at least 30–70 mo. The active rehabilitation program was started at least 4 mo after the acute onset.

In the control group, consisting of 92 patients, 27 patients (29.3%) died of recurrent myocardial infarction. Nine patients (17%) of those examined had suffered a second myocardial infarction. The mean age of this group at their last examination was 61.2 yr, and a mean of 11.9 yr had passed since their first coronary event. For 27 mortalities, the mean time since the first event until death was 8.1 yr.

In the group with the short-term rehabilitation program, 19 (32.7%) of the patients died due to recurrent myocardial infarction, three others died of other causes. The mean age of this group was 58.6 yr at the time of examination and 10.1 yr (mean value) passed since the first coronary event. The mean time since the first event until death was 7.3 yr; four patients suffered from reinfarction (6.8%).

In the group of patients who underwent continuous physical training during a period of 30–70 mo, four patients (9%) died of cardiac cause; three other patients died of cancer. In this group, five patients (13%) suffered a second myocardial infarction. Four of them had a superimposed infarction of the same wall damaged at the first event. The mean age of this group at the time of examination was 56 yr, and 9.6 yr had elapsed since the acute event. The mean duration of time since the first event until death was 7.7 yr. There was no difference in risk factors such as overweight, cholesterol, and smoking in the three groups.

Although the number of participants in our study is low, the findings are encouraging, but of course not conclusive. Rechnitzer et al.[54] found in a 7-yr follow-up that, in 77 patients who underwent physical training programs after myocardial infarction, 58% of the nonexercising controls died a cardiac death. The nonfatal recurrences rate was 3.03% for the exercising groups and 11.11% for the controls in the same period of time.

Another study published by Sanne[55,56] indicated that in a 3-yr follow-up, they could find no statistical difference in the mortality of two groups of patients after myocardial infarction. The patients were selected at random, one group exercising, the other without training.

In trying to clarify the importance of supervised rehabilitation programs as a secondary prevention measure in patients after myocardial infarction, one will find that it is hazardous to compare different groups of patients even though they are properly matched. The most important bias, as we see it, is in fact that the group who is involved in the supervised programs, visits the hospital or the institute, two or more times a week and the psychological impact of such a relationship between the patient and his "belonging" to a medical set-up is tantamount. This relationship gives the patient the feeling of security. Constant medical care and guidance may have an influence on the "life-style" of the patient, as to the change in his habits and often in his behavior patterns. Along with other risk factors to be controlled in such a program, it

Table 5. Morbidity and Mortality

| | Control Group | | | | Physical Conditioning | | | | | | | |
| | Without physical activity | | | | Short term (4 mo) | | | | Continuous | | | |
	N	Alive	Died	Reinfarction	N	Alive	Died	Reinfarction	N	Alive	Died	Reinfarction
N	92	64	27 (+1) 29.3%	9/53 16.9%	58	36	19 (+3) 32.7%	4 6.8%	44	37	4 (+3) 9.0%	5 13.1%
$\bar{x}$ age to day or at death (yr)		61.2 ±2.04	59.5			58.6 ±2.8	60			56.9 ±2.7	55.7	
Time lapse from first myocardial infarction (yr)		11.9	8.1			10.1	7.3			9.6	7.7	

Statistical evaluation: Test of differences between correlated proportions.[97] The difference in mortality between Groups I and II, as compared with Group III was highly significant (p < 0.0001).

seems at least possible, that there may be a prognostic influence of rehabilitation measures, in well selected groups of coronary patients. However, not much has been proved to date and the controversy on this subject is justified.

The Place of Coronary Artery Surgery as a "Rehabilitation Measure"

It is still too early to state definitely whether coronary surgery can prevent infarction in patients with stable or unstable angina. It seems that there is an agreement that, in patients with uncontrolled angina, coronary surgery should be considered. The results of lately published studies show that approximately 85% of the patients who survived the surgical procedure have relief of angina, and 60% have no further chest pain.[95] The results of objective testing after surgery show that the improvement seems to correlate fairly well with the patency of the bypass grafts. Nevertheless, it has been shown that improvement in exercise tolerance was achieved also in patients with nonfunctioning bypasses.

In the United States, the experience in patients after coronary surgery who undergo rehabilitation programs is much greater, and it is to be hoped that the next years will show if and when rehabilitation measures should be undertaken in such patients and whether such undertakings have any influence on the prognosis. As to the indication of transferring patients from rehabilitation programs to coronary surgery procedures, it is our opinion that the patient with constantly increasing angina and decreased exercise tolerance should be considered for surgery. In our experience, this is only a small percentage, approximately 5% of our patient material. Aronow and Stemmer[57] found that, in 40 patients with angina pectoris in which 20 underwent coronary bypass graft surgery and 20 other comparable patients were treated medically, 78% of the surgical patients and 53% of the medically treated had no angina after exercise. One year after the control period, 25% of the medically treated patients and 40% of the surgical patients not receiving digitalis had no postexercise ischemic ST segment depression. The authors suggest that the coronary bypass operation should only be considered if medical therapy fails to relieve disabling angina. Scholer[58] studied the hemodynamic response to exercise (bicycle ergometer) in 40 patients with saphenous vein bypass grafts, in 32 of whom all grafts were open. The most striking find-

ing was that patients with an angiographically normal left ventricle (LVN) and patent grafts, exhibited normal end-diastolic pressure (LVED) even during exercise. In this they differed from unoperated patients with LVN and coronary disease, whose LVED rose abnormally on exercise. In patients with LVN and clotted grafts the same pathologic alterations were observed. All patients with an abnormal ventricle display abnormal LV function even with patent grafts and in this respect do not differ from unoperated patients. Only 4 of 12 patients undergoing pre- and postoperative study showed clearly improved LV function during equivalent work loads, though there was a significant postoperative rise in work capacity in all cases. It seems to us that in the coronary patient with angina pectoris in which the angina cannot be controlled by medical treatment and/or rehabilitation measures coronary surgery should be undertaken. It is worthwhile mentioning that, in patients without functioning grafts, the PWC is sometimes increased after the unsuccessful operation and the anginal attacks are decreased. This phenomenon has been seen in one of our patients and has been reported by a personal communication to us by Caro.[59]

DISCUSSION

There is no definite evidence that physical activity may influence the natural cause of coronary heart disease (CHD). The possibility that physical training may prevent reinfarction and death has been brought up by a number of authors in the past two decades.

Early in the '50s a relation between physical inactivity and the increase in morbidity and mortality of coronary heart disease was found by epidemiological researchers, especially by Morris in the London Busmen Study, 1953[60,61] and his findings were confirmed 20 yr later.[62]

Other epidemiological studies such as by Zukel et al.[63] and others[64-66], showed that the incidence of CHD is less in individuals who are physically active and that an increase in habitual physical activity is beneficial. On the other hand, Keys[67] did not find a correlation between physical habits and CHD incidence.

In an extensive review, Fox and Haskell[68] discussed the pros and cons of their epidemiological research on this subject, and they came to the conclusion that, in primary prevention of coronary heart disease, much more evidence is needed, and many conclusive studies need be undertaken in order to establish whether physical activity can contribute to the prevention of CHD. In this respect, we wish to mention that many authors who are in favor of physical activity programs are referring to the well-documented study on animals by Eckstein[69] which demonstrated an effect of exercise and coronary artery narrowing to the extent that exercise accelerates and develops a coronary collateral circulation. Burt and Jackson[70] in their animal study could not confirm these findings.

As it can be seen, there are many controversies in connection with the influence of physical activity, and, despite the fact that the aforementioned may have a direct implication on primary prevention, we think that one should be aware of the many unsolved problems when discussing rehabilitation based on physical training. Here the crucial question should be asked: What is really achieved in introducing supervised rehabilitation programs?

It has been documented by our studies[9,21,23-25] and those of others[11,35,39,56,71-73] that supervised rehabilitation programs based on physical activities, have a beneficial influence on physiologic and psychological conditions in the coronary patient and this may have a natural impact on socioeconomic aspects.

The question has been raised by some authors[79,80] that the physiologic benefits observed in training programs may be due to placebo effect. Indeed, there are some strong arguments that the physiologic and/or the psychological improvements achieved in rehabilitation programs are due to placebo effect. This effect should never be underestimated and it should not be forgotten that a placebo effect may be stronger than a drug effect. Every clinician has made the observation that, on occasion, unexplained subjective and objective improvements occur in patients with severe coronary heart disease. Other patients have been found to improve their physical capability after an aortocoronary bypass operation and in which the bypass was not functioning. The improvements in the latter patients occasionally reach significance, especially when these patients suffered severe angina pectoris and were almost completely disabled prior to the operation.[58,59]

Only a few studies examined the placebo effect of physical training applied to coronary patients.

In one of these studies published in 1967 by Zohman and Tobis,[80] compressed air was administered by a mask. All the patients improved subjectively; in 50% of the patients there was an improvement in exercise testing, and in 20% there was improvement in EKG changes observed at the same work load. The results were not significantly different from those obtained during a short-term training period. In the study of Zohman and Tobis[80] the individuals included consisted only of patients with angina pectoris. In such a patient population, several testing procedures are needed in order to establish a real base line PWC since physical capabilities may change from day to day.

In another study Bergman and Varnauskas[79] made an attempt to evaluate the placebo effect in patients with coronary heart disease. The study included ten male patients—seven had severe angina pectoris and three had myocardial infarction. The placebo period lasted 4-6 wk, and the patient was given placebo tablets and was seen once a week in the outpatient department. After this placebo period a training period of 4-6 mo duration began. The patients trained for $\frac{1}{2}$ hr three times a week on a bicycle ergometer. After 4-6 wk of the training (as 4-6 wk after the placebo period) and at the completion of the training period, hemodynamic studies were done both at rest and at the work load chosen for each individual patient. The results were as follows: during the placebo period four patients considered themselves improved, five were unchanged, and one became worse. The exercise tests were mostly unchanged and one patient could carry out a higher work load.

Despite some evidence that a placebo effect may be involved, studies published to date have involved small numbers of patients and the reports published on this subject are not convincing. Nevertheless, one should not neglect certain facts which are of great importance in the consideration of the results of any treatment and especially in the patient–doctor relationship in a rehabilitation program. This relationship is a major determinant of placebo effect. In his paper on etiological factors in placebo effect, Shapiro[81] stated: ". . . the more effective the therapy will appear to be . . . this occurs when the patient displaces the interest from the therapy to himself and experiences the physician's interest in his treatment as a personal one. A vast array of psychological factors arise in the patient-physician relationship. Many hopes, ex-

EXERCISE	DESCRIPTION	FREQUENCY per min.	Cal./min.	H.R./min.
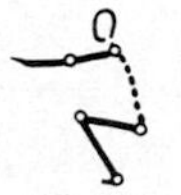	KNEE BENDING	37	7.1	134 ±10
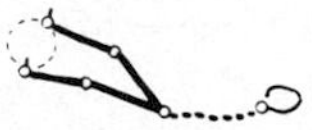	SUPINE CYCLING	50	3.5	104 ±10
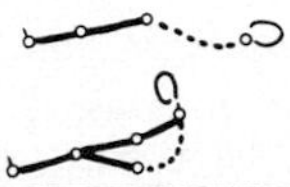	SHOULDER BRIDGE LIFTING HEAD AND SHOULDERS TO TOUCH THE OPPOSITE KNEE WITH THE HAND & VICE VERSA	16	3.3	96 ±9
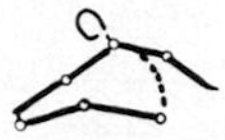	FINGERS TOUCHING THE TOES OF THE OPPOSITE LEG AND VICE VERSA	40	4.9	108 ±13
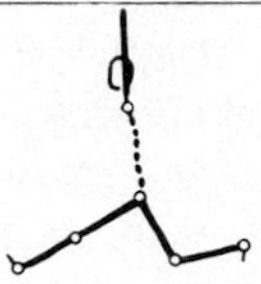	FROM STANDING TO KNEELING WITH THE OTHER LEG EXTENDED TO THE FRONT AND THE ARMS ELEVATED SIDEWARDS	16	6.8	130 ±10
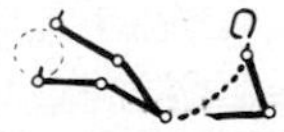	BACK-LYING ON ELBOWS AND CYCLING	20-24	4.8	107 ±13
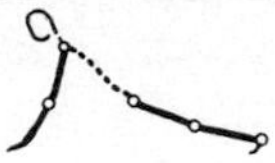	PUSH-UPS * MEASURED FOR 1 min. ONLY	18	4.3*	132 ±12
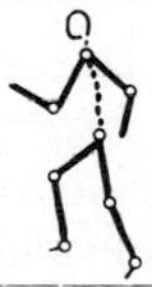	RUNNING ON THE SPOT (ONLY Lt. LEG COUNTED)	80	8.4	135 ±15
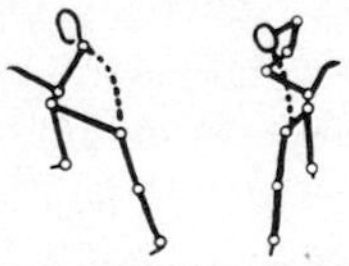	CROSS-OVERS OF Rt. ELBOW TO Lt. KNEE AND VICE VERSA	24	4.1	103 ±12

Fig. 13. Caloric expenditure of exercises.

pectations, fantasies, fears, feelings of guilt and inadequacy, etc., become involved in the relationship and treatment."

Exercise Causing Death

There are arguments indicating that the physical exertion and strenuous exercise may endanger the patient. Indeed, there are a number of reports on exercise causing cardiac death.[82,83] It is natural that the application of uncontrolled exercise even in "healthy" individuals above the age of 35 and of course in all patients with a history of cardiac disease of any kind should be avoided in all circumstances. We strongly suggest the so-called "pharmaco-dynamic concept of exercise."[11] The

indication and contraindication as well as dosage, precaution and signs of toxicity should be strictly observed. Therefore physical training programs should be based on the individual capability of the patient and the type of exercise should be adapted to his physical work performance. The caloric requirements of every program can be measured by open circuit spirometry, a method used during all the years of our program. Figure 13 is one example of our caloric measurements obtained in more than 50 patients after myocardial infarction. Such tables will enable a safe application of a program based upon exact exercise prescription.

Not only the exercises used in the training program should be measured but also actual work performance under field conditions should be determined. This can be done by open circuit spirometry and especially by using dynamic electrocardiography.[84] We have studied the physiologic response to driving in 250 coronary patients and compared the predominant emotional stress of driving under heavy traffic conditions with the exercise performance of the same patients under laboratory conditions.[85] Hellerstein et al.[86] have studied the sexual activity in the post coronary patient and in an unpublished study we have measured the heart rate and the EKG in an unselected group of our postinfarction patients during sexual activity. The information gained under field examinations and the knowledge of the caloric expenditure and the peak heart rate levels reached during exercise and other activities, will enable prevention of untoward events.[23] Bruce[87] indicated that there are many aspects as regards the prevention and control of complications. Exertional cardiac arrest can be avoided in most cases by proper precautions. Knowledge of the aerobic requirements, adjustment of the individual capacity and strict supervision are primary considerations. There are some arguments about the intensity of training programs needed to achieve training effects. We have found that a training program of 2–3 times per week is sufficient in order to achieve a physiologic improvement.[9,23] Pollack et al.[88] have shown that a training program of 2 days/wk, at different intensities in middle aged men, improves the cardiovascular function equally at the intensities of 80%–82% of maximal heart rate, which is equal to 70%–87% maximal oxygen uptake.

The Physical Training Program and its Influence on Acceleration and/or Development of Collaterals

There exists a hypothesis that physical activity will develop and/or accelerate a collateral circulation. To date insufficient evidence has been garnered to document this for the human heart. Eckstein[69] examined the connection of exercise and the development of coronary collateral circulation in an animal model. It was indicated that exercise may induce a coronary collateral circulation in animals with moderate and severe narrowing of the coronary arteries. His findings are rather unique so far and, to date, there is no study available to demonstrate that exercise has an influence on the development of coronary collateral circula-

tion in man. In other animal studies, Schaper and others[90] found that the acceleration of collateral formation is dependent on the pressure gradient between the entrance and the outlet of the collateral vessel. This is the crucial factor for the increase in flow through the collateral vessel. The first assumption for the development of a collateral circulation is local hypoxia. It has been found by Allison[91] and later by Forrester[92] in the postmortem examinations, that in a very high percentage collaterals were found in patients with coronary heart disease who had moderate to severe narrowing of the coronary arteries. Occasionally, collaterals were found in coronary patients who did not suffer from angina pectoris or had only a slight narrowing of their coronary arteries. There were only sporadic findings of collaterals in the postmortem of these who died from other causes and had an intact heart.

It is generally accepted that hypoxia is the strongest stimulus for the development and/or accelerated growth of collaterals. It is important to stress that there is no evidence that positively correlates the physical activities during life and the appearance of the collateral circulation as found at postmortem. Thus an influence of physical training in the accelerated formation of a coronary collateral circulation has not been established.

Furthermore, there is still a lack of understanding as to which mechanism is responsible for the significant physiologic improvement obtained in most patients undergoing rehabilitation programs. Despite preliminary findings indicating decreased mortality in some studies (0.8% per 100 man yr experience in the training group and 2.5% in the control[26] group, (3.5% in training groups and 6.8% in the matched control group),[54] definite evidence that a physical training program prevents reinfarction and death is still lacking. Astrand and Rodahl[93] indicate in their textbook as to the influence of physical activity on coronary heart disease. "Research in this area is very complicated and it may take 100 yr or more of intensive studies, particularly longitudinal and intervention type studies to demonstrate with certainty that there is or is not a connection between cardiovascular disease and inactivity."

In conclusion, there are many problems involved in the field of rehabilitation of coronary patients. These problems are of substantial importance and we refer mainly to the crucial question, whether rehabilitation procedures based on physical activities and/or comprehensive programs, can influence morbidity and mortality. On the other hand, there are some facts which have been established and these are:

Short term (4–5 mo) training programs started during the maintenance phase after myocardial infarction, or in well selected patients with coronary heart disease with and without angina, can improve and expedite the return to normal activities in patients who were unable to return to work on their own initiative after myocardial infarction because of improper medical guidance, anxiety, and chest pain. In our population, 65% of this population (below age 65) returned to work after a short rehabilitation program.

Physical capabilities as expressed by means of the functional work assessment can be improved significantly in coronary patients who undergo physical training programs if they return to work after an acute coronary episode or not.

If rehabilitation programs are implemented on the basis as a secondary prevention measure, such a program must be continued throughout the life of the patient. Despite a great number of unsolved questions, it is our belief that comprehensive programs should be instituted in well selected patients with CHD on a long term basis.

Physiologic and psychological improvements during rehabilitation programs have been reported many times and from different centers in the world. Our knowledge to date points only to the fact that the patient benefits from these improvements especially by a more balanced emotional stability, an increased work performance, reduction of drug dependency and a decrease of fear, anxiety and insecurity. Whether the exercise therapy involved in most programs will change the patients' destiny as to reinfarction and death remains an open question, despite the preliminary reports involving small groups of patients which demonstrate a decrease of mortality in patients after myocardial infarction who undergo continuous programs.

Coronary surgery may play an important role as a therapeutic measure to be undertaken mainly in these patients with angina, who cannot be controlled by conservative treatment and especially these patients in younger age groups. The future will show whether rehabilitation measures to be undertaken in patients after surgery can further influence the course of the disease.

Much more well controlled studies are needed in order to find the best methodology and the proper use of rehabilitation measures in patients with CHD. One should be aware that enthusiastic recommendations on one hand and inappropriate approaches, on the other hand, will cause much harm to a controversial discipline in cardiology, which despite the many unsolved problems, may find its way as a method of treatment in well selected patients with coronary heart disease.

REFERENCES

1. Kellermann JJ: Cardiac rehabilitation: An editorial view. G Ital Cardiol 3:617–624, 1973

2. World Health Organization Technical Report Series 270: Rehabilitation of patients with cardiovascular diseases, report of a WHO expert committee. 1964

3. WHO Working group: Program for the physical rehabilitation of patients with acute myocardial infarction. Freiburg/Br., March 1968

4. Kellermann JJ: Cardiac rehabilitation—What has been done and what should be done. Acta Cardiol 14 (Suppl): 61–68, 1970

5. Myocardial infarction: how to prevent, how to rehabilitate, in Council on Rehabilitation. Int Soc of Card, Mannheim, Boeniger 1973, p 148

6. Groden BM: The management of myocardial infarction: a controlled study of the effects of early mobilization. Cardiac Rehabil 1:13–16, 1971

7. Levine SA, Lawn B: Armchair treatment of acute coronary thrombosis. JAMA 148:1368, 1952

8. Brock L: Early ambulation of the post myocardial infarction patients. (B) Early reconditioning for post myocardial infarction patients. Spalding Rehabilitation Center, Chap 22. In Ref. 19, p 315

9. Kellermann JJ and Kariv I, et al: Rehabilitation of coronary patients, Cardiac Evaluation and Rehabilitation Institute: Tel Hashomer, Segal Press, 1970, p 102

10. Wenger NK: The use of exercise in the rehabilitation of patients after myocardial-infarction. J Sci Med Assoc 65 (Suppl) 1:66–68, 1969

11. Hellerstein HK: Exercise therapy in coronary disease. Bull N.Y. Acad Med. 44:1028–1047, 1968

12. Kellermann JJ, Modan B, Levy M, et al: Return to work after myocardial infarction. Geriatrics 23:151–156, 1968

13. Kellermann JJ, Mann A, Kariv I: Functional evaluation of cardiac work capacity by spiroergometry in patients with rheumatic heart disease. Arch Phys Med Rehabil 50:4;189, 1969

14. Bruce RA, Rowell LB, Blackman JR, et al: Cardiovascular function tests. Heart Bull. 14:9, 1965

15. World Health Organization Technical Report 388:

Exercise tests in relation to cardiovascular function, report of a WHO meeting. 1968

16. Scandinavian Committee on EKG classification: The "Minnesota code" for EKG classification. Acta Med Scand 183 (Suppl 481), 1967

17. Kellermann, JJ: Problems in exercise testing. Chest 59:124–125, 1971

18. Astrand PO: Experimental Studies of Physical Working Capacity in Relation to Sex and Age. Copenhagen, Munksgaard, 1952, p 137

19. Hellerstein HK, Hirsch EZ, Ader R, et al: Principles of exercise prescription in exercise testing and exercise training in CHD. Naughton JP, Hellerstein HK (eds) New York, Academic Press, 1973, p 131

20. Lange Andersen K: Work capacity of selected populations, in Baker PT, Weiner AS (ed): The Biology of Human Adaptability. Oxford, Clarendon, 1966

21. Kellermann JJ: Rehabilitation of coronary patients in cardiologia D'Oggi, in Puddu, Anguisolla (ed): Edizione Medico Scientifiche, Rome (in press)

22. Sarnoff SJ, Braunwald E, Weich GH, et al: Hemodynamic determinants of oxygen consumption of the heart with special reference to the tension time index. Amer J Physiol 209, 919, 1965

23. Kellermann JJ, Feldman S, Levi M, et al: Rehabilitation of coronary patients. J Chron Dis 20:10:815–821, 1967

24. Kellermann JJ, Mann A, Ledermann D, et al: The evaluation and rehabilitation of coronary patients in Cardiology—Current Topics and Progress. New York; London, Academic Press, 1970, pp 505–507

25. Kellermann JJ, Modan B, Feldmann S, et al: Evaluation of physical work capacity in coronary patients after myocardial infarction who returned to work with and without a medically reconditioning program. Physical Activity and Aging Medicine and Sport, vol 4. New York, Karger, Basel, 1970, pp 148–155

26. Kellermann JJ, Mann A, Eschar Y, et al: Mortality, morbidity and physical work capacity in coronary patients with and without physical conditioning, in Roskamm and Reindell FK (eds): Das Kranke Herz. Stuttgart; New York, Schattauer-Verlag, 1973 pp 501–506

27. Vuopala U: Resumption of work after myocardial infarction in Northern Finland. Acta Med Scand, 1972

28. Higgins LE, Pooler WS: Myocardial infarction and subsequent reemployment in Syracuse, New York. Amer J Publ Hlth 58:312, 1968

29. Sharland DE: Ability of men to return to work after cardiac infarction. B Med J 2:718, 1964

30. Master AM, Jaffe HL, Teich EM, et al: Survival and rehabilitation after coronary occlusion. JAMA 156:1552, 1954

31. Kolko S: A critique and evaluation of methodology in rehabilitation of cardiac patients. Utilization conference Sedars Sinai Medical Center, Los Angeles 1970, p 46–47

32. Frick MH: The effect of physical training in manifest ischemic heart disease. Circulation 4:433, 1969

33. Varnouskas EM: Peripheral hemodynamic effects of physical health and in ischemic heart disease, in De Haas JH, Hemker HC, Snellen HA (eds): Ischemic H. Disease Leyden, 1970, p 219

34. Bjernulf A: Hemodynamic aspects of physical training after myocardial infarction. Acta Med Scand (Suppl) 548, 1973

35. Kentala E: Physical fitness and feasibility of physical rehabilitation after myocardial infarction in men of working age. Ann Clin Res 4 (Suppl 91): 1–84, Helsinki, 1972

36. Frick MH, Katila M: Hemodynamic consequences of physical training after myocardial infarction. Circulation 36:192, 1968

37. Varnouskas E, Bergman H, Houk P, et al: Hemodynamic effects of physical training in coronary patients. Lancet 2:8, 1966

38. Kellermann JJ: Clinical aspects of cardiac rehabilitation. Bull Int Soc Cardiology 3:1–2, 1971

39. Broustet JP: La Readaptation de Coronariens. Paris, Sandoz Editions, 1973, pp 375

40. Naughton J, Bruhn JG, Lategola MT: Effects of physical training on psychologic and behavioral characteristics of cardiac patients. Arch Phys Med 49:131–138, 1968

41. Groden BM: Return to work after myocardial infarction. Scot Med J 12:297, 1967

42. Redwood DR, Rosing DR, Epstein SE: Circulatory and symptomatic effects of physical training in patients with coronary artery disease and angina pectoris. N Engl J Med 286:959–965, 1972

43. Kasch RW, Boyer JL: Changes in maximum work capacity resulting from six months training in patients with ischemic heart disease. Med Sci Sports 1:156–159, 1969

44. Sarnoff SJ, Braunwald E, Welch GH, Jr, et al: Hemodynamic determinants of O_2 consumption of the heart with special reference to the tension–time index. Am J Physiol 192:148–56, 1958

45. Sonnenblick EH: in Larsen OA, Malmborg RO (eds): O_2 consumption of the heart in coronary heart disease and physical fitness. Copenhagen, Munksgaard, 1971, pp. 89–92

46. Holmberg S, Serzysko W, Varnauskas E: Coronary circulation during heavy exercise in control subjects and patients with coronary heart disease. Acta Med Scand 190:465–480, 1971

47. Clausen JP, Larsen OA, Trap-Jensen J: Physical training in the management of coronary artery disease. Circulation 40:143, 1969

48. Wallace AG, Mitchell JH, Skinner NS, et al: Duration of the phases of left ventricular systole. Circ Res 12:611–619, 1963

49. Whitsett TL, Naughton J: The effect of exercise on systolic time intervals in sedentary and active individuals and rehabilitated patients with heart disease. Am J Card 27:352–58, 1971

50. Frick MH: Hemodynamic consequences of physical training after myocardial infarction. Circulation 37:192, 1968

51. Braunwald E, Ross J, Jr, Sonneblick EH: Mechanism of Contraction of Normal and Failing Heart. Boston, Little, Brown, 1968

52. Kellermann JJ: Physical conditioning in patients after myocardial infarction. Schweif Med Wschr 103:79–85, 1973

53. Kellermann JJ: Clinical implications of a rehabilitation programme in patients. Cardiac Rehabil 4:59, 1973

54. Rechnitzer PA, Packard HA, Panio AV, et al: Long term followup study of survival and recurrence rate following myocardial infarction in exercising and control subjects. Circulation 65:4:853–857, 1972

55. Sanne HM, Wilhelmsen L: Physical activity as prevention and therapy in coronary heart disease. Scand J Rehabil Med 3:47–56, 1971

56. Sanne H: Exercise tolerance and physical training in nonselected patients after myocardial infarction. Acta Med Scand 551 (Suppl):7–110, 1973

57. Aronow WS, Stemmer EA: Isovolumic contraction and left ventricular ejection times. Am J Card 26:238–40, 1970

58. Scholer Y, Gettiker K, Liese W, et al: Belastungs dynamik nach aorto-koronarem bypass. Schw Med Wschr 103:1822–1824, 1973

59. Caro C: (Personal communication) Rome, 1973

60. Morris JN, Heady JA, Raffle PAB, et al: Coronary heart disease and physical activity of work. Lancet 2:1053–1111, 1953

61. Morris JN, Heady JA, Raffle PAB: Physique of London busmen: Epidemiology of uniforms. Lancet 2:569, 1956

62. Morris JN, Chave SPW, Adam C, et al: Vigorous exercise in leisure-time and the incidence of coronary heart disease. Lancet 1:333–338, 1973

63. Zukel WJ, Lewis RH, Enterline PE, et al: A short term community study of the epidemiology of coronary heart disease. Am J Public Health 49:1630, 1959

64. Kannel WB: Habitual level of physical activity and risk of coronary heart disease. In Proceedings of the International Symposium on Physical Activity and Cardiovascular Health, reprinted in Can Med Assoc J 96:811, 1967

65. Stamler J, Lindberg HA, Berkson DM, et al: Prevalence and incidence of coronary heart disease in strata of the labor force of a Chicago industrial corporation. J Chronic Dis 11:405, 1960

66. Taylor HL, Klepetar E, Keys A, et al: Death rates among physically active and sedentary employees of the railroad industry. Am J Public Health 52:1697, 1962

67. Keys A: Physical activity and the epidemiology of coronary heart disease, in Brunner D, Jokl E (eds): Medicine and Sport, vol 4, (Physical Activity and Aging) Baltimore, Univ Park Pr, D. Brunner and E. Jokl. 1970, p 264

68. Fox SM, Haskell WL: Physical activity and the prevention of coronary heart disease. Bull NY Acad Med 44:950, 1968

69. Eckstein RW: The effect of exercise and coronary artery narrowing on coronary collateral circulation. Circ Res 5:230, 1957

70. Burt JJ, Jackson R: Sport Med (Torino) 5:203, 1965

71. Gottheiner V: Le sport apres infarctus du myocarde. Ann Cardiol Angeiol (Paris) 20:129, 1971

72. Naughton JP, Lategola M, Shanbour K: A physical rehabilitation program for cardiac patients: A progress report. Am J Med Sci 75:545, 1966

73. Clausen JP, Larson OA, Trap-Jensen J: Physical training in the management of coronary artery disease. Circulation 40:143;154, 1969

74. World Health Organization Technical Report Series 270:Rehabilitation of patients with cardiovascular disease, report of a WHO expert committee. 1964

75. WHO working group: A program for the physical rehabilitation of patients with acute myocardial infarction. Freiburg 4–6, 1968

76. Lange Andersen K, Shephard RJ, Denolin H, et al: Fundamentals of exercise testing. WHO Geneva: 27–32; 74–82, 1971

77. World Health Organization Technical Report Series 388: Exercise test in relation to cardiovascular function. Geneva, 1968

78. Acker JE: The cardiac rehabilitation unit: Experiences with a program of early activation. Circulation 44(Supp 11):11–119, 1971

79. Bergman H, Varnauskas E: Placebo effect in physical training of coronary heart disease, in Larsen OA, Malmborg RO (eds): Patients in CHD and physical fitness. Copenhagen, Munksgaard, 1971, pp 48–51

80. Zohman LR, Tobis JS: The effect of exercise training on patients with angina pectoris. Phys Med 48: 525–532, 1967

81. Schapiro AK: Etiological factors in placebo effect. JAMA 187:712–714, 1964

82. Jokl E, Melzer L: Acute fatal nontraumatic collapse during work and sport, in Jokl E, McClellan JT (eds): Exercise and Cardiac Death. S. Karger-Basel, 1971, p 5–18

83. James TN, Froggatt P, Marshall TK: Sudden death in young athletes. Op. Cit. pp 102–111

84. Holter NJ: New methods of heart studies. Science 134:1214–1220, Oct. 20, 1961

85. Kellermann JJ, Lederman D, Wortreich B, et al: Heart rate, blood pressure, and EKG during physical exertion and driving in healthy individuals and coronary patients, in Car Driving and Cardiovascular Disease. Report of a working group of the European Society of Cardiology Roma, Ed. CEPI 1971, pp 29–34

86. Hellerstein HK, Friedman EH: Sexual activity and the post coronary patient. Med Aspects Hum Sex 3:70, 1969

87. Bruce RA: Prevention and control of cardiovascular complications. Naughton JP, Hellerstein HK (eds), New York, Academic, 1973, pp 355–363

88. Pollock MI, Broida J, Kendrick Z, et al: Effect of training two days per week at different intensities on middle-aged men. Med Sci Sports 4:192, 1972

89. Malmkrona R., Soderholm B., Bjorntorp P., Myocardial infarction in younger age group; (2) Follow-up observations with special references to capacity for work. Acta Med Scand 171:59, 1962

90. Schaper W., Flameng W., Snoeckx L., et al: Der Einfluss Korperlichen Trainings auf den kollateral Kreislauf des Herzens Verh. Germany, Kreisl-Forsch, 1971, pp 37, 112

91. Allison RB, Rodriguez FL, Higgins EA, et al: Clinicopathologic correlations in coronary artherosclerosis. Circulation 27:170, 1963

92. Forrester JS, Kemp HG, Gorlin R: Distinctive characterization of the patients with myocardial infarction and no angina pectoris. Clin. Res. 16:229, 1968

93. Astrand PO, Rodahl K: Textbook of Work Physiology. New York, McGraw-Hill. 1970, pp 373–430

94. Fisher ST: Unmet needs in psychological evaluation of intervention programs. Naughton JP, Hellerstein HK (eds), New York, Academic, 1973, pp 289–296

95. Gott VL: Outlook for patients after coronary artery revascularization. Am J of Cardiol 33:431–437, 1974

96. Sheldon WC: Vein graft surgery in the treatment of coronary artery disease. Das Chronisch Kranke Herz. Stuttgart; New York, Schattaver-Verlag, 1973, pp 236–242

97. Guilford JP: Fundamental statistics in psychology and education. New York, McGraw-Hill, 1965, pp 188–189

Analysis of Epidemiologic Studies of Physical Inactivity as Risk Factor for Coronary Artery Disease

Victor F. Froelicher and Albert Oberman

A S MANY AS 8 MILLION ADULTS in this country exercise on a regular basis for cardiovascular fitness. Physicians and other health professionals, individually and through official organizations, actively promote physical exercise as a preventive and therapeutic measure for coronary artery disease. Yet, critically controlled studies are sufficiently rare in this area of investigation as to constitute a major shortcoming in defining the precise role of physical activity in coronary artery disease. The inherent danger of sudden death due to coronary artery disease during exercise,[1-5] and the magnitude of the economic cost and commitment of manpower, necessitate careful scrutiny of the evidence upon which the decision to promote vigorous exercise is based.

Numerous studies demonstrate the hemodynamic consequences of physical conditioning in normals of all ages and in persons with coronary artery disease; this subject has been reviewed by Katz[6] and Frick.[7] Consistent findings have included decreased heart rate at rest and during exercise allowing increased myocardial perfusion at any workload. Increases in maximal cardiac output and oxygen consumption have been demonstrated, suggesting that the heart is able to tolerate stress better. Also, the feasibility of rehabilitating selected postcoronary patients has been established.[8-10] The possible increase in work capacity is important in those in whom the quality of life is diminished by the physical limitations of their disease. However, an important unanswered question is whether or not these hemodynamic and functional changes increase the quantity of life. Psychologic improvement is often noted clinically, but the effect on morbidity and mortality is unknown.

Although experimental studies of the direct effect of physical activity on atherosclerosis are inadequate and contradictory,[11,12] many physicians, including ourselves, feel that physical conditioning can be helpful as part of a program aimed at modifying the major risk factors.[13-16] Various studies suggest that regular exercise can prevent the manifestations of coronary artery disease by other mechanisms including: (1) improved myocardial perfusion due to increased cardiac capillary-fiber ratio,[17,18] opening of collaterals,[19] and enlargement of the coronary arteries;[20,21] (2) metabolic and morphologic changes in peripheral and cardiac muscle;[22-25] (3) myocardial hypertrophy and increased contractility;[26] (4) effects on the coagulation system;[27-30] (5) decreased manifestations of the neurohumoral adrenergic system;[31] and (6) electrophysiologic changes in the myocardium that protect against fatal arrhythmias.[31] However, these are only postulated protective mechanisms that need confirmation.

Those interested in finding evidence to support the decision to promote exercise have turned to the epidemiologists for morbidity and mortality data. If the above postulated preventive and protective mechanisms are in effect, their results should be apparent in population studies. Proponents of physical exercise cite certain epidemiologic studies of coronary artery disease as confirmatory evidence for this approach, but there are a number of other studies that have shown no relationship of coronary artery disease to the level of physical activity. The major difficulties in this type of epidemiologic research have not always been recognized or adequately taken into account. Because the epidemiologic data is so crucial for the justification of the therapeutic and preventive use of exercise, the sole objective of this paper will be to review the population studies dealing with physical inactivity as a risk factor for coronary artery disease.

MATERIALS AND METHODS

This report is based upon the analysis of 35 published reports of original epidemiologic research relating to the proposed association between coronary artery disease and physical inactivity. It is not possible to review all of the

From the University of Alabama School of Medicine, Birmingham, Ala.

Victor F. Froelicher, M.D.: Major, United States Air Force Medical Corps, Aerospace Medical School (AFSC), Brooks Air Force Base, San Antonio, Texas; formerly Fellow in Cardiology, and Instructor in Medicine, University of Alabama School of Medicine, Birmingham, Ala. Albert Oberman, M.D., M.P.H.: Professor of Public Health and Epidemiology, and Associate Professor of Medicine, University of Alabama School of Medicine, Birmingham, Ala.

Table 1. Format for Grouping the Epidemiology Studies of Physical Activity and Coronary Artery Disease

A. Retrospective studies
    I. Large population studies utilizing death certificate and population data from an entire city, state or country, with activity level judged from the occupation listed on death certificates, and the end point coronary artery disease listed on a death certificate
        1. Mortality data for England and Wales
        2. Chicago mortality statistics
        3. California mortality statistics
    II. Studies involving analysis of data from a specific population with the activity level assessed by job classification and/or questionnaire, and with coronary artery disease listed on the death certificate or reported symptoms or coronary artery disease as the end point
        1. London busmen
        2. North Dakota
        3. Israel kibbutzim
    III. Studies of data from specific occupational groups with the activity level assessed by the standardized job title, and with coronary artery disease listed as the cause of death in industrial records as the end point
        1. South African railroad
        2. U.S. railroad
        3. U.S. postmen
    IV. Studies of specific populations with activity level assessed by occupation or questionnaire; diagnoses of acute myocardial infarct was the end point
        1. Health Insurance Plan of New York
        2. Canadian VA
        3. Malmo
    V. Prevalence or cross-sectional studies
        1. Peoples Gas Company
        2. U.S. railroad
        3. Evans County
    VI. Socioeconomic studies
        1. Baltimore
        2. Dupont
        3. Bell Telephone
B. Prospective studies
        1. Peoples Gas Company
        2. U.S. railroadmen
        3. Western Electric Company
        4. Los Angeles civil servants
        5. Seven countries
        6. London busmen
        7. San Francisco longshoremen
        8. Western collaborative group
        9. Gotesburg
       10. Framingham
C. Pathologic studies
        1. Westchester County, N.Y.
        2. Jaffa, Israel
        3. England
        4. Oxford
        5. Clarence DeMar—autopsy
D. Rehabilitation studies
        1. Cleveland program
        2. Tel-Aviv program

studies reported in the literature, thus we have chosen those most commonly cited, and those of particular instructive value. Fifteen retrospective studies, three prevalence studies, ten prospective studies, five pathologic studies, and two rehabilitation studies were reviewed. The studies are specifically analyzed regarding the experimental design with emphasis upon the following basic aspects:

(1) characteristics of the population studied, the population size, and the period of observation; (2) methodology of assessing the level of physical activity; (3) evaluation of the major risk factors and their influence, if known; and (4) diagnostic criteria for coronary artery disease.

The retrospective studies are grouped according to similarities of format in order to facilitate comparison and evaluation. A number of socioeconomic studies are included since they have been interpreted by some to lend evidence to the physical inactivity and coronary artery disease hypothesis, although physical activity itself was not assessed. The studies are classified as either positive or negative. The positive studies are those that have been interpreted as giving evidence for the hypothesis that physical activity protects against the manifestations of coronary artery disease, while those that show no relationship are categorized as negative studies. Lastly, the major pathologic and rehabilitation studies will be reviewed. Table 1 shows the format for grouping the studies, and Table 2 summarizes the results of the analysis of the studies.

RESULTS

Retrospective Studies

This first group includes three large population studies that have utilized death certificate and population data from an entire city, state, or country. The activity level was judged from the occupation listed on the death certificate, and the end point was coronary artery disease listed on death certificates.

Morris has presented the data from the occupational-mortality records for England and Wales, interpreting this data as support for the hypothesis that occupational physical inactivity is a risk factor for coronary artery disease.[32,33] Social class as used in these studies is based on the grading of occupation by its level of skill and role in production, and its general standing in the community.[34] Social class ranges from I, which includes leading professions such as physicians and stockbrokers, to Class V, which includes unskilled workers such as railroad porters and builders' helpers. The level of activity is based on the independent evaluation of the occupations by several industrial experts. The activity level of the last job held was found to be inversely related to the mortality from coronary artery disease as determined from death certificates. Some of the limitations of this study include imprecise diagnostic criteria, and bias due to the selection of the sick for less active jobs.

Stamler et al. analyzed the mortality statistics from Chicago for the years 1951 and 1953.[35] Both the cause of death and occupation were obtained from the death certificates and the occupations were broken down into five categories: (1) professional and semiprofessional workers, proprietors, managers, and officials; (2) clerical, sales, and kindred workers; (3) craftsmen, foremen, and operatives; (4) service workers; and (5) laborers. These categories were also combined as white collar workers (categories 1 and 2) and blue collar workers (categories 3, 4 and 5). The authors found no significant occupational group differences in age-specific coronary artery disease death rates for white males aged 45–64.

Breslow and Buell noted that British mortality reports indicated an excess mortality rate from coronary artery disease, with high social class based on occupation and also with decreasing physical activity of occupation, while studies in the United States failed to confirm this.[36] They proposed that comparing groups with similar general mortality would make apparent the protective effect of physical activity in agreement with the British studies. In order to demonstrate this, they analyzed census and death certificate data for California from 1949-1951. As other investigators have reported, they found inconsistencies in the records as to whether the last, the usual, or longest held occupation were reported. Nonetheless, they felt that the data revealed a gradient of decreasing mortality rate from coronary heart disease with increasing physical activity but only when occupational groups of similar general mortality were considered.

The following retrospective studies involved analysis of data from a specific population with activity level assessed by job classification and/or questionnaire, and with coronary artery disease listed on the death certificate or reported symptoms of coronary artery disease used as the end points.

Morris et al. presented data from a sequence of epidemiologic studies to support the following hypothesis:[33] "Men in physically active jobs have a lower incidence of coronary heart disease than men in physically inactive jobs. More important, the disease is not so severe in physically active workers, tending to present first in them as angina pectoris and other relatively benign forms, and to have a smaller early case fatality and a lower early mortality rate." The first study dealt with the drivers and conductors of the London Transport System. Thirty-one thousand white males aged 35-64 were included for analysis over a period of 18 mo in 1949-1950. The end points were coronary insufficiency, myocardial infarction, and angina as reported on sick leave records, and listing of coronary artery disease on death certificates. The age-adjusted total incidence was 1.5 times higher, and the sudden and 3-mo mortality was 2

Table 2. Summary of the Epidemiology Studies of Physical Activity and Coronary Artery Disease

Study	Primary Investigator	Approximate Population Size (Middle-aged Men)	Period of Observation	Method of Assessing Physical Activity	Evaluation of Risk Factors	Diagnostic Criteria for CAD*	Relationship of CAD to Physical Inactivity and Comments
Retrospective Studies							
England–Wales mortality	Morris	2,000,000	1930–1932 1949–1952	Occupation on D.C.†	No	CAD listed on D.C.	Positive but the diagnosis is based on death certificates, physical activity on the title of last occupation, and part of the data was obtained before the ECG was available for a diagnosis
Chicago mortality	Stamler	400,000	1951, 1953	Occupation on D.C.	No	CAD listed on D.C.	Negative but there is very little gradient in the activity level of the population
California mortality	Breslow	1,000,000	1949, 1951	Occupation on D.C.	No	CAD listed on D.C.	Positive but only after grouping the population according to general mortality
North Dakota	Zukel	20,000	1957	Occupation and questionnaire	Cigarette smoking only	Angina, coronary insufficiency, AMI,‡ CHF and sudden death due to CAD as reported in local medical records	Positive, but the questionnaire evaluating physical activity was found to be inaccurate by the authors
London Transport	Morris	31,000	1949–1950	Drivers vs. conductors	No (later done in followup)	AMI, angina, death due to CAD as reported in industrial records	Drivers had a higher incidence of CAD but this could be due to the selection of other risk factors within this group; later studies showed them to be heavier, and to have higher BP and serum cholesterol
Israel kibbutzim	Brunner	6,000	1946–1961	Sedentary—80% or more of job time sitting; active—all others	No	AMI, angina, death due to CAD as reported in industrial records	Positive, but no other risk factors evaluated

Location	Author	Number	Years	Method	Other risk factors controlled	Diagnostic criteria	Comments
U.S. railroad men	Taylor	100,000	1955–1956	Switchmen vs. clerks and executives	No	CAD listed on D.C.	Positive, but influenced by differential rate of job transfers; those with CAD transfer most often from active to inactive jobs
South African railroad men	Adelstein	20,000	1954–1959	Job titles	No	CAD listed on D.C.	Negative
Washington, D.C. postal employees	Kahn	1,500	1940–1962	Mail carriers vs. clerks	No	CAD listed on D.C.	Positive
HIP	Frank	301	1961–1963	Questionnaire	No	Acute MI	Positive but the activity questionnaire is influenced by bias and selective forces favoring such a relationship
Toronto VA	Shanoff	100	1960	Questionnaire	Yes	Acute MI	Negative for "habitual" physical activity
Malmo Hospital	Forssman	66	1958	Occupation	Yes	Acute MI	Negative but physical activity determined only by occupational title
Prevalence Studies Peoples Gas Co., Chicago	Stamler	1,500	1958	Occupation	Yes	Diagnostic ECG, AMI, sudden death, angina, coronary insufficiency, and CHF due to CAD	Positive but effects of differential job transfers obvious; those with CAD most often transfer from active to inactive jobs
U.S. railroad men	Taylor	2,000	1957–1959	Switchmen vs. clerks and executives	Yes	Diagnostic ECG and angina	Positive but effects of differential job transfers obvious—those with CAD most often transfer from active to inactive jobs
Evans County, Georgia	McDonough	1,000	1960	Occupation	Yes	Diagnostic ECG, angina, and history of MI	Positive but with similar biases as other prevalence studies.
Prospective Studies San Francisco	Paffenbarger	3,300	1951–1967	Cargo workers vs. clerks	Yes; except cholesterol	CAD listed on D.C.	Positive but no cholesterols obtained and there is a selective process for men to become clerks or cargo workers

(Continued)

Table 2. Summary of the Epidemiology Studies of Physical Activity and Coronary Artery Disease (Cont'd)

Study	Primary Investigator	Approximate Population Size (Middle-aged Men)	Period of Observation	Method of Assessing Physical Activity	Evaluation of Risk Factors	Diagnostic Criteria for CAD*	Relationship of CAD to Physical Inactivity and Comments
Framingham	Kannel	2,500	1949–1967	Questionnaire, physiologic measurements	Yes	CAD listed on D.C. diagnostic ECG changes symptomatic CAD	Positive but the physiologic parameters are of the uncertain relationship to physical activity
London transportation workers	Morris	687	1960–1965	Drivers vs. conductors	Yes	AMI diagnostic ECG changes, angina and sudden death	Positive but the drivers and the young recruits for bus driving had other risk factors for CAD
Gotesborg	Werko	834	1963–1967	Retrospective questionnaire	Yes	AMI diagnostic ECG changes and angina	Positive but the activity level was determined retrospectively
Western collaborative	Rosenman	3,180	1960–1965	Questionnaire	Yes	Diagnostic ECG changes, angina, AMI and death due to AMI	Positive; main emphasis on personality types
Seven Country	Keys	25,000	1960–1965	Questionnaire	Yes	Diagnostic ECG changes, angina, AMI and death due to AMI	Negative; very heterogeneous because of different culture and peoples studied
Los Angeles	Chapman	1,400	1949–1962	Questionnaire	Yes	AMI, angina, sudden death, coronary insufficiency	Negative but only job title used for activity level
U.S. railroad men	Taylor	2,000	1960–1965	Switchmen vs. clerks and executives	Yes	AMI, angina, sudden death due to AMI, and diagnostic ECG changes	Negative
Western Electric, Chicago	Paul	1,700	1957–1965	Job evaluation and title; and interview	Yes	AMI, angina and death due to CAD	Negative
Peoples Gas Co., Chicago	Stamler	1,240	1958–1965	Job title	Yes	CAD listed on D.C.	Negative but inadequate physical activity gradient within the population
Rehabilitation Studies Cleveland rehabilitation group	Hellerstein	254	1960–1967	Physical training with parameters of CV fitness measured	Yes; and appropriate treatment of risk factors	Death	Positive but volunteers and selection results in a healthier post infarction group

Study	Author	N	Years	Activity assessment		Method	Results
Israel rehabilitation group	Gottenheimer	1,103	1961–1966	Physical training with parameters of CV fitness measured	No	Death	Positive, but volunteers and selection results in a healthier postinfarction group
Pathological Studies							
National British Necropsy Series	Crawford and Morris	4,000	1954–1956	Last occupation	No	Macroscopic estimation	Negative; no difference in the degree of atherosclerosis or luminal obstruction among the activity levels; ischemic myocardial fibrosis appeared more common in inactive occupations
Israel Traumatic Death Autopsy Series	Mitrani	172	1968	Last occupation	No	Macroscopic estimation and calculation of luminal obstruction	Negative; no significant difference in atherosclerotic narrowing though there was slightly less in the active occupations
New York Medical Examiner Autopsy	Spain and Bradess	207	1957–1958	Last occupation	No	Macroscopic estimation	Negative; no difference in the degree of atherosclerosis between the activity levels
Oxford study	Rose	170	1962–1963	Last occupation	No	Degree of atherosclerosis not studied; macroscopic estimation of infarct size	Undiseased portion of RCA studied to judge size of coronary arterial tree; small RCA in infarction group; RCA tended to be larger in active occupations though data only suggestive
Autopsy of Clarence DeMarr	Currens and P.D. White	1	1958	Lifelong history of marathon running	No	Macroscopic estimation	Coronary arteries 2-3x normal diameter with mild atherosclerotic involvement but no luminal obstruction; rather than secondary to running, this could be genetically endowed and explain why he became a great runner

*CAD: Coronary artery disease; †D.C.: Death certificate; ‡AMI: Acute myocardial infarction; §RCA: Right coronary artery.

times higher in the driver group as compared to the conductor group. The authors suggested that this could be explained by differences in constitution, mental stress, or physical activity. The difference in physical activity was only inferred from knowing that one group drove the buses while the other group conducted on the double-decked vehicles. No attempt was made to quantitate the activity difference or to measure differences in off-the-job activity. In their original study, the authors did not investigate differences in selection in the two groups, but proceeded to a similar study with postmen and clerks, which also resulted in numbers that agreed with their hypothesis. Interestingly, though, in 1956 Morris published a paper subtitled "The Epidemiology of Uniforms," which reported that the drivers had greater girth than the conductors.[37] A later study in 1966 by Morris also showed that the drivers had higher serum cholesterols and higher blood pressures than the conductors.[38] Also, a study by Oliver documented that for some unknown reason, even the recruits for the two jobs differed by lipid levels and weight.[39] These differences put the drivers at increased risk to coronary artery disease for reasons other than an approximated difference in physical activity. Morris et al. realized that bias and other factors could be influencing their results, and they hoped to supersede these problems by performing a number of similar studies to corroborate their results. Unfortunately, there is no reason to think that the bias and selection could not reoccur.

Zukel et al. analyzed data from a population of 106,000 individuals living in six counties in North Dakota.[40] From the 20,000 males aged 35 or greater within this population, they found 228 men with coronary artery disease that became manifest during 1957. The data was obtained from reviewing death certificates, office visits, or hospital admissions reported by local doctors for acute myocardial infarctions, coronary ischemia, congestive heart failure due to coronary artery disease, or angina. Farmers had slightly less total coronary artery disease and one-half the infarctions and death from coronary artery disease. The authors did not relate this directly to differences in physical activity since they were aware of socioeconomic and environmental differences between the two groups. However, in their conclusions, they comment that physical activity was probably related to coronary artery disease, based on a questionnaire of physical activity administered to sur-

vivors of infarction and to matched controls. The following, though, is their frank assessment of this portion of their study:[40] "Unfortunately, interview information on physical activity appears to be very unreliable. Dividing hours of heavy physical work into 0, 1–6, 7 or more, only a 51 per cent agreement was found for 273 men for whom replicate information was obtained. Moreover, there was a tendency for men to report less heavy physical work in their usual occupation after their coronary attack than before."

Brunner has surveyed Jews of European origin living in the kibbutzim or collective settlements in Israel over the period of 1946–1961 with 5279 males aged 40–69 in the group as of 1961.[41] Coronary heart disease was determined from medical records of myocardial infarction, angina pectoris, and sudden death due to coronary artery disease. Sedentary workers, defined as those who spent 80 per cent or more of their time at work sitting, had 2.5–4 times the incidence of coronary artery disease as the nonsedentary workers (all others). Although Brunner believes that this population is ideal for study because their mode of life eliminates socioeconomic differences, no investigation of differences in risk factors was reported. Characteristics of the sedentary group other than physical activity could equally account for differences in the incidence of coronary artery disease.

These next retrospective studies involve data obtained from specific occupational groups with the activity level assessed by the standardized job title, and with coronary artery disease listed as the cause of death in the industrial records as the end point.

In a mortality study, Adelstein compared white South Africans working for the South African railroads as officers (clerks, administrators, high-paid executives) with employees (ranging from unskilled laborers to skilled artisans).[42] Mortality, secondary to coronary artery disease during 1954–1959 among these employees when age adjusted, did not differ from the general population. The categories of artisans, semiskilled, and others were analyzed with the physical demand of work within each group determined on a scale of five by four experienced, industrial health inspectors and the mean ratings used. Again, no significant differences were found in mortality from coronary artery disease and level of physical activity.

Taylor et al. have reported on the mortality of white males employed by the U.S. railroad industry.[43] The employees were separated by job title into three groups representing three levels of physical activity. Death certificates for the years 1955 and 1956 were analyzed by these groupings and the following age-adjusted rates were obtained: (1) clerks, light activity, 5.7 deaths/1000 man yr; (2) switchmen, moderate activity, 3.9 deaths/1000 man yr; (3) section men, heavy activity, 2.8 deaths/1000 man yr. They concluded that the data was consistent with the hypothesis that men in sedentary occupations have more coronary heart disease than those in occupations requiring moderate to heavy physical activity.

In planning a prospective study, the authors discovered a number of important points that pertained to their mortality study.[44,45] They found that the groups were not clearly separated by occupation as to the level of physical activity. Work analyses and further questioning revealed that some clerks consumed as many calories per day as section men, who presumably were working more vigorously. The most important finding was that men with coronary artery disease withdrew from the ranks of switchmen at a greater rate than from the ranks of sedentary clerks. It then became apparent that this bias in job transfers and retirement could explain the difference in mortality between the groups, rather than any protective influence exerted by physical activity.

Kahn gathered information from federal employee records to analyze mortality data on men who were appointed to positions in the Washington, D.C. Post Office from 1906-1940.[46] Of 2240 men so identified, 93% were determined as either dead or alive as of January 1962. The study was designed to test Morris' hypothesis by comparing the mortality data of sedentary clerks to active mail carriers. Kahn noted that the records showed that the carriers transferred to clerk positions much more frequently than clerks switched jobs. He adjusted for this effect by considering a subsample of men who did not change jobs. The data from this preselected group suggested that the clerks had 1.4-1.9 times the mortality from coronary artery disease than the carriers. The author mentions in his discussion that "It is entirely possible that the differences observed are only coincidentally related to physical activity differences and that indoor versus outdoor activity, differential proportion of cigarette smokers, original biases of selection, and so on are the really meaningful factors."

The following retrospective studies represent specific populations in which the activity level was assessed by occupation or questionnaire; diagnosis of acute myocardial infarction served as the end point.

Frank et al. have studied the 55,000 males aged 25-64 enrolled in the Health Insurance Plan of Greater New York (HIP).[47] In this group, 301 men were identified as having had an initial myocardial infarction between November 1, 1961 and April 30, 1963. An index for on-the-job and off-the-job activities was obtained by completion of a questionnaire during a personal interview after the infarction by the patients, or the wives of those who had died. The men were divided into three categories: least active, intermediate, and most active. The authors concluded that inquiry about customary physical activities on and off the job permitted delineation of a group of "least active" men who were much more likely to experience a clinically severe episode and die within 4 wks of its onset, than men who were relatively more active.

Keys has reported a number of inherent difficulties in this study.[48] He notes that many of the 301 men who provided incidence data on infarction were ill prior to infarction. Twenty-two per cent had manifestations of coronary artery disease, 19% had high blood pressure, and 10% were diabetic, and it would be expected that these people would be less active. Being both less active and at high risk for acute myocardial infarction, they represent a statistical bias for inactivity and subsequent myocardial infarction as well as for the severity of the infarction. Another difficulty was that the widows tended to underestimate the physical activity of their dead husbands.

Shanoff et al. have studied a group of men with documented myocardial infarction, randomly selected from the files of the Toronto VA Hospital matched to a group from the hospital files of patients admitted with nonchronic illnesses.[49] Within both groups, there were approximately 25 individuals for each decade from the fourth through the seventh for a total of 100 individuals per group. The individuals were questioned as to lifelong activity, with assessment of their physical activity in childhood, youth, and adult life. This type of questioning made available additional information because the two groups did not differ as to present activity or occupation but did differ as to habitual activity. In this study, coronary artery disease was not associated with habitual physical inactivity.

Forssman and Lindegard organized a study in

Malmo, a Swedish town of about 200,000 people.[50] The city is served by one hospital, and the study group was comprised of all male survivors of an acute myocardial infarction admitted to the hospital from 1948–1955 and whose age at the time of the study examination in 1956 was 55 or less. This included 66 men for whom healthy similar aged controls were randomly selected from the town. Occupational physical activity was determined by knowledge of the job rather than personal questioning. No difference in occupational physical activity between the controls and postinfarction group were determined.

The following three prevalence or cross-sectional studies represent a modification of the retrospective or case history approach. The main advantage is that the statistics on the studied disease are gathered at the time of the study. Thus, the end points can be well defined, and the methods for diagnosis standardized; unfortunately, selection continues to be a problem.

In 1958, a complete evaluation was performed on 1465 male employees of a utility company in Chicago.[51] Prevalence of coronary heart disease was determined by reviewing industrial health records for diagnostic electrocardiographic changes or history compatible with the manifestations of coronary artery disease. There was little difference in major risk factors between the activity level groups studied. Prevalence of coronary artery disease was lower in the blue collar workers than in the white collar workers, and in the nonsedentary than in the sedentary. However, Stamler warned that this data was confounded by such factors as differential rates of retirement among blue and white collar workers, and shifts from blue collar to white collar jobs after a coronary artery disease episode.

In 1957–1959, a sample of 3049 railroad men were randomly selected for study of the prevalence of risk factors in coronary artery disease.[43] Active switchmen and sedentary clerks and executives were included in order to have two different activity groups for comparison. Extensive screening was performed and the manifestations of coronary artery disease were well defined. The data on the 1948 men that submitted to the evaluation suggested that the switchmen had less coronary artery disease. However, Taylor points out the results were confounded by many factors. Of particular note was the fact that occupational mobility of the switchmen with coronary artery disease was

greater than that of clerks. He concluded that the majority of the factors affecting observed prevalence rates operated to exaggerate any true protective influences of physical activity.[45]

In 1960, the population of Evans County, Ga. was studied for the prevalence of coronary heart disease.[52] Coronary artery disease was defined as angina pectoris, history of a myocardial infarction, or diagnostic electrocardiographic findings. Definite and probable cases according to defined standards were used for statistical analysis. The study group included 1062 men consisting of almost equal numbers of high social class whites, low social class whites, and blacks. Within the study group there were 52 cases of coronary artery disease. Social class and occupational comparison among black males was not possible because they predominately were of low social class and in physically active occupations. Among white males, distribution of coronary artery disease by occupation suggested that those with higher activity had less prevalence of coronary artery disease. White males had three times the coronary artery disease as the black males, while high social class white males had two times as much as low social class white males, and five times as much as black males. Black males were felt to be more active by analysis of occupation and caloric consumption, but they also were thinner and had lower serum cholesterols. The authors concluded that physical activity appeared to be a major determinant of coronary artery disease prevalence. A recently reported 7-yr incidence study in Evans County found the incidence of coronary artery disease to be lower among professionals (94/1000) and highest among manual laborers and clerks (184/1000).[53] This contradictory result is interesting, especially since the two other prevalence studies were felt to be influenced by a bias which favored the physical activity hypothesis.

The following studies regarding socioeconomic differences and coronary artery disease mortality are reviewed because some authors have cited these as relating physical activity and coronary artery disease.

Lilienfild analyzed the statistics of certified deaths in Baltimore from 1949 through 1951.[54] Socioeconomic classes were determined from addresses on the death certificate on the basis that monthly rent has been shown to correlate with other socioeconomic indices like income, years of schooling, and occupation. This investigation showed no difference in the mortality rates for atherosclerotic cardiovascular disease among the five different socioeconomic groups distinguished.

Pell and D'Alonzo studied the 90,000 employees of the DuPont Chemical Company across the United States with regard to the incidence of coronary artery disease by job level.[55,56] The authors did not attempt to classify by level of activity, but rather by salary. From their data, it was demonstrated that the highest salaried group had the lowest incidence of coronary artery disease, the middle group the highest, with the lowest salaried group between the other groups. The data showed no difference in 5-yr survival between white and blue collar workers. The authors did not study the relationship of myocardial infarction to daily level of physical activity on or off the job.

Hinkle et al. studied 270,000 men employed by the Bell Telephone Company through 1964–65, analyzing morbidity and mortality as obtained from company health records.[57] Their primary goal was to test the hypothesis that striving, competitive, hard-working people were more likely to develop coronary heart disease. Their findings did not indicate that men of high level responsibility or with rapid promotions had an increased risk of coronary heart disease, but rather men with a college education had a lower incidence of coronary heart disease and less morbidity and mortality. They suggested that this was somehow due to socioeconomic differences.

Prospective Studies

In 1958, Stamler et al. began a prospective study of 1241 apparently healthy male employees of the Peoples Gas Company in Chicago.[58] By 1965, there were 39 deaths due to coronary artery disease. They found that the coronary artery disease mortality was higher in the blue collar workers (37 deaths/1000 men) with an estimated higher habitual activity at work, than in the white collar workers (20 deaths/1000 men). Stamler felt that this was consistent with the hypothesis that groups of men with similar findings with respect to the "cardinal risk factors" (hypertension, hypercholesterolemia, cigarette smoking, and excessive weight) will experience similar incidence and mortality rates for coronary heart disease irrespective of habitual physical activity of work. However, the population in general had a low level of physical activity, and lack of a gradient of physical activity limits the possibility of demonstrating an association of mortality and physical activity.

From 1956–1960, 687 healthy London busmen were examined for risk factors and coronary artery disease.[38] In 1965, they were reexamined and there were 47 cases of coronary artery disease diagnosed, including sudden deaths, myocardial infarction, electrocardiographic changes, and angina. Incidence rates per 100 men in 5 yr were 4.7 for conductors and 8.5 for drivers. However, the drivers were found to have significantly higher blood pressure and serum cholesterol than the conductors. Furthermore, classifying the conductors as an activity-protected group was inconsistent, since they had an incidence of coronary artery disease similar to sedentary London physicians.[38]

Taylor has studied the effects of occupational activity differences among railroad men.[43] Thirty units of men were randomly selected by chunk sampling from a population of 3049 men working for 20 northwestern railroads. Of this group, there were 860 sedentary clerks, 251 executives, and 837 active switchmen aged 40–59 when first examined from 1957–1959. Energy expenditure was estimated by activity and dietary analysis. It was found that the switchmen expended 600–1200 calories a day more than the sedentary groups. The groups did not differ by any of the major risk factors. After 5 yr of followup, no difference in coronary incidence rates between the two different activity levels was found.[48]

In 1951, examinations were performed on 3263 males aged 35–64, who worked as longshoremen in San Francisco.[59] Paffenbarger et al. recently presented the 16-yr followup mortality data. There were 44,595 man years observed with 291 deaths attributed to coronary artery disease on the death certificates. Two classes of workers differing by about 925 calories in work day expenditure were identified. The data suggested that the less active group had a 33 per cent higher coronary death rate. The authors note that longshoremen have an apprenticeship that selects men into the different activity levels. The two groups did not differ by blood pressure or cigarette smoking, but serum cholesterols were not measured and the difference in mortality possibly could be explained by this potent risk factor.

In 1957, 1719 white males aged 40–55 were randomly selected from the 20,000 employees of the Hawthorne Electric Works in Chicago.[60] After 8 yr of followup, there were 24 deaths due to coronary artery disease, 53 acute myocardial infarctions with survival, and 80 patients with the diagnosis of angina pectoris. Activity off the job was assessed by a personal interview. Approximate differences in caloric expenditure and intensity of work were determined for shop and office workers, and also with special means for two different classes of shop workers. The authors report no difference in coronary artery disease among the different levels of activity.

In 1949, 1403 healthy white males with a median age of 47 were randomly chosen from 20,200 Civil Servants in Los Angeles.[61] After an initial examination in 1951, periodic followup examinations and yearly questionnaires were completed. By 1962, a total of 177 new events of coronary artery disease as manifested by myocardial infarction, sudden death, angina pectoris, or coronary insufficiency were diagnosed. No differences in the incidence of coronary heart disease was observed according to socioeconomic class, or to level of physical activity as determined from job title.

The Western Collaborative Group study was initiated in 1961 with emphasis on psychological patterns.[62] Annual followup studies were obtained through 1965 on 3182 men, initially aged 35–59 and healthy at the onset. New coronary heart disease as manifested by symptomatic myocardial infarction, angina, and electrocardiographic changes was observed in 133 individuals. The customary exercise habits of each participant were obtained by personal interview. Nine hundred and sixty subjects were classified as exercising with reasonable regularity, i.e., they daily or almost daily indulged in some calisthenics, walking exercise, athletics, or equivalent physical activity. The remaining 2222 subjects admitted to only occasionally engaging in some form of physical activity. No differences in age or risk factors in these two groups were apparent, except that the exercising group had slightly lower triglyceride and cholesterol measurements. After 4.5 yr of followup, the annual incidence of coronary heart disease was 10/1000 for men without regular exercise habits, compared to 7.4/1000 in men with such habits. This difference was due to symptomatic myocardial infarction, since no difference was observed in the incidence of silent infarction, angina, or in recurring infarction. Fatal myocardial infarction occurred in 2/1000 men without regular exercise habits compared to 0.5/1000 with such habits.

The Seven Countries Coronary Artery Disease Study consists of collaborative groups from Japan, Yugoslavia, the U.S., Finland, Italy, Netherlands, and Greece.[63] This study involves chunk samples in which self-selection was minimized and complete examination coverage could be rendered to all men aged 40–59 in the geographically defined areas. The examinations and definitions were rigidly standardized, and coordinated by facilities at the University of Minnesota. Individuals were classified as sedentary, moderately active, or very active, as determined by a questionnaire for evaluating total physical activity. Data from the first 5 yr of followup, 120,000 man years observed, shows no difference in coronary artery disease incidence between physically active and sedentary men. This study is still in progress and the 10-yr analysis should be of much interest.

In 1963, Werko et al. began a study on a cohort consisting of one-third of all men born in 1913 in the industrial Swedish town of Gotesburg.[64] This cohort consisted of 834 males aged 50 without signs or symptoms of coronary artery disease. Over the next 4 yr there were 23 acute myocardial infarctions, 18 individuals with angina pectoris diagnosed, and 9 individuals with diagnostic electrocardiogram changes of a myocardial infarction. The symptomatic infarction group was questioned in order to retrospectively assess activity level on and off the job 1 yr prior to their infarction. Activity levels were categorized as light, moderate, or heavy. A random sample of healthy men of a comparable age were questioned in a similar fashion as to activity, and in comparison, this sample group was more active than those with infarctions.

In Framingham, Mass., approximately 5000 men and women aged 30–62 and free of clinical evidence of coronary artery disease at the onset, have been examined biennially since 1949. "The level of physical activity was crudely assessed using a 24-hour history of usual physical activity," and a physical activity index arrived at from five classifications of activity status.[65] A number of physiologic measurements hypothesized to be parameters of physical activity were determined for each participant, i.e., resting heart rate, vital capacity, hand grip strength, and relative weight. Coronary heart disease mortality was subsequently found to be higher in the cohorts with indices or measurements consistent with sedentary life style.[66]

Pathologic Studies

The results of 207 consecutive autopsies of otherwise healthy white males aged 30–60, who died suddenly and unexpectedly from accident, homicide, or suicide, were reported by Spain and Bradess.[67] The autopsies were done in the Medical Examiners Office of Westchester County, N.Y. All major branches of the coronary arteries were examined in cross section at 3-mm intervals. The estimated degree of reduction in luminal diameter by atherosclerotic lesions was used as the basic criteria for grading the degree of coronary atherosclerosis. The occupation of the individuals was determined from available information. All individuals who had a history or autopsy evidence of disease influencing atherosclerosis were excluded. They were separated by occupational title as active or sedentary with approximately 100 in each group. The authors found no significant differences in the degree of coronary atherosclerosis between those engaged in sedentary occupations and those engaged in physically active occupations.

Mitrani et al. have reported the results of consecutive specialized cardiovascular autopsies on 172 European-born Jews who were victims of traumatic death.[68] According to personal documents and some information obtained from relatives, 93 had led a sedentary life, and 79 were manual workers. Each coronary artery was cross sectioned at 1 cm distances to measure internal and external diameters. The percentage of narrowing of the vessels was calculated using these measurements. There was no significant difference between the active and inactive groups.

Morris and Crawford sent out requests to approximately 200 British pathologists to complete a standard questionnaire on a series of autopsies performed on men aged 45–70.[69] The pathologists were asked to give macroscopic estimates of the degree of coronary atheromata and fibrosis of the left ventricle and interventricular septum. The last occupation of the deceased was requested, and estimated as involving light, active, or heavy physical activity by the title. In this manner, the results of 3800 autopsies on individuals dying of causes other than coronary artery disease were gathered from 1954–1956. Ischemic myocardial fibrosis and complete coronary occlusion was commoner in lighter occupations, but coronary atheromata and narrowing were of equally high prevalence in all occupational groups.

Measurements were made from radiographs of injected coronary arteries obtained from two necropsy studies at the Radcliff Infirmary, Oxford.[70] Ninety-two cases without postmortem evidence of myocardial infarction were used as controls, while a group of 79 had evidence of acute or healed infarction. The right coronary artery measured in a nondiseased segment approximately one-half between its origin and the right heart border was assumed to reflect the diameter of all the coronary arteries. The physical activity of the last occupation was determined by job title as light, active, or heavy. The diameter of the right coronary artery in normals increased with age, but the infarction group showed a smaller diameter of the right coronary artery in each age group. The data was only suggestive that in the normals the right coronary artery diameter increased with activity of work, while in the infarction group it decreased with the activity of work. These differences were not statistically significant, and no determination of the degree of atherosclerosis was made.

Currens and White presented the cardiovascular autopsy results of Clarence DeMar, a famous long distance runner, who died of rectal carcinoma.[71] He was still actively involved in long distance running until shortly before his death at age 70. His coronary arteries were found to be 2–3 times normal size with some atherosclerotic involvement, but no narrowing.

Rehabilitation Studies

Hellerstein has reported his 7-yr experience in a prospective study of the effects of enhanced physical fitness on the development and course of coronary artery disease.[8] This program also aimed at modifying other risk factors by advising an antiatherogenic diet, abstinence from cigarettes, and weight reduction. The rehabilitation group included 254 patients with documented coronary artery disease, who remained in the exercise program. Over this 7-yr period, 11 subjects with coronary artery disease died with a death rate of 2/100 subject-years. In a matched group of conventionally treated subjects, the death rate was 5/100 subjects. Unfortunately, this study was not controlled and there was selection of a healthier patient group by the exclusion of those patients who could not tolerate the exercise program. Also, other risk factors were modified.

Gottheiner has reported data on the 1103 trainees with ischemic heart disease that remained in his rehabilitation program for 5 yr.[9] Initially, the group consisted of 1500, but nearly one-third dropped out. His program involved careful advancement through gradually more intensive exercise with testing prior to advancement to a higher stage. It culminates in competitive team games for those who have progressed to the upper fitness categories. The author suggests that the use of competitive sports maintains the participant's interest in the program. He reports a mortality rate of 3.5 percent over 5 yr compared to 12% in a comparable series of physically inactive postinfarction patients in Israel. Similar to other reported rehabilitation studies, there is selection of a healthier patient group by the loss of those unable to tolerate the exercise program.

DISCUSSION

We have reviewed the available data regarding physical inactivity as a risk factor for coronary artery disease, attempting to document the protective influence of physical activity. However, the results are both contradictory and inconclusive.

The majority of studies have dealt with occupational differences in retrospective studies. Although retrospective studies are attractive because the data are usually easily available, with resultant economy of time, effort, and cost, such an approach has many inherent difficulties. The information collected is frequently not standardized or complete; this is especially true in dealing with physical activity, a difficult factor to measure. Furthermore, the population base tends to be highly selected due to job transfers, retirement, or death, particularly as influenced by cardiovascular diseases. Frequently, confounding factors such as lipids, blood pressure, and other pertinent data are just not available. Some of these studies have impressive numbers of man years observed, but it should be realized that bias is not eliminated by increasing numbers. With limited depth of study, and reliance on poorly standardized information, the assessment of physical activity and the diagnosis of coronary artery disease is by necessity less precise.

Prospective studies are best for accurately determining preexisting risk and minimizing the likelihood of bias, but these studies are more expensive and difficult to perform. Although the data and methodology are much more precise in a prospective study, the present means for classifying the physical activity of an individual are vague and imprecise. Few, if any, prospective studies of large scale have employed the detailed methodology necessary to characterize the physically active individual either historically or physiologically.

Most studies have used occupation or job title alone to assess the level of physical activity; yet, when the last job held is considered, as is necessary

when job information is obtained from a death certificate, this may result in preselecting those with coronary artery disease in less active work, because the sick usually transfer to less demanding jobs. In most instances, men select their jobs for personal reasons, and those with illness, obesity, or chest pain will more likely obtain sedentary jobs. Also, individuals that differ by occupation may well differ by social and economic status and by other risk factors. Inaccuracies of physical activity assessment often become apparent when a job assumed to be of a certain activity level is investigated closely, or when the off-the-job activities are considered. Thus, job title without true assessment of energy expenditure or off-the-job activity make it difficult to truly classify individuals as active or inactive.

Assessing the level of physical activity by a questionnaire completed by the subject or by an interviewer tends to be grossly inaccurate. Some investigators have reported poor reproducibility of results when they have readministered their questionnaires.[40] Others have encountered problems with exaggeration or denial mechanisms, particularly in postinfarction patients, as well as the usual inconsistencies due to the limitations of understanding and memory. When questionnaires are administered to a population at risk, which includes individuals with angina, prodromes of coronary artery disease, or high risk disease such as hypertension and diabetes, a bias is introduced which tends to increase the association between physical inactivity and coronary artery disease. These individuals are at high risk to develop coronary artery disease and also likely to be less active. Data from such questionnaires would in fact relate physical inactivity to coronary artery disease when both are actually associated through a third factor such as diabetes. Diabetes would be associated with coronary artery disease and physical inactivity so that an apparent relationship between physical inactivity and coronary artery disease would be present but not meaningful.

The Framingham study has used heart rate, obesity, vital capacity, and hand grip strength as measurements reflecting the level of physical activity. [65,66] However, while these measurements may be related to the level of physical activity, the relationship is indirect and dependent upon other factors. For instance, vital capacity is closely related to height,[72] which in itself has been inversely associated with coronary artery disease,[38] conceivably accounting for the association of vital capacity and coronary artery disease. Other investigators have used caloric consumption, assuming a steady weight, to assess the level of physical activity. This method depends upon food questionnaires or dietary sampling, both of which have well-known limitations and methodologic problems.

A major problem with assessing physical activity is that if it truly does exert protective influence, the physiologic mechanism has not been defined. Hemodynamic and functional changes such as the "training effect,"[6,7] improved myocardial perfusion due to increased cardiac capillary to muscle fiber ratio,[17,18] opening of collaterals,[19] and enlargement of the coronary arteries,[20,21] are mechanisms supported by exercise studies. Metabolic and morphologic changes in peripheral and cardiac muscle,[22-25] including myocardial hypertrophy and increased contractility[26] have been demonstrated as effects of chronic exercise. Lowering of serum cholesterol,[14] blood pressure,[15] and body weight[16] as a result of physical activity could decrease the risk of developing coronary artery disease. Other possible mechanisms include modification of the coagulation system[27-30] and the neurohumoral adrenergic system.[31]

For instance, if the training effect is the mechanism of protection, certain considerations apply to epidemiologic studies that might not apply if other mechanisms were responsible. Attention to increased intensity and frequency of activity would be paramount because these factors are the most important in achieving the training effect.[73] Tests of the training effect such as maximal oxygen uptake and heart rate response to exercise would be of possible correlative and prognostic value, though consideration of these measurements as influenced by natural endowment as well as physical training is necessary.[74] Some investigators have suggested that the failure to find a protective influence due to physical activity is because so few middle-aged American men are physically fit, as determined by the maximal oxygen uptake test.[58] On the other hand, if the mechanism of action is through alteration of major risk factors, the additional attributes of physical fitness would be of less importance. In fact, it is uncertain what type of exercise is necessary to achieve the effects of many of the postulated mechanisms listed above.

End points used in the population studies have included angina, coronary insufficiency, acute myocardial infarction, diagnostic electrocardiographic changes, sudden death, and congestive heart failure believed to be due to coronary artery disease. In many of these studies, definitions and tests for these end points were not standardized and the investigators relied upon the diagnoses of many different physicians and information collected specifically for other reasons. The problems with diagnosis by death certificate are easily appreciated.[75,76] Such data is especially tenuous before the mid-1940s, when objective criteria from electrocardiograms were not available. Other difficulties arise in the coding of the death certificate and the selection of the underlying cause of death, as contrasted with immediate cause of death and other contributory conditions.

The pathologic studies have been of limited value because physical activity was estimated from the title of the last job, and because of the difficulty in determining the degree of atherosclerosis or the caliber of coronary arteries. The hypothesis that physical activity enlarges the coronary arteries in man has not been demonstrated, and the data presented is only suggestive. Even if there is an association between the size of the coronary arteries and the level of physical activity, it is conceivable that persons with large coronary arteries may be naturally selected into more vigorous habits and occupations. It is striking, though, that the three studies that investigated the degree of coronary atherosclerosis found little or no difference between their active and sedentary groups.[67-69]

With respect to the rehabilitation studies, there are now more than 80 physical activity programs in the United States for patients with coronary artery disease.[77] Investigators have shown that under proper supervision, exercise training can be carried out with reasonable safety in selected persons with coronary artery disease and with some assurance that the characteristic hemodynamic response of the trained state will be exhibited.[78,79] Importantly, the ability of these persons to tolerate physical stress will be increased, and a high proportion of them will be able to return to a more active life. It has been well documented that walking or cycling programs will increase the work level that an individual can reach without angina,[80,81] although this is possibly due to a more efficient circulatory response to exercise rather than enhanced myocardial perfusion or performance.[82,83]

Unfortunately, these studies have not been controlled, have depended upon volunteers, and are further selective by the loss of higher risk patients unable to stay in an exercise program. Volunteers with a disorder invariably do better in terms of morbidity and mortality than a randomly selected group.[84] Our local study of the influence of physical activity on coronary artery disease in a small, but well-controlled sample of ambulatory patients with manifest coronary artery disease, failed to show significant effects of physical activity on risk factors or measurements of fitness other than endurance after 1 yr.[85] The psychologic benefits of rehabilitation programs have been established,[8-10] but there is no evidence that they statistically lessen morbidity or mortality from coronary artery disease. A controlled study of the influence of physical activity on morbidity and mortality in postcoronary patients is especially needed since the usual risk factors do not seem to be significant.[86-88]

The influence of physical activity on coronary artery disease is a complex problem. Because of the multifactorial nature of coronary artery disease, large-scale controlled studies with large numbers of patients will be required to conclusively demonstrate any effects of physical activity. In order to see if the observed differences between activity groups or occupations are due to the level of activity or due to other factors, it is necessary to adjust for the other risk factors such as hypertension, hypercholesterolemia, cigarette smoking, and obesity. This is especially so since it has been shown that selective forces can concentrate these factors in a particular occupation or level of activity. Indirect associative studies and poorly controlled trials have suggested that physical activity may play a role in the prevention and therapy of coronary artery disease. It is entirely possible that further analytic studies and experimental trials will strengthen this association, but the available evidence remains speculative.

However, since there are inadequate data at this point to demonstrate that regular physical exercise reduces the morbidity and mortality of coronary artery disease, reasons against its recommendation must be considered. The danger of exercise in persons with coronary artery disease, even in those with silent disease, is well established.[1-5] Surprisingly, myocardial infarctions do not most commonly occur during exertion,[55,56] but this may be due to physiologic warnings that make persons

with coronary artery disease limit their activities. The admonishment to "get more exercise" may be enough to make a person ignore these warnings and exceed the limits of his myocardial perfusion.

Besides the mortality associated with exercise, there can be significant morbidity, especially in older individuals. Infarctions have been reported and one carefully supervised training study involving middle-aged men reported a 50% incidence of significant orthopedic problems.[89] Another consideration is the expense of facilities, equipment, and supervision for exercise. Priorities must be considered in establishing any preventive program for coronary artery disease. Analysis of the data regarding physical inactivity as a risk factor, although suggestive, remain tenuous and should not supersede efforts directed toward the major risk factors.

CONCLUSION

Population studies relating physical inactivity and coronary artery disease do not establish physical inactivity as a risk factor of comparable magnitude to hypercholesterolemia, cigarette smoking, and hypertension.[90] There are a number of inherent methodologic problems: difficulty in accurately assaying physical activity; inability to assess the type of exercise that is most protective; lack of a gradient of physical activity in the general population; and insufficient sample size to permit adjustment for confounding factors, or no available data regarding them. The pathologic studies are limited not only from difficulties in assaying physical activity prior to death, but also from imprecise measurement of atherosclerotic involvement and caliber of the coronary circulation. The studies reviewed have demonstrated no effect of physical activity on either atherosclerosis or the size of the coronary circulation. The rehabilitation programs appear to have merit, but the results obtained can be explained by patient selection. Unfortunately, large-scale controlled rehabilitation studies have not been reported.

A carefully planned clinical trial involving a high risk population with randomization into a program of physical activity might establish the relationship of physical activity and coronary artery disease. Such a study would be expensive, lengthy, difficult, and complicated by the multifactoral nature of coronary artery disease. There is sufficient evidence to justify such a trial, and possibly the clinical and investigational evidence suggesting that exercise is beneficial will be supplemented by evidence that it reduces morbidity and mortality.

Yet, since the danger of exercise in persons with coronary artery disease, even in those with silent disease, is well established,[1-5] the recommendation for patients and the public in general to exercise must be given cautiously, and definite guidelines should be observed.[91] Exercise therapy for patients should at first be carefully monitored, and the emphasis in prevention for the general public should be on the well-established risk factors, i.e., hypercholesterolemia, hypertension, and cigarette smoking.

REFERENCES

1. Pyfer HR, Doane BL: Cardiac arrest during exercise testing. JAMA 210:101, 1969

2. Cantwell JD, Fletcher GF: Cardiac complications while jogging. JAMA 210:130, 1969

3. Resnekov L: Jogging and coronary artery disease. JAMA 210:126, 1969

4. Bruce RA, Kluge W: Defibrillatory treatment of exertional cardiac arrest in coronary disease. JAMA 216: 653, 1971

5. Jokl E, McClellan JT: Exercise and cardiac death. In Medicine and Sport, Vol V. Baltimore, University Park Press, 1971

6. Katz LN: Physical fitness and coronary heart disease. Circulation 35:405, 1967

7. Frick MH: Coronary implications of hemodynamic changes caused by physical training. Amer J Cardiol 22: 417, 1968

8. Hellerstein HK: Effects of an active physical reconditioning intervention program on the clinical course of coronary artery disease. Mal Cardiovasc 10:461, 1969

9. Gottheiner V: Long-range strenuous sports training for cardiac reconditioning and rehabilitation. Amer J Cardiol 22:426, 1968

10. Zohman LR, Tobis JS: Cardiac Rehabilitation. New York, Grune & Stratton, 1970

11. McAllister FF, Bertsch R, Jacobson J, D'Alessio G: The accelerating effect of muscular exercise on experimental atherosclerosis. Arch Surg (Chicago) 80:54, 1959

12. Myasnikov AL: Influence of some factors on development of experimental cholesterol atherosclerosis. Circulation 17:99, 1958

13. Mann GV, Garrett HL, Farhi A, Murray H, Billings FT: Exercise to prevent coronary heart disease. An experimental study of the effects of training on risk factors for coronary disease in man. Amer J Med 46:12, 1969

14. Gustafson A: Effect of training on blood lipids. In Larsen OA, Malmborg RO (Eds): Coronary Heart Disease and Physical Fitness. Baltimore, University Park Press, 1971 p 125

15. Boyer JL, Kasch FW: Exercise therapy in hypertensive man. JAMA 211:1668, 1970

16. Carter JEL, Phillips WH: Structural changes in exercising middle-aged males during a 2-year period. J Appl Physiol 27:787, 1969

17. Bloor CM, Pasyk S, Leon AS: Interaction of age and exercise on organ and cellular development. Amer J Path 58:185, 1970

18. Tomanek RJ: Effects of age and exercise on the extent of the myocardial capillary bed. Anat Rec 167:55, 1970.

19. Eckstein RW: Effect of exercise and coronary artery narrowing on coronary collateral circulation. Circ Res 5:230, 1957

20. Tepperman J, Pearlman D: Effects of exercise and anemia on coronary arteries in small animals as revealed by the corrosion-case technique. Circ Res 9:576, 1961

21. Stevenson JA, Feleki V, Rechnitzer P: Effect of exercise on coronary tree size in the rat. Circ Res 15:265, 1964

22. Holloszy JO: Morphological and enzymatic adaptations of training—a review. In Larsen OA, Malmborg RO (Eds): Coronary Heart Disease and Physical Fitness. Baltimore, University Park Press, 1971, p 147

23. Penpargkul S, Scheuer J: The effect of physical training upon the mechanical and metabolic performance of the rat heart. J Clin Invest 49:1859, 1970

24. Oscai LB, Mole PA, Holloszy JO: Effects of exercise on cardiac weight and mitochondria in male and female rats. Amer J Physiol 220:1091, 1971

25. Banister EW, Tomanek RJ, Cvorkov N: Ultrastructural modifications in rat heart: responses to exercise and training. Amer J Appl Physiol 220:1935, 1971

26. Crews J, Aldinger EE: Effect of chronic exercise on myocardial function. Amer Heart J 74:536, 1967

27. Astrup T, Brakman P: Responders and non-responders in exercise-induced blood fibrinolysis. In Larsen OA, Malmborg RO (Eds): Coronary Heart Disease and Physical Fitness. Baltimore, University Park Press, 1971, p 130

28. Simpson MT, Hames CG, Meier D: An epidemiological study of platelet aggregation and physical activity. Circulation 43–44 (Suppl II):88, 1971

29. Epstein SW: Angina pectoris: Pathophysiology, evaluation, and treatment (Fibrinolysis). Ann Intern Med 75:272, 1971

30. Moxley TR, Brakman P, Astrup T: Resting levels of fibrinolysis in blood in inactive and exercising men. J Appl Physiol 28:549, 1970

31. Raab W: Preventive Myocardiology. Springfield, Ill, Charles C Thomas, 1970, p 22

32. Morris JN: Epidemiology and cardiovascular disease of middle age. Parts I, and II. Mod Conc Cardiovasc Dis 29:625, 1960

33. Morris JN, Heady JA, Raffle PA, Roberts CG, Parks JW: Coronary heart-disease and physical activity of work. Lancet 2:1111, 1953

34. Morris JN, Heady JA, Raffle PA, Roberts CG, Parks JW: Health and social class. Lancet 1:303, 1959

35. Stamler J, Kjelsberg M, Hall Y: Epidemiologic studies on cardiovascular-renal diseases: I. Analysis of mortality by age-race-sex-occupation. J Chronic Dis 12: 440, 1960

36. Breslow L, Buell P: Mortality from coronary heart disease and physical activity of work in California. J Chronic Dis 11:421, 1960

37. Morris JN, Heady JA, Raffle PA: Physique of London busmen. Lancet 2:569, 1956

38. Morris JN, Heady JA, Raffle PA, Kagan A, Pattison DC, Gardner MJ: Incidence and prediction of ischaemic heart disease in London busmen. Lancet 2:553, 1966

39. Oliver RM: Physique and serum lipids of young London busmen in relation to ischaemic heart disease. Brit J Intern Med 24:181, 1967

40. Zukel WJ, et al: A short-term community study of the epidemiology of coronary heart disease. Amer J Public Health 49:1630, 1959

41. Brunner D: The influence of physical activity on incidence and prognosis of ischemic heart disease. *In* Raab W (Ed): Prevention of Ischemic Heart Disease. Springfield, Ill, Charles C Thomas, 1966, p 1

42. Adelstein AM: Some aspects of cardiovascular mortality in South Africa. Brit J Prev Soc Med 17:29, 1963

43. Taylor HL, Klepetar E, Keys A, Parlin W, Blackburn H, Puchner T: Death rates among physically active and sedentary employees of the railroad industry. Amer J Public Health 52:1697, 1962

44. Taylor HL, Blackburn H, Brozek J, Parlin RW, Puchner T: Railroad employees in the United States. Acta Med Scand Suppl 460:55, 1966

45. Taylor HL, Blackburn H, Brozek J, Parlin RW, Puchner T: Occupational factors in the study of coronary heart disease and physical activity. Canad Med Ass J 96:825, 1967

46. Kahn HA: The relationship of reported coronary heart disease mortality to physical activity of work. Amer J Public Health 53:1058, 1963

47. Frank CW, Weinblatt E, Shapiro S, Sager R: Physical inactivity as a lethal factor in myocardial infarction among men. Circulation 34:1022, 1966

48. Keys A: Physical activity and the epidemiology of coronary heart disease. *In* Brunner D (Ed): Physical Activity and Aging. Medicine and Sport, Vol IV. Baltimore, University Park Press, 1970, p 250

49. Shanoff HM, Little JA: Studies of male survivors of myocardial infarction due to "essential" atherosclerosis. I. Characteristics of the patients. Canad Med Ass J 84:519, 1961

50. Forssman O, Lindegard B: The post-coronary patient. A multidisciplinary investigation of middle-aged Swedish males. J Psychosom Res 3:89, 1958

51. Stamler J, Lindberg HA, Berkson DM, Shaffer A, Miller W: Prevalence and incidence of coronary heart disease in strata of the labor force of a Chicago industrial corporation. J Chronic Dis 11:405, 1960

52. McDonough JR, Hames CG, Stulb SC, Garrison GE: Coronary heart disease among Negroes and Whites in Evans County, Georgia. J Chronic Dis 18:443, 1965

53. Hames CG, Heyden S, Cassel JC, Bartel A, Tyroler HA: Prevalence versus incidence of ischemic heart disease in relation to physical activity-Evans County, Georgia Study. Presented at Conference on Cardiovascular Disease Epidemiology, San Diego, Calif, March 1, 1971

54. Lilienfeld AM: Variation of mortality from heart disease. Public Health Rep 71:545, 1956

55. Pell S, D'Alonzo CA: Immediate mortality and five-year survival of employed men with a first myocardial infarction. New Eng J Med 270:915, 1964

56. Pell S, D'Alonzo CA: A three-year study of myocardial infarction in a large employed population. JAMA 175:463, 1961

57. Hinkle LE, Whitney LA, Lehman EW, Dunn J, Benjamin B: Occupation, education, and coronary heart disease. Science 161:238, 1968

58. Stamler J, Berkson DM, Lindberg HA, Whipple TT, Miller W, Hall Y: Long-term epidemiologic studies on the possible role of physical activity and physical fitness in the prevention of premature clinical coronary heart disease. *In* Brunner D (Ed): Physical Activity and Aging. Medicine and Sport, Vol IV. Baltimore, University Park Press, 1970, p 274

59. Paffenbarger RS, Laughlin ME, Gima AS, Black RA: Work activity of longshoremen as related to death from coronary heart disease and stroke. New Eng J Med 282:1109, 1970

60. Paul O: Physical activity and coronary heart disease. II. Amer J Cardiol 23:303, 1969

61. Chapman JM, Massey FJ: The interrelationship of serum cholesterol, hypertension, body weight, and risk of coronary disease. J Chronic Dis 17:933, 1964

62. Rosenman RH: The influence of different exercise patterns on the incidence of coronary heart disease in the western collaborative group study. *In* Brunner D (Ed): Physical Activity and Aging. Medicine and Sport, Vol IV. Baltimore, University Park Press, 1970, p 267

63. Blackburn H, Taylor HL, Keys A: Coronary heart disease in seven countries. Circulation 41 (Suppl 1):154, 1970

64. Werko L: Can we prevent heart disease? Ann Intern Med 74:278, 1971

65. Kannel WB: Habitual level of physical activity and risk of coronary heart disease: The Framingham Study. Canad Med Ass J 96:811, 1967

66. Kannel WB, Gordon T, Sorlie P, McNamara P: Physical activity and coronary vulnerability: The Framingham Study. Cardiol Digest 6:28, 1971

67. Spain DM, Bradess VA: Occupational physical activity and the degree of coronary atherosclerosis in "normal" men. Circulation 22:239, 1960

68. Mitrani Y, Karplus H, Brunner D: Coronary atherosclerosis in cases of traumatic death. *In* Brunner D (ed): Physical Activity and Aging. Medicine and Sport, Vol IV. Baltimore, University Park Press, 1970, p 241

69. Morris JN, Crawford MD: Coronary heart disease and physical activity of work. Brit Med J 2:1485, 1958

70. Rose G, Prineas RJ, Mitchell JR: Myocardial infarction and the intrinsic calibre of coronary arteries. Brit Heart J 29:548, 1967

71. Currens JH, White PD: Half a century of running. New Eng J Med 265:988, 1961

72. Comroe JH, Forster RE, Dubois AB, Briscoe WA, Carlsen F: The Lung. Chicago, Year Book, 1966, p 10

73. Roskamm H, Reindell H: Optimum patterns of exercise for healthy adults. *In* Brunner D (Ed): Physical Activity and Aging. Medicine and Sport, Vol IV. Baltimore, University Park Press, 1970, p 19

74. Mitchell JH, Blomqvist G: Maximal oxygen uptake. New Eng J Med 284:1018, 1971

75. Moriyama IM, Baum WS, Haenszel WM, Mattison B: Inquiry into diagnostic evidence supporting medical certifications of death. Amer J Public Health 48:1376, 1958

76. James G, Patton RE, Heslin AS: Accuracy of cause-of-death statements on death certificates. Public Health Rep 70:39, 1955

77. American Heart Association: Exercise Programs for Cardiacs: Directory New York, American Heart Association.

78. Frick MH, Katila M: Hemodynamic consequences of physical training after myocardial infarction. Circulation 37:192, 1968

79. Bergman H, Varnauskas E: The hemodynamic effects of physical training. *In* Brunner D (Ed): Physical Activity and Aging. Medicine and Sport, Vol IV. Baltimore, University Park Press, 1970, p 138

80. Kattus AA: Diagnosis, medical and surgical management of coronary insufficiency. Ann Intern Med 69:114, 1968

81. Kaufman JM, Anslow RD: Treatment of refractory angina pectoris with nitroglycerin and graded exercise. JAMA 196:151, 1966

82. Clausen JP, Trap-Jensen J: Effects of training on the distribution of cardiac output in patients with coronary artery disease. Circulation 42:611, 1970

83. Detry JR, Rousseau M, Vandenbrocke G, Kusumi F, Brasseur L, Bruce R: Increased arteriovenous oxygen difference after physical training in coronary heart disease. Circulation 44:109, 1971

84. Brusis OA, Gibson TC: Risk factors in volunteers for "coronary prevention programs." Circulation 43 and 44 (Suppl II):85, 1971

85. Oberman A, Schnaper HW: Unpublished data

86. Shanoff HM, Little JA, Csima A: Studies of male survivors of myocardial infarction. XII. Relation of serum lipids and lipoproteins to ten-year survival. Canad Med Ass J 103:927, 1970

87. Frank CW: The course of coronary heart disease: Factors relating to prognosis. Bull NY Acad Med 44:900, 1968

88. Oberman A, Jones WB, Riley CP, Reeves TJ, Turner ME, Sheffield LT: Natural history of coronary artery disease. Bull NY Acad Med. In press

89. Kilbom A, Hartley LH, Saltin B: Physical training in sedentary middle-aged and older men. I. Medical evaluation. Scand J Clin Lab Invest 24:314, 1969

90. Stamler J: Acute myocardial infarction—progress in primary prevention. Brit Heart J 33 (Suppl):145, 1971

91. Cooper KH: Guidelines in the management of the exercising patient. JAMA 211:1663, 1970

Cardiocirculatory Responses to Muscular Exercise in Congestive Heart Failure

Dean T. Mason, Robert Zelis, John Longhurst, and Garrett Lee

THE PURPOSE of this review is to delineate current knowledge of the cardiocirculatory adjustments that accompany physical exercise in clinical congestive heart failure. To provide the necessary background information for understanding such a discussion, it is first important to concisely consider the cardiac and peripheral circulatory responses operative in normal individuals during exertion. Thus, the first section describes the normal responses of the heart to muscular exercise and those of the systemic vasculature to physicial stress. Then, proceeding from this fundamental information, the principal portion of this review is focused on the series of systematic studies, largely carried out in our laboratories, to elucidate the cardiocirculatory mechanisms in the congestive heart failure state.

NORMAL CARDIAC RESPONSES TO DYNAMIC EXERCISE

The cardiac responses in normal subjects to exercise are now acknowledged to involve interactions of alterations in heart rate, contractility, preload, and impedance. The relative roles of each of these factors in regulating cardiac output are, to a great extent, dependent upon the conditions comprising the manner of physical exertion. It is the current belief that rise in cardiac output occurring during moderate exercise in the supine position results principally from an increase in heart rate.[1] Conversely, improvement of cardiac output during heavy exertion in the erect posture is accompanied by marked elevation of stroke volume.[2] In addition, myocardial contractility is increased and aortic impedance is reduced, thereby facilitating ventricular emptying under all conditions of dynamic exercise. The increase in heart rate is primarily due to adrenergic stimulation, while parasympathetic withdrawal is also influential. Augmentation of the sympathetic nervous system accounts for the increase in inotropism, while the elevation of stroke volume is attributable to operation of the Frank–Starling mechanism in consort with the increased contractile state. The reduction in ventricular impedance is due to decrease in total peripheral vascular resistance.

While the normal heart usually decreases in size during exertion, the Frank–Starling mechanism is still operative but is masked by the opposing effects on cardiac diameter of tachycardia, elevated myocardial contractility, and lowered impedance to ventricular ejection.[3] Thus, the normal response of the heart to exercise constitutes the integrated effects of all four of the aforementioned determinants of cardiac output: heart rate, contractility, preload, and impedance. Although mild exertion can be accomplished by the action of only one or two of these variables, the considerable rise in cardiac output required during maximal levels of muscular activity necessitates the operation of all four of these determinants of ventricular performance.

NORMAL PERIPHERAL CIRCULATORY RESPONSES TO DYNAMIC EXERCISE

Systemic Arterial System

Although the many factors that govern blood flow in the regional circulations are not necessarily similar in quality or degree, certain physical principles apply to each of the vascular beds.[4] Thus, blood flow to an organ is determined by the ratio of the driving pressure (the difference between the arterial and venous pressures) to the resistance to flow offered by the vessels. In general, regional flow is regulated by alterations in vasomotor tone, which in turn are controlled by intrinsic humoral and neural influences. It is important to remember that calculated vascular resistance does not necessarily equate with vasomotor tone, but rather is a

From the Section of Cardiovascular Medicine, University of California at Davis, School of Medicine, Davis, Calif., and Sacramento Medical Center, Sacramento, Calif.

Supported in part by Research Program Project Grant HL-14780 from the National Heart, Lung and Blood Institute, National Institutes of Health, Bethesda, Md. and research grants from California Chapters of the American Heart Association, Dallas, Texas.

Reprint requests should be addressed to Dean T. Mason, M.D., Professor and Chief, Department of Cardiovascular Medicine, University of California, School of Medicine, Davis, Calif. 95616.

complex function of the cross-sectional area of the arteriolar bed. Furthermore, changes in arteriolar resistance may be either active or passive. The fact that resistance to blood flow is related critically to the radius of the arterioles is expressed in the Poiseuille relationship, which indicates that blood flow is proportional to the fourth power of the radius. Thus, relatively large adjustments in vascular resistance may be brought about by small changes in the radius of the arterioles. Since the arterioles in the peripheral circulation are connected in parallel rather than in series, the total resistance in a single organ is approximately equal to the resistance in a single vessel divided by the number of vessels in parallel. In view of the fact that blood vessels are distensible and not rigid tubes, increasing the transmural pressure across the arteriolar wall will reduce the resistance opposing flow. The distending force pushing the arteriole outward is balanced by the restraining force of tension developed within the vessel wall. Expressed in terms of the Laplace equation, this tension is proportional to the product of the transmural pressure and the vessel radius. At very low intraluminal pressures, usually about 20 mm Hg for arterioles, the elastic and muscular forces in the vessel wall exceed the distending force so that the vessel collapses and flow ceases.

The local control of vasomotor tone of the arterioles is achieved principally by vasodilation produced by metabolic products and anoxia. The cerebral circulation is particularly sensitive to changes in carbon dioxide tension, while the coronary and skeletal muscle beds adjust to alterations in oxygen tension of the blood. It is of interest that the pulmonary arterioles respond in an opposite manner to changes in these blood gases. The resistance of the arterioles is also regulated by sympathetic vasoconstrictor fibers. Vasoconstriction is produced by augmentation of reflex sympathetic nervous activity, and vasodilation occurs as a result of increased local metabolic vasodilator influences and decreased sympathetic vasoconstrictor impulses. It should be remembered that in the peripheral vascular beds, receptors for the adrenergic nervous system situated at the effector cell are separated into two types: activation of the alpha-adrenergic receptors results in arteriolar constriction, while activation of the beta-adrenergic receptors induces arteriolar dilatation. In the regional circulations, these adren-

ergic receptors are not equally partitioned, either as to receptor type or as to absolute number of receptors. Thus, the arterioles of the coronary and cerebral beds appear to contain relatively few adrenergic receptors, while the vascular beds in most other areas possess abundant receptors. Importantly, in the arteriolar bed of skeletal muscle, humorally transported norepinephrine acts on both alpha- and beta-receptors, while neuronally released norepinephrine stimulates only alpha-receptors. Although certain regional circulations exhibit little reflex activity, the afferent pathways for the reflex control of arteriolar tone are situated in the carotid and aortic arch baroreceptors[5] and chemoreceptors, the ventricular chambers, in the low-pressure areas of the intrathoracic vascular bed, and in somatic nerve fibers in exercising skeletal muscle.

Resting Regional Blood Flow

The distribution of the cardiac output in the major organs of the body in normal subjects is shown in Fig. 1.[6] The largest of these vascular beds is the splanchnic bed. By infusing bromsulphthalein and applying the Fick principle, it has been shown that hepatic blood flow approximates 25% of the total cardiac output in fasting subjects at rest, while the oxygen uptake of this region makes up a similar fraction of the total oxygen consumption of the body. This proportionally equal uptake of oxygen to blood flow is characteristic of the splanchnic circulation; all other organs exhibit a disproportionate relation between oxygen consumption and regional flow. The second largest of the peripheral circulations is the renal circulation, which receives approximately 20% of the cardiac output. The study of renal blood flow has been based on the renal clearance of a substance, such as sodium para-aminohippurate, removed in one passage through the kidney. Since the oxygen saturation of blood from the renal vein is only slightly less than that of arterial blood, the oxygen consumption of the kidney is small compared to its blood flow. The cerebral circulation has been investigated by measuring the rate of uptake by the brain of an inert foreign gas, such as nitrous oxide. From these studies, it has been determined that the brain receives about 12% of the cardiac output but consumes a greater proportion of oxygen (20% of the total oxygen consumption of the body). Coronary

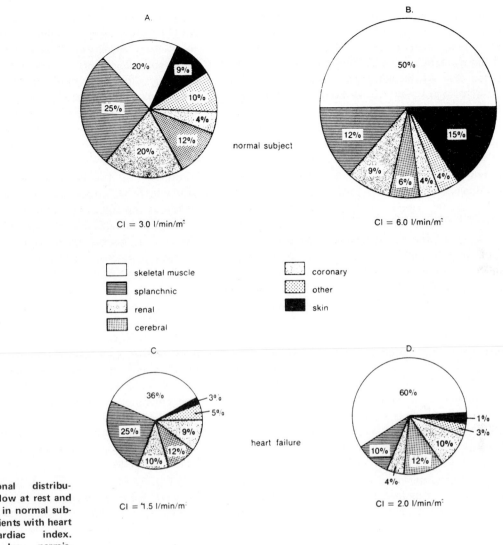

Fig. 1. Regional distribution of blood flow at rest and during exercise in normal subjects and in patients with heart failure. CI, cardiac index. (Reproduced by permission.[16])

blood flow has been measured by a similar technique, utilizing the myocardial uptake of inhaled nitrous oxide or injected radioactive krypton.[85] Although the heart is supplied with only 4% of total body flow, it consumes nearly three times this percentage of the oxygen utilized by the body. Thus, the coronary arteriovenous oxygen difference is greater than that occurring in any vascular bed, and coronary sinus blood normally contains less oxygen than any other venous effluent.

Knowledge of the blood flow to skeletal muscle has been obtained from studies on the forearm and leg employing the plethysmographic technique.[7] In this method, obstruction to venous out-

flow from the limb is produced suddenly, and the change in volume of the extremity, which is proportional to arterial inflow, is measured. Since epinephrine iontophoresis can eliminate the cutaneous circulation temporarily, the amount of blood flow partitioned between muscle and skin can be calculated. Further, the determination of deep and superficial venous oxygen content of the limbs also has been used to follow relative changes in muscle and skin flow. Skeletal muscle blood flow is approximately 20% of the cardiac output, while these tissues utilize about 30% of the total oxygen uptake of the body. Thus, the musculature consumes a greater share of oxygen than any other organ system in the body and, like the cardiac and cerebral circulations, extracts a large amount of oxygen relative to blood flow. Since the primary function of the cutaneous circulation is the regulation of body temperature, the rate of blood flow to the skin is very labile. However, in terms of percentage for the body as a whole, this regional bed receives a flow that is nearly five times that of its oxygen consumption. Thus, the low metabolic requirements relative to blood flow of the skin are similar to those of the kidney, and it is these circulations that are constricted selectively when the cardiac output falls.

Regional Blood Flow During Exercise

The distribution of the cardiac output in normal subjects during muscular exercise has received considerable attention recently (Fig. 1).[6] It is now recognized that the augmented blood flow to exercising muscles is accomplished not only by an increase in the total cardiac output, but also by redistribution of blood flow. With moderate to severe exercise, blood flow to active skeletal muscles rises, accompanied by an elevation of coronary blood flow, while splanchnic and renal flow remain at precontrol levels despite increased vasoconstriction in these visceral beds.[8] Blood flow to nonexercising skeletal muscles is diminished during moderate to strenuous activity.[9] The cerebral circulation is maintained during moderate activity, but when maximal exercise is performed, there is a tendency for this flow to become slightly reduced as a result of the fall in arterial carbon dioxide tension that accompanies hyperventilation. The circulation in the skin varies with the intensity and duration of exercise.[9] At the onset of exercise, flow declines, but in order to eliminate heat, the cutaneous flow rises as activity continues. However, with maximal exercise, this augmented flow to the skin is often delayed until after the exercise is terminated.[9] Thus, vasodilation occurs in the arteriolar beds of exercising skeletal muscle and the heart, while vasoconstriction takes place in the gut and kidney and, to a lesser extent, in the skin and resting muscle. The mechanisms by which the redistribution of regional flow is accomplished are not completely understood, but it is not unreasonable to assume that, with the marked increase in cardiac output occurring during severe exertion, local flow in exercising muscles is augmented in response to the accumulation of vasodilator metabolites, perfusion is maintained in certain

visceral organs despite vasoconstriction, and blood flow to some areas is reduced with the overall result being reduction of total peripheral vascular resistance accompanied by moderate elevation of blood pressure. This view implies that the generalized reflex sympathetic discharge occurs in all of the regional circulations, but in certain organs, this action is overridden by vasodilator influences.

Systemic Venous System

Although it has been appreciated for many years that the basic function of the venous system is the return of blood to the heart, only recently have satisfactory methods become available for the assessment of changes in tone of the capacitance vessels.[10] These methods for the study of venous tone or distensibility are based on establishing the pressure–volume characteristics of the capacitance bed in the forearm, calf, or hand. It is now established that the veins participate actively, through reflexes mediated by the sympathetic nervous system, in maintaining normal circulatory function and can constrict in response to physiologic stimuli to preserve venous pressure and to augment venous return. Thus, in response to emotion, cold environment, norepinephrine, hyperventilation, muscular exercise, and the assumption of upright posture, venoconstriction occurs in certain regional beds,[11] accompanied by a shift of blood in the systemic venous reservoir toward the central circulation. In general, the veins respond to sympathetic and humoral effects less rapidly and quantitatively than do the arterioles. Little information is available concerning the location of the afferent limb of the reflex that is capable of initiating changes in venomotor tone. There is some evidence to suggest that such receptors might exist in low-pressure vascular compartments within the chest. The effects of stimulation of the carotid baroreceptors on venous tone indicate that skeletal muscle is only minimally innervated, while the cutaneous circulation demonstrates marked venoconstriction.[12]

Additional Compensatory Mechanisms During Exercise

Besides the aforementioned cardiocirculatory adjustments during exercise, certain other normal mechanisms help in augmenting oxygen delivery to metabolizing tissues. These additional systems include: (1) increased oxygen extraction from

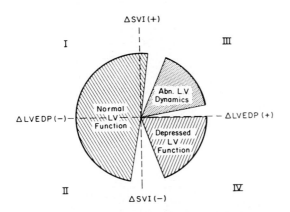

Fig. 2. The patterns of left ventricular response to supine muscular exercise. Normal left ventricular (LV) function (quadrants I and II, hatched area) includes a variable change in stroke volume, usually an increase, and a fall or no change in LV end-diastolic pressure (LVEDP). Abnormal left ventricular dynamics (quadrant III, stippled area) is associated with an increase in stroke volume index (SVI) and an increase in LVEDP. Depressed LV function (quadrant IV, hatched area) is characterized by no change or a fall in SVI and an increase in LVEDP. (Reproduced by permission.[1])

blood perfusing exercising skeletal muscle causing widening of the arteriovenous oxygen difference; (2) augmentation of the lower extremity, thoracic, and respiratory muscles by pumping increased venous return to the heart; (3) some enhanced oxygen-carrying capacity of the arterial blood resulting from splenic contraction by increasing circulatory red cell mass; and (4) rightward displacement of the hemoglobin-oxygen dissociation curve thereby facilitating unloading of oxygen from red blood cells to the peripheral tissues.

CARDIAC RESPONSES TO DYNAMIC EXERCISE IN CONGESTIVE HEART FAILURE

Although studies in which cardiac output is related to total oxygen consumption indicate the degree to which the output of the heart is capable of satisfying increased metabolic demands of exercise, they are not helpful in differentiating loading from inotropic factors that may limit the cardiac output response. A useful method for qualitative evaluation of these factors is the study of left ventricular performance by determination of the effects of supine exercise on cardiac output, stroke volume or stroke work, and left ventricular end-diastolic pressure.[1] The integrity of ventricular performance in response to the stress of muscular exercise can be analyzed within the

framework of alterations of the position of ventricular function curves.[13] Thus, augmentation of sympathetic activity during exercise normally increases myocardial contractility and thereby alters the shape and position of the ventricular function curve, so that its ascending slope is steeper and elevated compared to the control curve. In contrast, patients with ventricular failure exhibit a depressed and flat curve with little change or a fall in cardiac performance despite the development of high levels of end-diastolic pressure. Thus, the failing ventricle does not appear to be able to increase its contractile state appropriately to the positive inotropic stimulation of the myocardium accompanying muscular exercise.

A simplified and valid means of assessment of these exercise data has been the comparison of the change from resting levels of stroke volume and end-diastolic pressure[1,14-16] (Fig. 2). In normal subjects during exercise, the end-diastolic pressure does not exceed 12 mm Hg and usually falls or rises by no more than 2 mm Hg accompanied by a rise in stroke volume. In contrast, patients with abnormal myocardial contractility exhibit a fall in stroke volume despite excessive increments in end-diastolic pressure that reach total levels of greater than 12 mm Hg.[1] An intermediate response consisting of a rise in stroke volume accompanied by excessive elevation of end-diastolic pressure is considered to be due to abnormal ventricular compliance or to a lesser impairment of ventricular contractility with increased use of the Frank–Starling principle to achieve an appropriate rise of cardiac output.

PERIPHERAL CIRCULATORY RESPONSES TO EXERCISE IN CONGESTIVE HEART FAILURE

Systemic Arterial System

It is clear that a state of arteriolar (Fig. 3) and venous constriction is characteristic of human congestive heart failure.[7,16-20] This vasoconstriction compensates for the reduced performance of the heart in support of central and peripheral circulatory function. The increase in total systemic vascular resistance provides a peripheral circulatory mechanism by which arterial pressure is maintained in the face of a low cardiac output.

The effects of heart failure on the dynamics of the arteriolar bed in the forearm have been char-

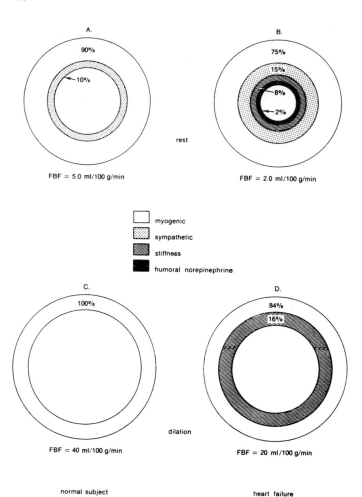

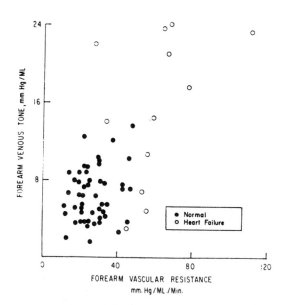

Fig. 3. Diagram represents the components of vascular resistance in the arterioles of the forearm at rest (A and B) and during maximal vasodilation (C and D) in a normal patient (A and C) and in a patient with heart failure (B and D). Components expressed as percentage of radius of arteriolar lumen, value estimated from changes in blood flow induced by certain interventions, and based on the Poiseuille relationship that indicates flow varies directly as the fourth power of the inner radius of the vessel. FBF, forearm blood flow. (Reproduced by permission.[18])

Fig. 4. Relation between forearm venous tone and forearm vascular resistance in normal subjects and in patients with congestive heart failure. (Reproduced by permission.[17])

acterized in recent studies employing plethysmographic techniques. In patients exhibiting heart failure, the forearm vascular resistance is significantly greater than in normal subjects (Fig. 4).[17] Since the total peripheral vascular resistance is elevated abnormally in heart failure, a state of arteriolar constriction exists in the entire systemic vascular bed, including the forearm. This arteriolar constriction in heart failure is produced mainly by increased sympathetic nervous activity[17] and by a stiffness component in the arteriolar wall (Figs. 5-8).[21] In contrast to the failing myocardium,[22] there are increased labile stores of norepinephrine in the arteriolar beds of skeletal muscle in patients with heart failure (Fig. 9).[23] The altered mechanical properties of the arterioles in heart failure result from increased sodium and water content in the vessel itself (Figs. 10 and 11)[24,25] and are responsible, in part, for the decreased arteriolar dilator capacity that has recently been demonstrated in these patients,[21] as well as the increased